Multiple Sclerosis and CNS Inflammatory Disorders

NEUROLOGY IN PRACTICE:

SERIES EDITORS: ROBERT A. GROSS, DEPARTMENT OF NEUROLOGY, UNIVERSITY OF ROCHESTER MEDICAL CENTER, ROCHESTER, NY, USA

JONATHAN W. MINK, DEPARTMENT OF NEUROLOGY, UNIVERSITY OF ROCHESTER MEDICAL CENTER, ROCHESTER, NY, USA

Multiple Sclerosis and CNS Inflammatory Disorders

EDITED BY

Lawrence M. Samkoff, MD
Associate Professor of Neurology
Neuroimmunology Unit
Department of Neurology
University of Rochester School of Medicine and Dentistry
Rochester, NY, USA

Andrew D. Goodman, MD
Professor of Neurology
Chief, Neuroimmunology Unit
Department of Neurology
University of Rochester School of Medicine and Dentistry
Rochester, NY, USA

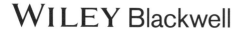

Library of Congress Cataloging-in-Publication Data

Multiple sclerosis and CNS inflammatory disorders / edited by Lawrence M. Samkoff, Andrew D. Goodman.
    p. ; cm.
  Includes bibliographical references and index.
  ISBN 978-0-470-67388-1 (pbk.)
  I. Samkoff, Lawrence M., 1958– editor. II. Goodman, Andrew D., 1952– editor.
  [DNLM: 1. Multiple Sclerosis.   2. Central Nervous System Diseases–immunology.
3. Neurogenic Inflammation–physiopathology. WL 360]
  RC377
  616.8′34–dc23
                                        2014007073

A catalogue record for this book is available from the British Library.

Set in 9.5/12.5pt Utopia by SPi Publisher Services, Pondicherry, India
Printed and bound in Malaysia by Vivar Printing Sdn Bhd

1 2014

Contents

Contributors

Brenda Banwell MD
Department of Pediatrics (Neurology)
The Hospital for Sick Children
Toronto, Ontario, Canada

Allen C. Bowling MD
Colorado Neurological Institute
Englewood, CO, USA

Leigh E. Charvet PhD
Department of Neurology
Stony Brook Medicine
Stony Brook, NY, USA

Jeffrey A. Cohen MD
Mellen Center for Multiple Sclerosis
Treatment and Research
Neurological Institute, Cleveland Clinic
Cleveland, OH, USA

Anne H. Cross MD
Department of Neurology
Washington University School of
Medicine
St Louis, MO, USA

Mark Freedman MSc, MD, FAAN, FRCP(C)
Multiple Sclerosis Research Unit
University of Ottawa
Ottawa, Ontario, Canada

María I. Gaitán MD
National Institute of Neurological
Disorders and Stroke
National Institutes of Health
Bethesda, MD, USA
and
Dr. Raúl Carrea Institute for
Neurological Research
FLENI, Buenos Aires, Argentina

Barbara Giesser MD
Department of Neurology, MS Division
UCLA School of Medicine
Los Angeles, CA, USA

Andrew D. Goodman MD
Neuroimmunology Unit
Department of Neurology

University of Rochester School
of Medicine and Dentistry
Rochester, NY, USA

Benjamin M. Greenberg MD, MHS
Department of Neurology and
Neurotherapeutics
and
Department of Pediatrics
University of Texas
Southwestern
Dallas, TX, USA

Megan H. Hyland MD
Neuroimmunology Unit
Department of Neurology
University of Rochester School
of Medicine and Dentistry
Rochester, NY, USA

Mohsen Khoshnam MD
Multiple Sclerosis Research Unit
University of Ottawa
Ottawa, Ontario, Canada

Benzi Kluzer MD
Department of Neurology
University of Colorado
Denver, CO, USA

George H. Kraft MD, MS
Department of Rehabilitation Medicine
and Neurology
Institute for Stem Cell and
Regenerative Medicine
University of Washington
Seattle, WA, USA

Lauren B. Krupp MD
Department of Neurology
Stony Brook Medicine
Stony Brook, NY, USA

Eric Logigian MD
Department of Neurology
University of Rochester
Medical Center
Rochester, NY, USA

Marcelo Matiello MD, MSc
Department of Neurology
Massachusetts General Hospital
and Brigham and Women's Hospital
Harvard Medical School
Boston, MA, USA

Nesanet S. Mitiku MD, PhD
Departments of Rehabilitation Medicine
and Neurology
and
Corinne Goldsmith Dickinson Center for
Multiple Sclerosis
Icahn School of Medicine at
Mount Sinai
New York, NY, USA

Callene Momtazee MD
Department of Neurology, MS Division
UCLA School of Medicine
Los Angeles, CA, USA

Ellen M. Mowry MD, MCR
Department of Neurology
Johns Hopkins University
Baltimore, MD, USA

Paul O'Connor MD
Division of Neurology
Institute of Medical Science
and
St Michael's Hospital
University of Toronto
Toronto, Ontario, Canada

Erica Patrick MD
Department of Neurology
University of Rochester Medical Center
Rochester, NY, USA

Laura Piccio MD, PhD
Department of Neurology
Washington University School
of Medicine
St Louis, MO, USA

Daniel S. Reich MD, PhD
National Institute of Neurological
Disorders and Stroke
National Institutes of Health
Bethesda, MD, USA

David J. Rintell EdD
Partners Multiple Sclerosis Center
Brigham and Women's Hospital
and
Partners Pediatric MS Center
Massachusetts General Hospital
Harvard Medical School
Boston, MA, USA

Jessica Robb MD
Neuroimmunology Unit
Department of Neurology
University of Rochester School
of Medicine and Dentistry
Rochester, NY, USA

Dalia Rotstein MD
Division of Neurology
Institute of Medical Science
and
St Michael's Hospital
University of Toronto
Toronto, Ontario, Canada

Sabahattin Saip MD
Department of Neurology
Cerrahpaşa School of Medicine
Istanbul University
Cerrahpaşa, Turkey

Lawrence M. Samkoff MD
Neuroimmunology Unit
Department of Neurology
University of Rochester School of
Medicine and Dentistry
Rochester, NY, USA

Alexius E. G. Sandoval MD
Maine Rehabilitation Outpatient Center
Bangor, ME, USA

Thomas F. Scott MD
Department of Neurology
Drexel University College of Medicine
and
Allegheny MS Treatment Center
Pittsburgh, PA, USA

Aksel Siva MD
Department of Neurology
Cerrahpaşa School of Medicine
Istanbul University
Cerrahpaşa, Turkey

Sonya U. Steele MSc
Department of Neurology
Johns Hopkins University
Baltimore, MD, USA

Robert Thompson Stone MD
Department of Neurology
University of Rochester
Medical Center
Rochester, NY, USA

Brian G. Weinshenker MD, FRCP(C)
Department of Neurology
Mayo Clinic
Rochester, MN, USA

Series Foreword

The genesis for this book series started with the proposition that, increasingly, physicians want direct, useful information to help them in clinical care. Textbooks, while comprehensive, are useful primarily as detailed reference works but pose challenges for uses at the point of care. By contrast, more outline-type references often leave out the "hows and whys"—pathophysiology, pharmacology—that form the basis of management decisions. Our goal for this series is to present books, covering most areas of neurology, that provide enough background information to allow the reader to feel comfortable, but not so much as to be overwhelming, and to associate that with practical advice from experts about care, combining the growing evidence base with best practices.

Our series will encompass various aspects of neurology, with topics and the specific content chosen to be accessible and useful.

Chapters cover critical information that will inform the reader of the disease processes and mechanisms as a prelude to treatment planning. Algorithms and guidelines are presented, when appropriate. "Tips and Tricks" boxes provide expert suggestions, while other boxes present cautions and warnings to avoid pitfalls. Finally, we provide "Science Revisited" sections that review the most important and relevant science background material, and references and further reading sections that guide the reader to additional material.

We welcome feedback. As additional volumes are added to the series, we hope to refine the content and format so that our readers will be best served.

Our thanks, appreciation, and respect go out to our editors and their contributors, who conceived and refined the content for each volume, assuring a high-quality, practical approach to neurological conditions and their treatment.

Our thanks also go to our mentors and students (past, present, and future), who have challenged and delighted us; to our book editors and their contributors, who were willing to take on additional work for an educational goal; and to our publisher, Martin Sugden, for his ideas and support, for wonderful discussions and commiseration over baseball and soccer teams that might not quite have lived up to expectations. We would like to dedicate the series to Marsha, Jake, and Dan, and to Janet, Laura, and David. And also to Steven R. Schwid, MD, our friend and colleague, whose ideas helped to shape this project and whose humor brightened our lives; but he could not complete this goal with us.

Robert A. Gross
Jonathan W. Mink
Rochester, NY, USA

Preface

The treatment of multiple sclerosis (MS) has been revolutionized by the expanding armamentarium of disease-modifying agents that have been developed over the past two decades. These advances have resulted from the rapidly increasing understanding of the pathogenesis of MS. It is in this context that we have undertaken to compose a text to assist the practicing neurologists in training in the day-to-day care of patients with MS and MS-like inflammatory disorders of the central nervous system (CNS), with a review of the essential basic science and clinical principles needed to provide that care.

Chapters 1 and 2 provide an excellent overview of the basic science, epidemiology, and pathophysiology of MS, focusing on immunologic, genetic, and environmental factors. Chapters 3 and 4 present the diagnostic approach to MS, with emphasis on current criteria that incorporate clinical, laboratory, and MRI data to fulfill the classic definition of MS as a disorder disseminated in time and space. Chapter 5 reviews the rapidly changing therapeutic landscape for relapsing MS, which includes not only the original first-line injectable drugs (interferon beta and glatiramer acetate) but also monoclonal antibody infusions and oral agents. Chapter 6 then discusses treatment strategies for patients with progressive forms of MS, a population that is arguably underserved by available medications. MS can also be differentiated on the basis of sex and age of presentation, with disease-specific features in women, men, and children that are expertly reviewed in Chapters 7 and 8.

Despite the great advances in MS disease modifying therapy, they generally do not relieve already established symptoms. In fact, most people with MS are burdened with permanent and often fluctuating or worsening symptoms. Chapters 9–13 detail the management of the wide array of physical and neuropsychiatric MS-associated symptomatology, focusing on pharmacologic, alternative medicine, cognitive-behavioral, and rehabilitative approaches to patient care.

The diagnosis of MS implies that other diseases that mimic MS have been reliably excluded. The last section of the book, covered in Chapters 14–18, addresses other primary and secondary CNS inflammatory disorders that can be confused with MS, highlighting their differentiating features and treatment options.

Throughout the book, we have strived to include easy-to-read "Tips and Tricks" and "Science Revisited" boxes, and algorithms to emphasize important and practical information that can be useful in the clinic. We thank our chapter authors for their superb contributions to this effort. We are grateful for the assistance of the staff at Wiley Publishing, and for the valuable comments of series' editors, Dr. Robert Gross and Dr. Jonathan Mink, in the production of this textbook. We deeply appreciate the enduring support of Sharon and Jordan, and of Terry, Adam, and Sarah, and we dedicate this book to them. It is our hope that this text will be a valuable addition to the bookshelves of clinicians caring for patients with MS and related illnesses.

Lawrence M. Samkoff, MD
Andrew D. Goodman, MD

Etiology

Sonya U. Steele and Ellen M. Mowry

Department of Neurology, Johns Hopkins University, Baltimore, MD, USA

Background

Multiple sclerosis (MS) is a chronic inflammatory disease of the central nervous system (CNS) characterized by the breakdown of the insulating myelin sheath that covers the nerve axons in the CNS and subsequent degeneration of axons. The process leads most commonly to intermittent neurological symptoms followed, over time, by progressive neurological symptoms in many patients. MS affects approximately 400,000 people in the USA and more than 2.1 million people worldwide, but the incidence has increased in the last five decades, particularly in women (3.6/100,000 person-years) compared to men (2.0/100,000 person-years) (Alonso & Hernan 2008; National Multiple Sclerosis Society 2012). While the etiology of MS is not understood in detail, it is unlikely to be the result of a single causative event. Instead, converging evidence suggests that MS is caused by an abnormal autoimmune response in genetically susceptible individuals after specific environmental exposures. Thus, it is not a heritable disease in the classic sense, but a complex disease that emerges from genes interacting with other genes and genes interacting with the environment. The factors thought to mediate the risk of MS are subject to intense ongoing research and include genetic, immunologic, infectious, and environmental contributors. The aim of this chapter is to review the current data on MS risk factors, with particular emphasis on those that may be modifiable on a personal or population level.

> ### ✋ CAUTION!
>
> Over the years, many different causes for MS have been suggested, several of which have led to unfounded angst in those living with or at risk for developing MS. Here are some of the most popular theories that have not been proven to date (National Multiple Sclerosis Society 2012):
> - Owning a dog or other small pet (canine distemper)
> - Allergies
> - Exposure to heavy metals (e.g., mercury, lead, or manganese)
> - Physical trauma
> - Aspartame

Genes

Familial aggregation is a well-recognized phenomenon in MS, and family and twin studies have long shown evidence for a strong genetic component underlying MS. This is illustrated by the 25–30% concordance among monozygotic twins, the 5% concordance among same-sex dizygotic twins, and the 3.5% concordance among nontwin siblings (Gourraud *et al.* 2012). However, the inheritance of MS cannot be explained by a simple genetic model, and

Multiple Sclerosis and CNS Inflammatory Disorders, First Edition. Edited by Lawrence M. Samkoff and Andrew D. Goodman.

neither the familial recurrence rate nor twin concordance supports the presence of a Mendelian trait. Rather, susceptibility is polygenic, with each gene contributing a relatively small amount of the overall risk. More than likely, genetic heterogeneity (different susceptibilities among individuals) also exists. Additionally, epidemiological data strongly hint at a parent-of-origin effect in MS: maternal half-siblings having double the risk for MS compared to paternal half-siblings (2.35% vs. 1.31%), while the risk for MS in maternal half-siblings compared to their full siblings does not differ significantly (Gourraud et al. 2012). The mechanism of the increased risk conferred maternally remains to be elucidated, but epigenetic mechanisms such as DNA methylation or histone modification may play a role (Handel et al. 2010).

🔬 SCIENCE REVISITED

Maternal parent-of-origin effect

Mendelian traits are controlled by a single locus and involve the transmission of one allele from both mother and father to a diploid offspring. This simple rule may not be followed in MS and other complex disorders, in which not only do multiple genes appear to contribute to susceptibility, but genomic imprinting may play an important role. Imprinting is an epigenetic process through which the expression of a gene is dependent on the sex of the parent from whom it was inherited. In other words, imprinted alleles are silenced such that the genes are either expressed only from the nonimprinted allele inherited from the mother or the father. Epidemiological data hint at a maternal parent-of-origin effect in MS. The mechanism of the increased risk conferred maternally remains to be elucidated, but epigenetic mechanisms that regulate genomic function (such as DNA methylation, RNA-associated silencing, and histone modifications) have been strongly implicated. Examples of other imprinted genetic disorders include Prader–Willi/Angelman syndrome and Russell–Silver syndrome.

The first direct evidence for a relationship between genes and MS susceptibility came in 1972, when MS was shown to be associated with the human leukocyte antigen (HLA) on chromosome 6p21 (encoding proteins involved in presenting peptide antigens to T cells) (Gourraud et al. 2012). This association was later fine-mapped to a specific locus, HLA-DRB1 of the class II gene HLA-DRB1 (Gourraud et al. 2012). Although the HLA-DRB*1501 haplotype exerts the strongest genetic effect in MS (heterozygosity conferring an odds ratio (OR) of 2.7 and homozygosity of 6.7), the association is not straightforward. In fact, a number of HLA-DRB1 haplotypes are both positively and negatively associated with the disease, differ in magnitude of effect, and either act on their own or greatly alter risk in combination with another haplotype (Kallaur et al. 2011). For example, HLA-DRB1*08 only modestly increases MS risk, but in combination with HLA-DRB1*15, it more than doubles the risk associated with a single copy of the latter (Kallaur et al. 2011). On the other hand, HLA-DRB1*14 carries such a protective effect that it completely abrogates the increased risk of HLA-DRB1*15 (Kallaur et al. 2011). And whereas association of MS with HLA-DRB1*15 has long been known in Northern Europe, in other regions, such as Sardinia, HLA-DRB1*0301, HLA-DRB1*0405, and HLA-DRB1*1303 are more commonly associated with MS (Kallaur et al. 2011). In fact, the relative frequencies of susceptibility and protective HLA haplotypes, which vary between countries, may play important roles in determining the risk of the disease.

It has been estimated that the HLA locus accounts for 20–60% of the genetic susceptibility in MS, leaving a large portion of the genetic component of MS (still) to be explained. In 2007, the International Multiple Sclerosis Genetics Consortium (IMSGC) completed the first MS genome-wide association study (GWAS) using trios (an affected individual and both their parents) from the UK and the USA (Gourraud et al. 2012). In addition to the HLA-DRB1 region, two new risk loci were identified: the genes for interleukin-7 receptor alpha (IL-7RA) and interleukin-2 receptor alpha (IL-2RA), which have since been replicated. These genes code for the alpha chain of the IL-7 or IL-2 receptors, which promote lymphocyte growth and differentiation. MS-associated variants in the *IL-2RA* gene contribute to the production of soluble IL-2RA, a biomarker of peripheral inflammation. The IL-7/IL-7RA interaction is important for memory T-cell maintenance and development and proliferation and survival of B and T cells; the protective haplotype is associated with less soluble IL-7RA; the risk allele thus likely produces a change in function (Gregory *et al.* 2007).

The most recent GWAS data from the IMSGC demonstrate at least 102 SNPs exerting a modest effect (OR, 1.06–1.22) (Gourraud *et al.* 2012). Most of the loci harbor genes with pertinent immunological roles, including several genes associated with other autoimmune disorders, consistent with the autoimmune hypothesis of MS etiology. Most notably, the results of the GWAS implicate genes coding for cytokine pathways (CXCR5, IL-2RA, IL-7R, IL-7, IL-12RB1, IL-22RA2, IL-12A, IL-12B, IRF8, TNFRSF1A, TNFRSF14, TNFSF14) and for costimulatory (CD37, CD40, CD58, CD80, CD86, CLECL1) and signal transduction (CBLB, GPR65, MALT1, RGS1, STAT3, TAGAP, TYK2) molecules of immunological relevance (Gourraud *et al.* 2012). Of interest, at least two genes (KIF1B, GPC5) not involved in the immune system but instead with neuronal growth and repair mechanisms may also be associated with MS. These genes may influence the potential of remyelination of lesions, and their discovery gives a hint to a disturbance of repair mechanisms in addition to autoimmune processes in MS.

Still relatively little is known about how the identified MS risk variants exert their effects at the molecular and cellular levels. Their incomplete penetrance and moderate individual effects probably reflect interactions with other genes, posttranscriptional regulatory mechanisms, or significant environmental and epigenetic influences. Further genetic and functional studies are required to pinpoint the functionally relevant genes and pathways, to understand how these influence risk, and to determine if the genes themselves, or the downstream effects thereof, can be modified to alter MS risk.

Gender effects: Genetic or biologic?

MS is more prevalent in females than males, and this female predominance appears to have increased markedly over the past 100 years. Interestingly, the preponderance of females among MS patients is even seen in the pediatric MS population, especially after about the age of 10 years. The mechanisms underlying these observations are still incompletely understood, and most investigations have focused on the role of gonadal hormones. However, several other factors may be of key relevance, such as intrinsic biological differences in the male and female immune system and CNS, genetic and epigenetic factors, maternal microchimerism, and differences in environmental exposures for males and females (e.g., higher numbers and changing roles of women in the workforce, outdoor activity, dietary habits, and alterations in menarche and in the age of childbearing).

The role of the environment

Genetic factors account only partially for MS susceptibility, as illustrated by the twin concordance data. Moreover, even among families, MS risk is known to be strongly influenced by location, season of birth, and the childhood environment. The environment thus appears to play an important role in setting thresholds for genetic penetrance. Further, recent increases in MS incidence are too rapid to be the result of genetic alterations and must, therefore, reflect differential exposure to environmental factors (Alonso & Hernan 2008). In particular, the rising worldwide incidence and increasing female to male preponderance have focused interest on environmental factors that may influence MS risk.

Environmental MS risk factors: The major players

All of the environmental factors involved in MS are not yet known, but accumulating evidence lends strong support to several candidates, most notably sunlight and/or vitamin D exposure, Epstein–Barr virus (EBV), and cigarette smoking (Ascherio & Munger 2007a, b), with unconfirmed or hypothetical support for obesity, diet, and altered gut microbiota as risk factors. These factors could conceivably act to alter susceptibility to MS at any point in life from conception (or even before) to the onset of disease.

Geography

The uneven geographical distribution of MS is central to understanding the role of environment. The prevalence of MS increases with distance from the equator (Ascherio & Munger 2007b) and is greater in areas with temperate rather than tropical climates. Within regions of temperate climate, MS incidence and prevalence increase with latitude. Some of these observations may be explained by the non-random geographic distribution of racial/ethnic groups within these risk areas, such that what appears to be a latitudinal effect may be confounded by the genetic backgrounds of those who live in the various regions (i.e., racial/ethnic groups with a higher burden of risk alleles may be those who happen to live in regions of higher prevalence). However, migration studies demonstrate that moving from a region of high to low risk, or vice versa, leads to the adoption of the risk of the new region, especially if the migration occurred at a young age (Ascherio & Munger 2007b) such that at least part of the latitudinal gradient must be due to environmental differences.

One of the strongest correlates of latitude is the duration and intensity of sunlight. Thus, it is not surprising that an inverse correlation between MS prevalence and sunlight was already noted in early ecological studies; among US veterans, the average annual hours of sunshine and the average December daily solar radiation at place of birth were strongly inversely correlated with MS (Ascherio & Munger 2007b). Furthermore, several retrospective studies have demonstrated that sun exposure during childhood and adolescence as well as outdoor activity as an occupational exposure is inversely related to MS susceptibility (Ascherio & Munger 2007b). The protective effects of sunlight are thought to be mediated by ultraviolet radiation (UVR), possibly via vitamin D (see section Vitamin D).

Migration studies and timing of environmental effect

While early migration studies suggested that migration prior to age 15 is critical to altering the risk of MS (Ascherio & Munger 2007b), more recent data suggest that the critical age period might even extend into the third decade. These intriguing findings suggest that MS risk factors may operate in childhood and beyond puberty, suggesting a more prolonged period of vulnerability (but notably also for potential intervention). There may also be transgenerational epigenetic modifications that influence MS risk, which could potentially be influenced by factors such as diet or sex hormones (Ascherio & Munger 2007b). Studies in UK migrants followed from gestation to the third decade of life suggest risk increases in the subsequent generation (Elian et al. 1990). Gestational or early life timing as a vulnerable period is also suggested by a marginally significant excess risk in dizygotic twins compared with nontwin siblings, coupled with evidence for maternal effects. More direct evidence comes from studies of month of birth in several northern countries, which have latitude-correlated increased risks for spring births and decreased risks for late fall births (Willer et al. 2005). The polarity of this distribution reverses in the southern hemisphere. Moreover, unaffected sibling controls differ in birth-month distribution from the general population as much as their affected brothers and sisters did but in the opposite direction (Willer et al. 2005). Since serum concentrations of vitamin D fluctuate in parallel with seasonal changes in exposure to ultraviolet B (UVB) light, this month of birth effect might reflect maternal end-of-winter deficiencies in vitamin D or in UVB itself. Taken together, these striking findings suggest that risk might be influenced in each of the periods of gestation, childhood, adolescence, and early adulthood. In addition to uncertainties regarding the exact timing of an exposure, it is unclear if exposure needs be discrete or prolonged. Since MS incidence peaks in early adulthood and then declines, risk cannot be determined by age-related mutations. Nevertheless, these data do not rule out a type of environmental imprinting, or that susceptibility (and resistance) could be entrained by cumulative exposures of (more than one) factors in the environment.

Vitamin D

It has become increasingly clear that vitamin D has a wide role in physiology and, importantly, also in disease. Evidence is mounting in support of vitamin D deficiency underlying risk for several autoimmune diseases. The pleiotropic actions of vitamin D, including immunomodulatory functions, lend strong support to the hypothesis that this hormone is important in the etiology of MS.

SCIENCE REVISITED

Vitamin D

The main source of vitamin D in humans is skin exposure to sunlight (hence its nickname, the *sunshine vitamin*), although it can also be obtained through the diet (e.g., through oily fish such as salmon, tuna, and mackerel, as well as cod liver oil) and from supplements. Previtamin D3 is formed in the skin upon exposure of 7-dehydrocholesterol to UVB radiation and is then converted to vitamin D3. Vitamin D from sun exposure and diet is hydroxylated (predominantly) in the liver to produce calcidiol (25(OH)D), the major circulating form of vitamin D. Since calcidiol is biologically inert, it requires further hydroxylation (predominantly) in the kidney to form the physiologically active form of vitamin D, calcitriol (1,25(OH)2D), a lipid-soluble secosteroid. Calcitriol is generally not used as an indicator of vitamin D status because it has a short half-life (15 h), and serum concentrations are closely regulated for purposes of calcium homeostasis. Calcitriol mediates its biological effects by binding to the vitamin D receptor (VDR), which is principally located in the nuclei of target cells and acts as a transcription factor that modulates gene expression. Vitamin D also affects the immune system, and VDRs are expressed in several cells involved in innate and adaptive immune responses, including monocytes, dendritic cells, and activated T and B cells.

For most people, skin exposure to sunlight is the major source of vitamin D and the most important predictor of vitamin D status. Several observations support that vitamin D insufficiency is a risk factor for MS: (1) MS prevalence increases as distance from the equator increases (corresponding with a decrease in sunlight exposure) (Ascherio & Munger 2007b); (2) those who migrate adopt the risk of the new area (Kurtzke *et al.* 1985); (3) UVB radiation (the main source of vitamin D) and skin cancer are inversely correlated with MS risk (Ascherio & Munger 2007b); (4) vitamin D intake significantly decreases the risk of MS (Munger *et al.* 2004); and (5) vitamin D levels inversely correlate with risk of MS later in life (Munger *et al.* 2006).

The strongest evidence for a role for vitamin D comes from a, nested case-control study among US military personnel showing that higher vitamin D levels conferred a lower subsequent risk of MS (Munger *et al.* 2006). Further evidence to support a protective effect of vitamin D on MS risk comes from the longitudinal Nurses' Health Study: those with intake of vitamin D of at least 400 international units (IU)/day had a relative risk (RR) for MS of 0.59 compared with those who did not take supplemental vitamin D (Munger *et al.* 2004). Although confounding by unknown factors cannot be excluded, these cohort data strongly support a protective effect of vitamin D on MS risk. Ecological studies in coastal fishing areas in Norway have shown that inhabitants of these areas have lower MS prevalence than their neighbors dwelling in inland agricultural communities, which may be explained by their greater consumption of fatty seafood and cod liver oil, both rich in vitamin D (Kampman *et al.* 2007).

There is also functional evidence associating vitamin D and MS. There is a vitamin D response element (VDRE) close to the promoter region of HLA-DRB1, and calcitriol (the active form of vitamin D) modulates the expression of the particular allele most consistently associated with increased risk of MS, HLA-DRB1*1501 (Ramagopalan et al. 2009). While the in vivo functional consequence of this finding is yet to be determined, it does form a conceptual basis for an environment–gene interaction in the determination of MS risk. The HLA-DRB1*15 risk allele also interacts with the season of birth such that the reported relationship with risk of MS appears to be predominately driven by those carrying at least one copy of the DRB1*15 risk allele (Ramagopalan et al. 2009). In addition, a recent GWAS found association with genetic regions containing vitamin D metabolism genes—CYP24A1 and CYP27B1 (Gourraud et al. 2012)—providing more evidence for the potential role for vitamin D in MS. However, some data suggest that UV light may exert effects on MS risk independent of vitamin D status, such that some or all of the geographic distribution of MS thought to be due to UV-determined vitamin D levels could in fact be due to another UV-mediated mechanism.

Infection

That MS might be triggered by infection is supported by presence of high concentrations of a number of IgGs in the cerebrospinal fluid (CSF) of more than 90% of MS patients that are not present in the blood (oligoclonal bands), indicative of immune activation. Indirect support for a role of infection in MS is that viruses have been associated with other human and experimental demyelinating diseases. Although dozens of pathogens have been investigated as MS risk factors, it is still not clear which, if any, are definitively etiologic. That being said, there is strong support for EBV infection as important to disease risk in many MS patients.

⬡ SCIENCE REVISITED

Epstein–Barr virus

EBV, also known as human herpesvirus-4 (HHV-4), belongs to the gamma-herpesvirus family, which includes herpes simplex virus and cytomegalovirus. EBV is present in all populations and infects over 90% of individuals at some point in their life. Its discovery dates to the early 1960s, where it was isolated in lymphoma cells cultivated from tumor biopsies obtained from African children with jaw tumors. Primary infection usually occurs through contact with infected saliva and is asymptomatic in young children, but in up to 40% of adolescents and adults, it results in the symptomatic illness infectious mononucleosis (IM), an acute and usually self-limited lymphoproliferative disease. Since EBV preferentially infects B lymphocytes and persists lifelong in a transcriptionally quiescent state in circulating memory B cells, it goes largely undetected by the immune system. By immortalizing autoreactive B cells, which act as professional antigen-presenting cells, it is thought that EBV may drive persistent autoimmunity, possibly through antigen mimicry, immortalization of B-cell clones, and cytotoxic T-cell dysfunction against viral-infected B cells.

Epstein–Barr virus

A link between EBV and MS was first proposed to explain the striking similarity between the epidemiology of IM and that of MS in terms of age, geographical distribution, socioeconomic status, and ethnicity (Ascherio & Munger 2007a). IM, like MS, is rare in developing countries and, more generally, in conditions of poor hygiene, in which virtually all children are infected with EBV in the first years of life (prior to the age at which symptomatic infection with EBV, or IM, occurs). In contrast, IM is common in Western countries, in which about 50% of individuals escape early EBV infection and acquire it during adolescence and young adulthood. In these countries, MS risk is two- to threefold higher among individuals with history of IM (Ascherio & Munger 2007a).

Although more than 90% of the general population appears to encounter EBV at some point in life, several lines of evidence highlight its possible role in the pathogenesis of MS. Large, independent studies have shown that nearly all (>99%) adults with MS are seropositive for antibodies directed against EBV, while the seropositivity rate is slightly lower in unaffected adults. The strongest evidence for the association with MS, however, comes from a nested case-control study of healthy individuals infected with EBV, whose subsequent MS risk increases by severalfold with increasing serum titers of anti-Epstein–Barr nuclear antigen (EBNA) complex and anti-EBNA-1 antibodies (Ascherio & Munger 2007a). These data show that EBV seroconversion predates MS onset. A history of EBV-induced IM increases the risk of developing MS, particularly in individuals who develop IM after the age of 15 years. Given the observation that EBV-negative individuals (likely to be exposed to the highest levels of hygiene) have the lowest risk of MS makes the hypothesis that good hygiene during childhood may predis-pose both to MS and to a later contact with EBV and therefore IM unlikely (Ascherio & Munger 2007a). However, whether the link between MS and EBV infection is actually causal or merely represents an association continues to be debated. In adults who are sero-negative for EBV, there seems to be virtually no risk of developing MS (Ascherio & Munger 2007a). However, while a recent investigation of pediatric MS patients showed that EBNA-1 seropositivity is associated with an increased risk of developing MS, not all individuals with MS were positive for EBV, suggesting that infection with EBV is not necessary for all cases of MS (Waubant et al. 2011).

It is important to note that IM is also not sufficient to cause MS; since the large majority of individuals are infected with EBV, but only a relatively small percentage will ever get MS, other genetic and environmental factors must be critical for MS development. Indeed, the HLA-DRB1*1501 allele has been shown to interact with high levels of EBV antibodies in its association with greater risk of MS (De Jager et al. 2008). Evidence suggests that there may be a synergistic effect of vitamin D and IM on MS risk, possibly by an alteration of the initial education of the immune system or of the subsequent immune response to EBV infection in vitamin D deficient states or by EBV itself potentiating the effects of vitamin D deficiency, leading to autoimmunity.

Other viruses

While several studies of adult MS have attempted to link other viruses to MS risk, the results have been inconclusive. On the other hand, the pediatric MS study described earlier found that, independent of EBV status, remote infection with CMV was associated with a lower risk of developing MS and that HSV-1 status interacted with HLA-DRB1 in predicting MS, such that HSV-1 positivity was associated with a greater MS risk in those without a DRB1*15 allele and a reduced risk in those who were DRB1*15 positive (Waubant et al. 2011). These results need confirmation, but the totality of data suggests that there might be a complex interplay between various viral infections acquired during childhood and MS risk.

Smoking

Cigarette smoking has been shown to sizably increase susceptibility to MS in multiple studies (Ascherio & Munger 2007b). The most recent meta-analysis examining the effect of past or current smoking on MS susceptibility reported an RR between 1.3 and 1.8 associated with smoking (Ascherio & Munger 2007b). The smoking effect appears to be independent of gender (Hedstrom et al. 2009)) as well as of latitude and ancestry (Ascherio & Munger 2007b). The risk of MS increases with cumulative doses of cigarettes. Even children ever exposed to parental smoking have been found to have a higher risk of developing MS (Mikaeloff et al. 2007).

The mechanism relating cigarette smoking to MS risk is unclear. Smokeless tobacco (snuff) use has not been found to increase the risk of MS (Hedstrom *et al.* 2009), suggesting that the effect does not appear to be mediated solely by nicotine, but perhaps by components of the actual cigarette smoke, such as nitric oxide, which has putative roles in demyelination and axonal loss. Animal models have also indicated that smoke exposure affects several facets of the immune system, including innate immunity, B and T lymphocytes, and natural killer cells, so a direct impact of smoking on immune function is possible. Recent studies are just beginning to shed light on how smoking interacts with other factors in influencing MS risk.

⚙ SCIENCE REVISITED

Cigarette smoking

Cigarette smoking is the most important preventable cause of premature disability and death in much of the world. Smokers have a higher prevalence of common diseases such as chronic obstructive pulmonary disease (COPD) and atherosclerosis, as well as some autoimmune diseases. How smoking may be related to the increased incidence of MS is unclear. The link may depend on the immunomodulatory effects of smoking, a direct effect of cigarette smoke components on the blood–brain barrier, or directly toxic effects on the CNS. A low-grade systemic inflammatory response is evident in smokers: elevated levels of C-reactive protein (CRP), interleukin-6, fibrinogen, as well as increased counts of WBC have been reported. Furthermore, coagulation and endothelial function markers like fibrin d-dimer, hematocrit, blood and plasma viscosity, circulating adhesion molecules, tissue plasminogen activator antigen, and plasminogen activator inhibitor type I are altered in chronic cigarette smokers.

Combining risk factors

While genetic and environmental risk factors clearly act together to influence MS risk, they have rarely been studied concomitantly, and much remains to be discovered about their respective contributions to or possible interplay in disease susceptibility. To date, the most comprehensive attempt at mathematically modeling risk factors to improve the prediction of MS was that by De Jager and colleagues, who attempted to combine 16 genetic risk loci, sex, smoking, and anti-EBNA-1 titers into a prediction model (De Jager *et al.* 2009). Overall, their data suggest that information obtained from MS susceptibility loci might provide useful if incorporated into clinical algorithms that contain other information, such as detailed immunological characterizations and environmental risk factors. More studies in large cohorts are needed to better understand the combined predictive power of risk factors.

Conclusion

Understanding the etiology of MS requires solving the complex genetics underlying the disease as well as advancing the understanding of the environmental components of its etiology. More information is needed on how the growing set of genetic susceptibility factors is affected by environmental risk factors such as EBV infection, smoking, and vitamin D status. Advances in genetics, immunology, and cell biology are greatly adding to the understanding of MS, and large national and international collaborations are underway to characterize the precise nature and extent of the multifaceted interactions between these known risk factors, as well as uncovering yet unknown ones. In recent years, the emphasis has increasingly been on identifying modifiable risk factors and translating these findings to the clinic. Thus, low circulating levels of vitamin D and cigarette smoking, clearly modifiable, are promising targets for the prevention and treatment of MS.

Acknowledgment

Dr. Mowry is funded by NIH K23NS067055.

References

Alonso, A. & Hernan, M.A. (2008) Temporal trends in the incidence of multiple sclerosis: a systematic review. *Neurology*, **71** (2), 129–135.

Ascherio, A. & Munger, K.L. (2007a) Environmental risk factors for multiple sclerosis. Part I: the role of infection. *Annals of Neurology*, **61** (4), 288–299.

Ascherio, A. & Munger, K.L. (2007b) Environmental risk factors for multiple sclerosis. Part II: Noninfectious factors. *Annals of Neurology*, **61** (6), 504–513.

De Jager, P.L., Simon, K.C., Munger, K.L., Rioux, J.D., Hafler, D.A. & Ascherio, A. (2008) Integrating risk factors: HLA-DRB1*1501 and Epstein-Barr virus in multiple sclerosis. *Neurology*, **70** (13 Pt 2), 1113–1118.

De Jager, P.L., Chibnik, L.B., Cui, J. *et al.* (2009) Integration of genetic risk factors into a clinical algorithm for multiple sclerosis susceptibility: a weighted genetic risk score. *Lancet Neurology*, **8** (12), 1111–1119.

Elian, M., Nightingale, S. & Dean, G. (1990) Multiple sclerosis among United Kingdom-born children of immigrants from the Indian subcontinent, Africa and the West Indies. *Journal of Neurology, Neurosurgery & Psychiatry*, **53** (10), 906–911.

Gourraud, P.A., Harbo, H.F., Hauser, S.L. & Baranzini, S.E. (2012) The genetics of multiple sclerosis: an up-to-date review. *Immunological Reviews*, **248** (1), 87–103.

Gregory, S.G., Schmidt, S., Seth, P. *et al.* (2007) Interleukin 7 receptor alpha chain (IL7R) shows allelic and functional association with multiple sclerosis. *Nature Genetics*, **39** (9), 1083–1091.

Handel, A.E., De Luca, G.C., Morahan, J. *et al.* (2010) No evidence for an effect of DNA methylation on multiple sclerosis severity at HLA-DRB1*15 or HLA-DRB5. *Journal of Neuroimmunology*, **223** (1–2), 120–123.

Hedstrom, A.K., Baarnhielm, M., Olsson, T. & Alfredsson, L. (2009) Tobacco smoking, but not Swedish snuff use, increases the risk of multiple sclerosis. *Neurology*, **73** (9), 696–701.

Kallaur, A.P., Kaimen-Maciel, D.R., Morimoto, H.K., Watanabe, M.A., Georgeto, S.M. & Reiche, E.M. (2011) Genetic polymorphisms associated with the development and clinical course of multiple sclerosis (review). *International Journal of Molecular Medicine*, **28** (4), 467–479.

Kampman, M.T., Wilsgaard, T. & Mellgren, S.I. (2007) Outdoor activities and diet in childhood and adolescence relate to MS risk above the Arctic Circle. *Journal of Neurology*, **254** (4), 471–477.

Kurtzke, J.F., Beebe, G.W. & Norman, J.E., Jr (1985) Epidemiology of multiple sclerosis in US veterans: III. Migration and the risk of MS. *Neurology*, **35** (5), 672–678.

Mikaeloff, Y., Caridade, G., Tardieu, M., Suissa, S. & KIDSEP study group (2007) Parental smoking at home and the risk of childhood-onset multiple sclerosis in children. *Brain*, **130** (Pt 10), 2589–2595.

Munger, K.L., Zhang, S.M., O'Reilly, E. *et al.* (2004) Vitamin D intake and incidence of multiple sclerosis. *Neurology*, **62** (1), 60–65.

Munger, K.L., Levin, L.I., Hollis, B.W., Howard, N.S. & Ascherio, A. (2006) Serum 25-hydroxyvitamin D levels and risk of multiple sclerosis. *JAMA*, **296** (23), 2832–2838.

National Multiple Sclerosis Society (2012). *What causes MS?* http://www.nationalmssociety.org/about-multiple-sclerosis/what-we-know-about-ms/who-gets-ms/index.aspx [accessed on January 14, 2012].

Ramagopalan, S.V., Link, J., Byrnes, J.K. *et al.* (2009) HLA-DRB1 and month of birth in multiple sclerosis. *Neurology*, **73** (24), 2107–2111.

Waubant, E., Mowry, E.M., Krupp, L. *et al.* (2011) Common viruses associated with lower pediatric multiple sclerosis risk. *Neurology*, **76** (23), 1989–1995.

Willer, C.J., Dyment, D.A., Sadovnick, A.D. *et al.* (2005) Timing of birth and risk of multiple sclerosis: population based study. *BMJ*, **330** (7483), 120.

2

Immunopathogenesis of Multiple Sclerosis

Anne H. Cross and Laura Piccio

Department of Neurology, Washington University School of Medicine, St Louis, MO, USA

What does the neuropathology of MS tell us about its pathogenesis?

Multiple sclerosis (MS) is a common, chronic central nervous system (CNS) disease characterized pathologically by inflammation, demyelination, and axonal loss. CNS pathology of MS suggests an immune-driven reaction to a CNS antigen. In addition to mononuclear inflammatory cell infiltration, the majority of active MS lesions contain antibodies, complement, and soluble immune mediators such as cytokines, chemokines, and free radicals. CNS pathology reveals not only injury to myelin but injury to axons, neurons, and oligodendrocytes. The cellular composition of MS lesions comprises primarily macrophages and T lymphocytes; both CD4 (*helper*) and CD8 (*cytotoxic*) T cells are present. To a lesser degree, B lymphocytes, plasma cells, and other types of cells such as gamma-delta T cells are also found within lesions and within the normal-appearing white matter. Polymorphonuclear cells are conspicuously absent. The neuropathology of MS suggests an autoimmune pathogenesis. However, thus far, no CNS component has been found to be the primary *self*-target of MS pathogenesis. If MS is an autoimmune disease, whether all people with the disease would also have the same autoantigen target is probably unlikely. Moreover, the pathology in active MS lesions is heterogeneous, suggesting either variation in the immune responses and/or the inciting events among individual patients.

> ☼ **SCIENCE REVISITED**
>
> MS has been traditionally viewed as a white matter disorder. However, it is now well accepted that MS lesions can also affect the gray matter, including both deep gray matter structures and cortical gray matter.

Gray matter pathology

For many years, it has been known that the gray matter, especially the deep gray structures such as the thalamus, can be affected by MS. However, a surprising new finding is that the cortical gray matter is affected in MS, often to a great extent. These gray matter lesions tend to be smaller than white matter MS lesions and are more difficult to detect with standard clinical imaging techniques. Demonstration of cortical MS lesions by histology is particularly difficult, but cortical demyelination is clearly apparent using specific myelin stains. Most studies indicate that cortical MS lesions are less inflammatory than white matter lesions. A study of biopsies of white matter lesions that incidentally included cortical gray in the specimen found that 40% had cortical gray MS lesions upon closer inspection. Given that the cortical gray components of these biopsies were small and random, it is plausible that a far greater proportion of the patients would have harbored cortical pathology if more regions had been examined.

Multiple Sclerosis and CNS Inflammatory Disorders, First Edition. Edited by Lawrence M. Samkoff and Andrew D. Goodman.
© 2014 John Wiley & Sons, Ltd. Published 2014 by John Wiley & Sons, Ltd.

Evidences supporting MS as an immune-mediated disease:

- MS neuropathology: presence of immune system cells including T and B lymphocytes, plasma cells, antibodies, and complement.
- MS genetics: the vast majority of genes associated with risk of MS are related to the immune system.
- MS animal model: EAE shares many similarities with MS and is induced by immunization with myelin proteins.
- MS therapies: drugs effective in reducing MS relapses all target the immune system.

Multiple sclerosis as an autoimmune disease

Much evidence supports that MS is a disorder in which the immune response aberrantly targets CNS antigens, leading to CNS pathology. This viewpoint is based on several factors. Genetic associations almost exclusively involve immune system genes, including a strong association of MS with certain HLA class II genes. HLA class II-bearing cells process and present antigens to T cells for the CD4$^+$ subtype. Thus, the manner in which HLA class II might increase risk of MS would presumably occur via its role in the processing and presentation of self-antigens to autoreactive T cells. The beneficial effect of drugs that alter the immune system, such as natalizumab and fingolimod, which affect trafficking of T lymphocytes, also supports an immune mechanism. Similarities of pathology, clinical course, and response to therapies of MS and the commonly used animal model experimental autoimmune encephalomyelitis (EAE) also support an autoimmune mechanism in MS. The EAE model is induced by immunization with any of several different myelin proteins. Despite the convergence of several lines of evidence in favor of an abnormal immune response in the pathogenesis of MS, formal proof that MS is an autoimmune disease is lacking.

Candidates for the self-antigen in multiple sclerosis

Because of the circumstantial evidence favoring an autoimmune etiology of MS, investigators have sought to identify a *self-antigen* that is the target of MS pathogenesis. The greatest focus has been on myelin proteins. T cells reactive to self-myelin proteins, including myelin basic protein (MBP), myelin oligodendrocyte glycoprotein (MOG), and myelin proteolipid protein (PLP), are readily found in MS patients' blood. However, the peripheral blood of healthy controls harbors T cells reactive with the same myelin proteins, and in frequencies similar to MS patients.

Thus, differences in the properties of myelin-reactive T cells in MS versus controls have been sought. Studies using several different methodologies have found that myelin-reactive T cells have been currently or previously activated in MS compared with controls. For example, increased numbers of T cells that recognized MBP and PLP and that expressed interleukin (IL)-2 receptors, a sign of activation, were reported in peripheral blood of MS patients compared with controls. Myelin-reactive T cells in peripheral blood harbor more mutations, a sign of prior proliferation, in MS than control subjects. T cells reactive with MBP, PLP, or MOG from MS patients expressed more Kv1.3 potassium channels per cell, a marker of effector memory T cells, than did T cells from control subjects.

Antigen spreading

Although these studies support that MS patients harbor more previously activated T cells directed against myelin antigens than do controls, they do not necessarily indicate autoimmunity as the *primary* pathogenic mechanism. Targeting of the immune responses to self-antigens may be the consequence of *antigenic spreading*. Here, the concept is that an initial CNS insult results in the liberation of CNS components and subsequently leads to secondary immune responses to these self-antigens, including myelin proteins. For example, MBP is not expressed on surface of myelin sheaths and would only be accessible to immune cells upon myelin destruction. Even when responses to several distinct self-antigens are found in an individual with MS, the initiating event might still have been to a single CNS antigen.

An infection could also incite autoimmunity within the CNS. That such a phenomenon is possible has been conclusively shown using a viral animal model, Theiler's murine encephalomyelitis. This virus-induced CNS demyelinating model is initiated by intracerebral inoculation with Theiler's virus in mice. Initial myelin destruction due to virus and virus-specific T cells is followed by a chronic progressive phase, in which autoreactive T cells that target myelin proteins are the cause of destruction. Presumably, the latter T cells are activated due to myelin destruction in which their target proteins (self-antigens) are accessible for processing and presentation to T cells.

Epitope spreading

Epitope spreading is a phenomenon that represents a subset of *antigen spreading*. Conclusive evidence for epitope spreading in mammals derives from EAE and other autoimmune models of MS. For example, after EAE initiation by immunization with a small peptide component of the CNS myelin antigen, MBP, different regions of the same protein (MBP) become major targets of the ongoing autoimmune response. During the relapsing–remitting course of EAE, T cells specific not only for the initiating MBP peptide but for additional regions of the same protein (epitope spreading) can become activated and mediate relapses in the model. Presumably, a similar phenomenon could occur in MS patients. It has been speculated that one reason why early treatment seems to be most effective in control of MS disease activity is that early treatment can prevent relapses and the tissue destruction that leads to epitope and antigen spreading. More than just CNS tissue destruction is needed to induce chronic, relapsing demyelination, as evidenced by multiple well-performed studies refuting any association of head trauma or stroke with subsequent MS.

> ### ⚗ SCIENCE REVISITED
>
> The *outside-in* hypothesis of MS pathogenesis suggests that immune cells are activated in periphery and then migrate into the CNS where they participate in tissue damage.
>
> The *inside-out* hypothesis implies that a fundamental abnormality exists within the CNS and this subsequently recruits inflammatory cells from the peripheral blood.

Outside-in versus inside-out?

The initial pathogenic events remain unknown. Two opposing mechanistic viewpoints exist, one stating that the initiation of the MS lesion is via an *outside-in* and the other upholding an *inside-out* mode of onset. The opposing mechanisms each have support based on neuropathology studies in MS. However, it should be kept in mind that studies of MS pathology can vary, depending upon the timing, sites, and preservation of tissue sampling; thus, interpretations may be erroneous if samples are not representative. The *outside-in* hypothesis suggests that the fundamental abnormality begins outside the CNS and proceeds into the CNS for lesion development. The *inside-out* mode implies that a fundamental abnormality exists within the CNS, behind the blood–CNS barrier, which subsequently recruits inflammatory cells from the peripheral blood. Such a paradigm is seen in the disease adrenoleukodystrophy (ALD). In ALD, a genetic mutation in the *ABCD1* gene resulting in abnormal white matter causes secondary CNS inflammation and demyelination. One proponent of the *inside-out* version has described early loss of oligodendrocytes without concomitant lymphocyte or macrophage invasion in some acute MS lesions, interpreting these findings as support that the MS disease process began in the CNS, with secondary immune cell recruitment.

Imaging studies have been inconclusive regarding the *inside-out* versus *outside-in* theories.

In careful studies using monthly MRIs, gadolinium enhancement was the very earliest evidence of new lesions in almost 100% of new T2-weighted white matter lesions. Because gadolinium enhancement indicates loss of the blood–CNS barrier integrity and moreover has been shown in limited numbers of studies to correlate closely with cellular inflammation in MS lesions, enhancement at lesion onset best supports the *outside-in* idea. Imaging support for *outside-in* is by no means airtight. Studies using several different nonstandard imaging modalities, such as MR spectroscopy and magnetization transfer, have indicated that abnormalities in CNS may be present months prior to the development of actual gadolinium enhancement and lesions seen by T2-weighted MRI. These studies lend some support to an *inside-out* mechanism. Current imaging techniques cannot fully answer the question of whether the MS lesion begins within the CNS itself or is initiated from the periphery.

Lymphocyte trafficking into the CNS

In either the *outside-in* or the *inside-out* mechanism, immune cells abnormally enter the CNS. Focal changes in vascular permeability including increased expression of cell adhesion molecules by the endothelium are believed to mediate the increased leukocyte trafficking into the CNS. Leukocyte migration through the blood–CNS barrier represents an important step in MS pathogenesis. This multistep process occurs in sequential interactions at postcapillary venules of different adhesion molecules and chemokines (see the following text) expressed on endothelial cells and immune cells. A key adhesion molecule implicated in leukocyte trafficking into the CNS is the α4β1 integrin (VLA-4, very late activating antigen), which is expressed on the lymphocyte surface and interacts with an adhesion molecule (vascular cell adhesion molecule-1, VCAM-1) expressed on the endothelium. The importance of this interaction is supported by the profound effect in decreasing MRI and clinical activity of natalizumab, a monoclonal antibody directed against VLA-4.

Chemokines are small cytokines that regulate migration of immune cells including leukocyte migration into the brain. When present on the surface of the brain endothelium, chemokines mediate leukocyte arrest through binding to specific chemokine receptors on the leukocytes. They also drive leukocyte transendothelial migration and locomotion within the tissue along chemoattractant gradients. Altered levels of chemokines and their receptors have been reported in MS peripheral blood cells, in MS cerebrospinal fluid (CSF), and in CNS lesions of MS. Taken together, these findings support a role of chemokines in MS pathogenesis.

Lymphocyte trafficking is also the presumed mechanistic target of the first oral medication available for MS patients, fingolimod. Fingolimod is a sphingosine-1-phosphate receptor modulator, which functionally acts as an antagonist and which leads to retention of lymphocytes within lymphoid tissue. This results in a profound decrease in circulating lymphocytes and thus the inability of the cells to gain access to the CNS.

Role of T cells in MS

Current evidence favors CD4+ autoreactive T cells as central players in MS pathogenesis. This idea is strongly supported by studies with the EAE animal model, in which the disease can be transferred into naïve recipient mice with myelin-reactive CD4+ T cells. After activation, naïve CD4+ T cells differentiate into one of several subsets with differing functions. Th1 CD4+ T cells produce proinflammatory cytokines such as of interferon (IFN)-γ that are considered critical in MS pathogenesis (IFN-γ treatment of MS led to disease exacerbation). Th17 cells are a distinct subset of CD4+ T cells that produce the proinflammatory cytokines IL-17A and IL-17F. Both Th1 and Th17 CD4+ T cells are independently capable of inducing the EAE mouse model of MS. The presence of IL-17 in MS lesions and increased IL-17 expression in blood and CSF of MS patients have been demonstrated. Additionally, high serum IL-17 concentrations may identify a subset of relapsing–remitting MS patients with a disease subtype that is less responsive to therapy with IFN-β than Th1-predominant MS.

Other subsets of T cells have been implicated in the regulation of the autoimmune and inflammatory responses in MS. These include Th2 cells and regulatory T (Treg) cells that secrete anti-inflammatory cytokines such as IL-4, or IL-10, and TGF-β, respectively. Mechanisms of suppression by Treg cells are poorly understood and may involve cell–cell interactions as well as secretion of regulatory cytokines. Some evidence suggests that Treg cell functions are altered in MS.

CD8+ T cells are also present in inflammatory MS lesions. One hypothesis would be that MS lesion formation is initiated by Th1 and Th17 cells, while amplification and damage are mediated by CD8+ T cells.

⚗ SCIENCE REVISITED

A key role for B lymphocytes in the pathogenesis of MS lesion development has been uncovered using monoclonal antibodies that specifically delete B cells.

Role of B cells and humoral immunity

B cells and humoral immunity have been implicated in MS pathogenesis, mainly because of the presence of oligoclonal bands (OCBs) and increased levels of immunoglobulins (Igs) specific to the CSF in more than 90% of MS patients. B cells, plasma cells, Igs, and complement deposition are typically present in MS lesions and often found in the normal-appearing white matter as well. New and strongly persuasive evidence supporting a central role of B cells in MS pathogenesis is the rapid effectiveness of B cell depletion in reducing disease activity in patients with relapsing MS. Several recent studies have shown the clinical efficacy of depleting circulating B cells with monoclonal antibodies targeting CD20, a surface marker that is expressed solely on mature B cells (rituximab and ocrelizumab).

MOG and MBP are myelin proteins that are often a target for antibodies, but their relevance to disease pathogenesis remains controversial. Many investigators believe that the antibodies targeting myelin proteins are the result rather than the cause of CNS pathology in MS.

On the other hand, CSF antibodies do associate with MS prognosis, suggesting that the antibodies may relate to pathogenesis. Increased concentrations of CSF antibodies and excessive CSF free kappa light chains correlate with MS worsening and poor prognosis. IgM and IgG in the CSF typically demonstrate a pattern of limited clonality, referred to as OCBs because of the banding pattern observed when concentrated CSF is electrophoresed. Higher numbers of CSF OCBs at MS onset are associated with poorer clinical outcome. CSF antibodies against neurofilaments, which are cytoskeletal components of axons, have been reported in the progressive forms of MS, and presence of antibodies to neurofilament in the CSF of MS patients is correlated with cerebral atrophy on MR imaging. Axon damage is common in MS lesions, and cerebral atrophy in MS patients is thought to reflect diffuse axonal loss. Implied by these studies is that antibodies to axonal neurofilaments as well as other CNS components might be pathogenic, although these data are only circumstantial evidence.

Role of microglia and macrophages

Microglia are considered the resident macrophages of the CNS and are quickly activated by injury or pathogens. Microglia provide functions similar to other tissue macrophages, including phagocytosis, antigen presentation, and production of cytokines, eicosanoids, complement components, excitatory neurotransmitters (glutamate), proteinases, and free radicals. Currently, there are no unique histochemical markers that distinguish intrinsic microglia from macrophages that have invaded the brain during inflammation. Based on the pathology of active lesions, macrophages/microglia actively participate in myelin breakdown in MS; phagocytosis of myelin proteins in the lesions by these cells is considered a reliable indicator of ongoing demyelinating activity.

In addition, activated microglia and macrophages express molecules critical for antigen presentation to T cells, including HLA class II and B7-1 and B7-2 molecules. Activated microglia produce a wide range of factors, many of which are likely to be pathogenic, such as prostaglandins, nitric oxide, oxygen free radicals, IL-1β, and TNF-α. Although many microglial products are proinflammatory, some may also have neuroprotective roles. Several lines of evidence demonstrate that microglia can be involved in neuroprotection by the secretion of soluble mediators that trigger neural repair and regeneration.

Role of other cells: Dendritic cells and astrocytes

Dendritic cells (DCs) are professional antigen-presenting cells typically residing in skin and other areas of contact with the external environment that take up and carry antigen to lymphoid tissues. In addition, DCs have several innate functions, such as the production of cytokines and the response to a spectrum of environmental cues by extensive differentiation and maturation. DCs are absent from the normal brain parenchyma but present in normal meninges, choroid plexus, and CSF. They likely play a key role in immune surveillance in the CNS. CNS inflammation is accompanied by recruitment and/or development of DCs in affected brain tissue. Important concepts have emerged lately regarding DCs in MS. DCs accumulate in the CSF and CNS in MS and EAE, and in this context, they are thought to be involved in the regulation of autoimmune responses directed against myelin antigens. Presence of DCs has been demonstrated in parenchymal lesions and meninges of MS patients with evidence of engulfment of myelin components and the potential for antigen presentation to T cells. Thus, CNS-infiltrating DCs may be important for sustaining local T cell activation and expansion.

Astrocytes are the most abundant cell population in the CNS. Among their many roles is to provide physical and metabolic support for neurons. One of the most important functions of these glial cells is their contribution to the formation of the blood–CNS barrier. Astrocytes form the *glia limitans*, a membrane that surrounds the perivascular (Virchow–Robin) spaces. Immune cells that invade the CNS during neuroinflammation, first, must cross the endothelial with its specialized tight junctions, then traverse the Virchow–Robin spaces, and subsequently interact with astrocytes of the *glia limitans* to penetrate into the CNS parenchyma. Astrocytes have potential roles in MS, some of which may be beneficial and others detrimental. Astrocytes might contribute to the limitation of neuroinflammation through the induction of apoptosis in infiltrating T cells, which has been shown in cultures of mouse T lymphocytes, and through proliferation and cellular enlargement to produce gliosis, which functions as a physical and biological barrier to limit the expansion of MS lesions. Gliosis may also limit CNS repair. Expression of antigen-presenting molecules (HLA B7-1 and B7-2) has been demonstrated on astrocytes after stimulation by proinflammatory cytokines, but formal demonstration of a role in antigen processing and presentation to T cells by astrocytes in MS is lacking. Astrocytes are capable of producing various cytokines and toxic molecules, including nitric oxide, that can cause damage.

Role of cytokines

Cytokines are soluble proteins acting in complex networks that have important roles in all phases of immune responses and inflammatory reactions. Proinflammatory cytokines are believed to play roles in MS pathogenesis in several ways, including (1) peripheral immune activation, (2) enhancement of trafficking of activated immune cells into the CNS, and (3) direct damage to oligodendrocytes, myelin, and/or axons. On the other hand, anti-inflammatory cytokines are likely to be beneficial in MS. Altered cytokine profiles have been found in the CNS and in the peripheral blood of

MS patients compared to healthy individuals. Major proinflammatory cytokines implicated in MS include IFN-γ, IL-2, and TNF-α, whereas anti-inflammatory cytokines implicated in MS included IL-10 and TGF-β.

IFN-γ is not only critical in the differentiation of Th1 cells, but also produced by Th1 cells. Its functions include activation of mononuclear cells, but IFN-γ also has regulatory functions (described mainly in animal systems including EAE), including anti-T cell proliferative activity and induction of T cell apoptosis. Of interest, a small clinical trial done in the late 1980s suggested that treatment of MS with recombinant IFN-γ resulted in relapses.

IL-2 acts on CD4$^+$ and CD8$^+$ T cells and is critical for T cell growth, differentiation, survival, and cytokine production. Produced by T cells, it can act in an autocrine manner, by signaling through receptors of the same T cell and further stimulating its own production. IL-2 is important to the development of Tregs as well as other T cells. It was the first cytokine to be shown to be increased in MS. The receptor for IL-2 is CD25, the target of the monoclonal antibody daclizumab, which has shown promising early results in studies of relapsing MS.

TNF-α is another proinflammatory cytokine that may play a role in MS pathogenesis. Numerous studies have reported elevation of TNF-α in CSF and in serum and of TNF-α-secreting blood mononuclear cells in MS patients compared to controls. Because of its potent proinflammatory proprieties, it was hypothesized that TNF-α would be detrimental to patients with MS, but strikingly, drugs that block TNF-α actually lead to worsening of MS. The reason for this is unclear, but perhaps within the context of the CNS, TNF-α has neuroprotective or anti-inflammatory properties. Of note, antibodies to TNF-α ameliorate mouse EAE, demonstrating that the EAE model is an imperfect model for MS.

IL-10 is a major anti-inflammatory cytokine, with its main effect being to inhibit the production of proinflammatory cytokines. IL-10 acts to regulate the immune system by suppressing expression of HLA class II, adhesion molecules, and costimulatory molecules on monocytes/macrophages and DCs. A number of studies have evaluated IL-10 in MS, with contradictory results. Decreased or elevated numbers of PBMC secreting IL-10 and lower serum levels of IL-10 have been reported in MS. Therefore, the role of IL-10 in MS is currently not known. Of note, IL-10 levels in blood were increased after initiation of the immunomodulatory drug, IFN-β.

TGF-β is a cytokine that may be involved in suppression of inflammation late in the chronic stages of disease. However, in the relapsing–remitting early phase of MS, TGF-β may heighten inflammation, as it does in EAE models of MS. TGF-β expression together with IL-6 may drive a Th17 response, a situation expected to perpetuate chronic tissue damage.

What might trigger autoimmunity?

The trigger(s) of the presumed autoimmune process in MS is unknown. Although association of MS risk with genetic markers such a HLA-DRB1*1501 suggests a genetic influence, this association is neither sufficient nor necessary. An environmental trigger seems probable. Infectious and noninfectious triggers have been proposed. The strong association of MS with prior exposure to Epstein–Barr virus (EBV) has stimulated much speculation related to its potential ability to trigger MS. In this regard, EBV peptides have been shown to cross-activate T cells recognizing myelin antigens (*molecular mimicry*), which is a plausible explanation for the link. Peptides of other infectious agents have similar molecular mimic abilities.

Further Reading

Axtell, R.C., de Jong, B.A., Boniface, K. *et al.* (2010) T helper type 1 and 17 cells determine efficacy of interferon-beta in multiple sclerosis and experimental encephalomyelitis. *Nature Medicine*, **16** (4), 406–412.

Benveniste, E.N. (1997) Role of macrophages/microglia in multiple sclerosis and experimental allergic encephalomyelitis. *Journal of Molecular Medicine*, **75** (3), 165–173.

Cannella, B. & Raine, C.S. (1995) The adhesion molecule and cytokine profile of multiple sclerosis lesions. *Annals of Neurology*, **37** (4), 424–435.

Cross, A.H. & Waubant, E. (2011) MS and the B cell controversy. *Biochimica et Biophysica Acta*, **1812** (2), 231–238.

Engelhardt, B. (2008) Immune cell entry into the central nervous system: involvement of adhesion molecules and chemokines. *Journal of the Neurological Sciences*, **274** (1–2), 23–26.

Henderson, A.P., Barnett, M.H., Parratt, J.D. & Prineas, J.W. (2009) Multiple sclerosis: distribution of inflammatory cells in newly forming lesions. *Annals of Neurology*, **66** (6), 739–753.

Kidd, D., Barkhof, F., McConnell, R., Algra, P.R., Allen, I.V. & Revesz, T. (1999) Cortical lesions in multiple sclerosis. *Brain*, **122** (Pt 1), 17–26.

Lucchinetti, C.F., Popescu, B.F., Bunyan, R.F. *et al.* (2011) Inflammatory cortical demyelination in early multiple sclerosis. *The New England Journal of Medicine*, **365** (23), 2188–2197.

McFarland, H.F. & Martin, R. (2007) Multiple sclerosis: a complicated picture of autoimmunity. *Nature Immunology*, **8** (9), 913–919.

Sawcer, S., Hellenthal, G., Pirinen, M. *et al.* (2011) Genetic risk and a primary role for cell-mediated immune mechanisms in multiple sclerosis. *Nature*, **476** (7359), 214–219.

Serafini, B., Rosicarelli, B., Magliozzi, R. *et al.* (2006) Dendritic cells in multiple sclerosis lesions: maturation stage, myelin uptake, and interaction with proliferating T cells. *Journal of Neuropathology and Experimental Neurology*, **65** (2), 124–141.

Sospedra, M. & Martin, R. (2005) Immunology of multiple sclerosis. *Annual Review of Immunology*, **23**, 683–747.

Vanderlugt, C.L., Begolka, W.S., Neville, K.L. *et al.* (1998) The functional significance of epitope spreading and its regulation by co-stimulatory molecules. *Immunological Reviews*, **164**, 63–72.

Williams, A., Piaton, G. & Lubetzki, C. (2007) Astrocytes--friends or foes in multiple sclerosis? *Glia*, **55** (13), 1300–1312.

Wucherpfennig, K.W. (2001) Structural basis of molecular mimicry. *Journal of Autoimmunity*, **16** (3), 293–302.

3

Diagnostic Process

Dalia Rotstein[1,2] and Paul O'Connor[1,2]

[1]Division of Neurology, Institute of Medical Science, University of Toronto, Toronto, Ontario, Canada
[2]St Michael's Hospital, University of Toronto, Toronto, Ontario, Canada

Introduction

Multiple sclerosis (MS) is a chronic disease characterized by multiple demyelinating attacks on the brain or spinal cord. In this chapter, we will discuss the phenotypes of MS, including the most common, relapsing–remitting MS (RRMS), in which there are clinical attacks of distinct neurological symptoms followed by complete or partial improvement. This is the trademark clinical history of MS, and it is accompanied by the characteristic MRI appearance of multiple white matter lesions, with new lesions developing over time. However, another classic feature of the disease is its variability among individuals in the number of relapses and extent of disability progression, which can make it challenging to prognosticate and sometimes to make a firm diagnosis. Fortunately, whereas MS was once solely a clinical diagnosis, MRI has allowed us to identify the disease with more confidence and earlier in the disease's evolution. We will review the 2010 McDonald criteria, the latest consensus guidelines for diagnosis. We will conclude with a discussion of several conditions that may mimic the symptoms of MS and should be considered early in the diagnostic workup. Ancillary tests, including CSF studies and antiaquaporin-4 neuromyelitis optica (NMO) serum antibody testing, may be helpful where diagnostic dilemmas arise.

Clinical features of MS

Defining MS

MS is a primary chronic disease of the central nervous system (CNS) that typically presents in early adulthood. It involves multiple attacks on the brain and/or spinal cord that are separated in space and in time. *Sclerosis* refers to the plaques or focal areas of demyelination that are the pathological substrate of the disease. The 2010 revised McDonald criteria define an attack as "patient-reported symptoms or objectively observed signs typical of an acute inflammatory demyelinating event in the CNS, current or historical, with duration of at least 24 h, in the absence of fever or infection." Demyelination may occur in areas that do not give rise to expression of symptoms as well as in neurologically eloquent areas that lead to the attacks or relapses experienced by patients. These *silent attacks* are most easily appreciated on MRI imaging. Clinical relapses in MS are therefore sometimes referred to as the *tip of the iceberg*, as there often are considerably more demyelinating lesions that can be visualized on imaging than one would expect from the clinical history.

Multiple Sclerosis and CNS Inflammatory Disorders, First Edition. Edited by Lawrence M. Samkoff and Andrew D. Goodman.

☆ **TIPS AND TRICKS**

Clinical attacks are the *tip of the iceberg* in MS. Demyelinating lesions may occur that do not give rise to clinical symptoms. MRI can help to predict the likelihood of future relapses after a first attack by providing a more complete picture of the number and extent of previous lesions.

Indeed, one of the classic features of MS is the great variability that exists among affected patients in clinical manifestations, disability progression, and lesion load. The lesions in MS are thought to result from an autoimmune reaction against the CNS. Recent infectious illness and immune activation, such as during the postpartum period, are known to provoke relapses.

MS disease courses

During an MS relapse, symptoms develop over hours to days then usually persist for weeks before improving. The majority of untreated MS patients experience the occasional clinical relapse every 1–2 years followed by remission with partial or complete recovery (Figure 3.1). This pattern is known as RRMS and affects 85% of those initially diagnosed with MS. Eventually, relapses become less frequent and then cease altogether. Around the same time, disability begins to steadily accumulate. This phase is known as secondary progressive MS (SPMS). There are two other main disease courses in MS: primary progressive MS (PPMS) and progressive relapsing MS (PRMS).

Declining mobility often helps to mark where RRMS ends and SPMS begins. Over time, patients may progress from ambulating with minor difficulty to needing a cane to walk to using a walker to requiring a wheelchair to being bedbound. Pre-existing deficits, such as impairments in vision, balance, and bladder control, tend to worsen during this stage of the disease. Bulbar dysfunction can occur as an advanced manifestation, and aspiration pneumonia or asphyxia can cause mortality.

It can be challenging to define when RRMS transitions into SPMS because relapses may continue even as neurologic disability starts to accumulate. Median time from first symptoms to walking with a cane has been estimated to be between 15 and 30 years with wide variation among studies. More recent studies have shown longer times to walking with a cane, which may reflect benefits from the disease-modifying therapies introduced in the 1990s. By some reports, 15% of people with MS appear to have a more *benign* or nonprogressive course, even many years after the disease's onset.

☆ **TIPS AND TRICKS**

Factors that predict poor outcome in RRMS include higher relapse rate, early onset of clinical progression, shorter interval to the second relapse, greater level of disability within the first 5 years of the disease, and the involvement of more systems (i.e., motor, sensory, cerebellar, etc.).

About 15% of patients experience an insidious onset of symptoms, with slow but inexorable progression in neurologic impairment. This is the hallmark of PPMS. In the majority of cases, patients present with a spastic paraparesis, often with asymmetric signs. Other common symptoms that may be evident on presentation or develop later include gait difficulties, weakness, ataxia, bladder dysfunction, sexual dysfunction, and sometimes cognitive issues. As in RRMS, it can be helpful to elicit characteristic clinical features like worsening with heat, exercise, and infection. However, history does not reveal episodes of unprovoked acute neurologic worsening.

In contrast to RRMS, which predominantly affects women, there is no gender imbalance among those diagnosed with PPMS. Patients are typically about 10 years older at onset compared to RRMS. Disability accumulates more rapidly, but there remains significant variability in the rate of progression as with RRMS. Poor prognostic features include spinal cord lesions, early brainstem or cerebellar lesions, male gender, and younger age at onset. Although MRI findings are

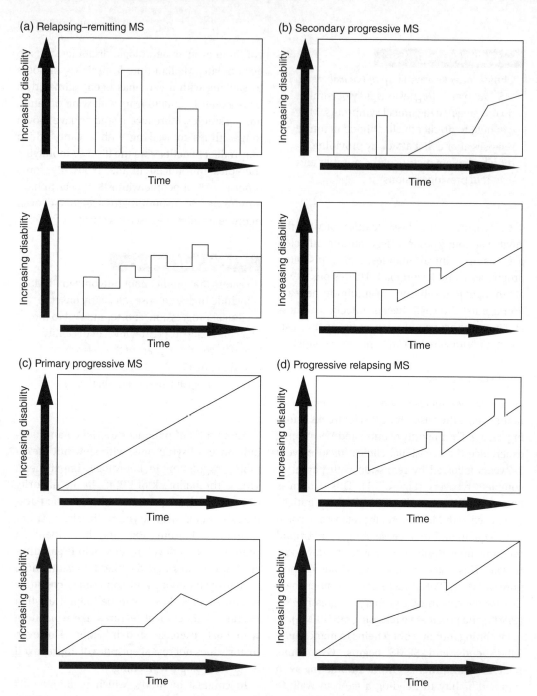

Figure 3.1 Disease courses of MS. These drawings illustrate how disability evolves with time in the different courses of the disease. (a) In RRMS, subjects may have complete recovery from intermittent relapses, or they may have partial recovery with some residual disability. (b) Subjects may have progressive disability without relapses in SPMS, or they may have some continuing relapses early in SPMS superimposed on an underlying progressive course. (c) PPMS can progress at a steady rate or may fluctuate in terms of rate of decline, in either event without any clear relapses. (d) In PRMS, there are both relapses and progressive decline from the onset of the disease, and recovery from relapses may be partial or complete. Source: Lublin and Reingold (1996). Reproduced with permission of Lippincott Williams & Wilkins.

similar to RRMS, the cerebral lesion burden and the prevalence of gadolinium-enhancing lesions are typically less than is seen in RRMS and SPMS. MRI is essential in the diagnosis of PPMS as it rules out other important differential diagnoses—structural lesions, cervical spondylopathy, leukodystrophy, and nutritional deficiencies (e.g., vitamin B12 or copper deficiency)—that may be difficult to distinguish on the basis of clinical presentation alone.

> ## ✋ CAUTION!
>
> Before making a diagnosis of PPMS, consider ruling out these common mimics: structural lesions, cervical spondylopathy, and vitamin B12 deficiency.

Approximately 5% of patients present with PRMS. These patients have distinct relapses, in which recovery may be incomplete, after an initial progressive course. Nevertheless, they continue to demonstrate slowly accumulating neurologic disability from disease onset.

There is a fifth categorization of MS disease types that is in fact a precursor to MS. The clinically isolated syndrome (CIS) refers to a single demyelinating attack. The majority of patients with CIS will go on to have a second attack, thus meeting criteria for clinically definite MS. A minority will never have another attack. MRI imaging has allowed us to predict the risk of conversion to MS on the basis of multiple white matter lesions in characteristic locations on MRI. In the Optic Neuritis Treatment Trial, there was an overall 50% risk of converting to clinically definite MS 15 years after an isolated optic neuritis. If there were one or more lesions on the MRI, the risk was 72%.

The 2010 *McDonald* diagnostic criteria allow more cases of first demyelinating attacks to be more expeditiously diagnosed as MS. The diagnosis can be made on the basis of a single clinical attack if there is an asymptomatic gadolinium-enhancing lesion and at least one other lesion. Alternatively, a second scan performed at any point following the first that demonstrates a new T2 lesion can be considered as proof of *dissemination in time* (DIT).

Occasionally, a first demyelinating attack can be quite fulminant, and it can be difficult to distinguish between a CIS foreshadowing MS and another pathological demyelinating process such as acute disseminated encephalomyelitis (ADEM) or NMO. The Marburg variant of MS refers to a fulminant form of the disease that is often fatal. Imaging shows large, enhancing lesions with mass effect. Tumefactive MS denotes a large, demyelinating lesion difficult to distinguish from tumor on the basis of imaging alone. It may present in a fulminant manner and be considered as an example of a Marburg variant MS or may present with more focal features. Magnetic resonance spectroscopy can be helpful in making the diagnosis, but sometimes brain biopsy is necessary.

Common symptoms in MS

A first demyelinating attack can often be quickly identified by its characteristic pattern of onset, the age of the subject, and symptoms involved. MS attacks usually occur in individuals between ages 15 and 50. The onset of symptoms is subacute over several hours to days. Symptoms then typically plateau, although they may persist for weeks to months before improving. Symptoms must persist for at least 24 h to be considered an attack consistent with MS. An attack may consist of one main clinical symptom or multiple symptoms.

Occasionally, the development of symptoms will represent a pseudoexacerbation rather than a new lesion. Pseudoexacerbations may be incited by infections, such as a UTI, or by overexertion. A transient worsening or appearance in symptoms with heat is known as *Uhthoff's* phenomenon. Patients will often complain of visual blurring, fatigue, or pain during a hot shower or on a very hot day. This finding was first described by Uhthoff in 1890 in the context of worsening of vision in subjects with optic neuritis after exercise. The pathophysiology of Uhthoff's is likely related to conduction block at

Table 3.1 Common Presenting Symptoms in MS

Most Common Presenting Symptoms	Other Symptoms
Sensory disturbance	Diplopia
Visual loss	Vertigo
Weakness	Bladder dysfunction
Ataxia	Gait disturbance
	Lhermitte's sign
	Pain
	Fatigue
	Headache

elevated temperatures. The threshold for conduction block is lower in demyelinated nerves because of current leakage along the full length of the axon.

Common presenting symptoms of MS are listed in Table 3.1. Sensory loss or disturbance is the most common presenting complaint. The most classic description is of numbness, tingling, and *pins and needles* sensations in the limbs. However, patients may also complain of a limb feeling heavy, cold, swollen, or as if it is vibrating. Some patients describe bilateral limb changes or a band-like sensation around the torso suggesting a spinal cord lesion localization. Spinal cord lesions in MS are often partial and in the posterior cord, with asymmetric examination findings.

Visual loss secondary to optic neuritis is the next most common presentation of MS. The affected eye or brow area can be painful, especially with lateral movement. The subject may also complain of photophobia. Color vision is altered, with loss of red–green contrast. Reds are often described as darker or muddier for the impaired eye. There may be a visual field cut, although the field loss is usually central. On examination, the deficit in visual acuity may range from minimal to complete loss of light perception. In general, optic neuritis associated with MS leads to a good recovery in visual acuity. In patients with visual loss that remains fixed, alternative diagnoses should be sought. NMO is another demyelinating disease in which optic neuritis has a much poorer prognosis.

⚠ CAUTION!

Optic neuritis that recovers poorly is less likely to be typical MS.

On fundoscopy, blurred disc margins will be seen in approximately one-third of cases. Later, the disc may appear pale due to atrophy of the optic nerve. The pallor is often best appreciated in the temporal aspect of the disc. In more than two-thirds of cases, the lesion in the optic nerve is retrobulbar and is not visible on fundoscopy.

A relative afferent papillary defect, also known as the Marcus Gunn pupil, may be present. This finding is most easily elicited in a dark room using the swinging flashlight test.

Weakness often affects the legs first. Examination findings can be subtle but should conform with a pyramidal distribution. Other upper motor neuron (UMN) signs that illustrate corticospinal tract involvement include hyperreflexia, clonus, and extensor plantar responses. As with sensory symptoms, when motor symptoms are bilateral, a spinal cord localization is implicated.

Posterior fossa symptoms, such as diplopia, ataxia, and vertigo, are other common presenting complaints. Diplopia in MS can be related to a lesion in one of the nuclei of cranial nerve (CN) III, IV, or VI; to a lesion in one of the fascicles of these cranial nerves; or to a lesion in the medial longitudinal fasciculus (MLF), an internuclear ophthalmoplegia (INO). The INO is most often associated with MS, although it can occasionally be seen in other disorders. The classic exam findings consist of an ipsilateral deficit in adduction and a contralateral abducting nystagmus. These deficits may be sufficiently subtle that all that is seen is slowing of adducting saccades. Unlike with a third nerve palsy, convergence is preserved.

Ataxia is usually associated with a lesion in the cerebellum or the cerebellar outflow pathways. Other cerebellar signs can be present including nystagmus, hyper- or hypometric saccades, scanning speech, and intention tremor. Ataxia can impair ambulation more than weakness, especially early in the disease. Patients may also complain of vertigo, frequently misdiagnosed as peripheral in origin. The presence of vertical or multidirectional nystagmus is indicative of central localization.

Other symptoms of MS can be associated with individual relapses but may also occur between attacks. Many people with MS report bladder and bowel dysfunction. Urinary urgency is the most common symptom; it results from uninhibited detrusor contraction. A hyperactive bladder can also cause urinary frequency, nocturia, and urge incontinence. Constipation and bowel urgency may also be present. Cognitive impairment commonly becomes evident as the disease progresses, although can also be an initial presenting complaint. It is highly unusual to observe cortical cognitive deficits such as aphasia and neglect. Neuropathic pain is suffered by many with MS and can even be a presenting symptom of the disease. Pain syndromes associated with MS include trigeminal neuralgia, L'hermitte phenomenon, paroxysmal tonic spasms, and dysesthetic limb pain. These are discussed elsewhere in this book.

Diagnostic evaluation of MS

MRI

MRI is undoubtedly the most helpful investigation in diagnosing MS. This is covered in more detail in another section of this book.

In general, MS lesions are typically asymmetrical in distribution, ovoid in shape, and greater than 5 mm in diameter. They occur in characteristic areas: the periventricular subcortical white matter, centrum semiovale, corpus callosum, cerebellum, brainstem, and juxtacortical white matter. Supratentorial lesions are best seen as hyperintensities on the FLAIR sequence, but in the posterior fossa, the T2 sequence is usually most revealing. A sagittal FLAIR can be very useful to identify *Dawson's fingers*, linear, flame-like hyperintense streaks that run perpendicular to the lateral ventricles along the path of the deep medullary veins. Dawson's fingers are highly specific for MS, but not truly pathognomonic, as they can be seen in some other inflammatory processes.

The T1 sequence is useful in viewing *black holes*, areas of hypointensity that can persist or resolve over a period of months. Persistent holes suggest chronic axonal loss. A gadolinium-enhanced T1 series can help to identify recent plaques. Contrast uptake can be detected within approximately 30–40 days of acute CNS attack with blood–brain barrier breakdown. Not all new lesions enhance with gadolinium. Sensitivity can be increased by using higher dose gadolinium (two to three times the regular dose). The pattern of enhancement is typically homogenous or in an open ring bordering the lesion. Occasionally, closed ring enhancement may be observed, which can pose a diagnostic dilemma over a demyelinating versus neoplastic etiology.

The MRI is highly sensitive for MS, though it is not specific. It can be difficult to distinguish between demyelinating lesions and leukoaraiosis, particularly in older individuals and those with a history of migraine headaches. The size of the lesions can be helpful, as demyelinating lesions are typically larger, >5 mm. The distribution of lesions is also important, as it is rare for ischemic lesions to directly abut the ventricles or to appear in the corpus callosum. A spinal cord MRI can be essential in differentiating demyelinating disease from leukoaraiosis, as it is more specific than brain MRI. MS-related spinal cord lesions are typically asymmetrical, longitudinally oriented lesions, located in the posterior aspect of the cord. They usually should span fewer than two vertebral segments. Longer lesions should raise the question of other demyelinating etiologies, particularly NMO. Table 3.2 lists features that may help discriminate between MS and other disease processes based on brain MRI.

Revised McDonald criteria for diagnosis of MS

The International Panel on the Diagnosis of Multiple Sclerosis, chaired by Dr. W. I. McDonald, first published a new set of criteria for diagnosing MS in 2001 that incorporates the use of

Table 3.2 MRI Features That Suggest Against a Diagnosis of MS

Symmetrical lesions
Diffuse white matter involvement
Unilateral lesions
Enhancement of all lesions
Absence of periventricular or corpus callosum lesions
Large and infiltrating brainstem lesions
Hemorrhage
Ill-defined lesion margins
Lesions <5 mm
Multiple basal ganglia lesions

Table 3.3 Differential Diagnosis of MS

Etiology	Disease
Inflammatory	Neurosarcoidosis
	SLE
	Behçet disease
	Sjögren syndrome
Infectious	HIV
	Lyme disease
	Neurosyphilis
	PML
	Cat scratch disease
	HTLV-1 and HTLV-2
Neoplastic	Lymphoma
	Paraneoplastic disorders
Vascular	Leukoaraiosis
	CNS vasculitis
	Spinal dural AV malformation
	Susac syndrome
	Stroke
Metabolic	Vitamin B12 deficiency
	Central pontine myelinolysis
Congenital disorders	Leukodystrophy
	Mitochondrial disease
	Spinocerebellar ataxia
	CADASIL
	Arnold–Chiari malformation
Nonorganic/ psychiatric	Conversion disorder
	Somatization disorders

MRI data in the assessment of lesion DIT and dissemination in space (DIS). In 2010, the International Panel published a second revision to the McDonald criteria, which are also discussed in detail in another chapter of this book. Along with allowing for earlier diagnosis, their stated goals included ensuring *applicability across populations*, particularly pediatric, Asian, and Latin American populations, in whom MS may present and evolve differently from the traditional Caucasian population studied. Both the DIS and DIT criteria were considerably simplified, without compromising sensitivity or specificity. The new criteria permit the diagnosis of MS based on only two or more lesions in at least two characteristic regions. In addition, MS can be diagnosed on the basis of a single MRI in certain situations. The authors emphasized that these criteria should only be applied after a first attack where the patient presents with typical symptoms and MRI appearance. It remains imperative to consider a differential diagnosis and order appropriate investigations to exclude other diagnoses.

⚓ CAUTION!

The 2010 McDonald criteria should only be applied after a first attack with symptoms and MRI appearance typical of MS.

With the 2010 criteria, a diagnosis of MS remains possible with a convincing history of at least two clinical attacks, although MRI can be useful in confirming the diagnosis. If there has been only one clinical attack, evidence of both DIS and DIT must be proven to establish a diagnosis of MS. PPMS may be diagnosed where there are no attacks, but progression from onset (Table 3.3). These criteria for PPMS have been adapted to harmonize with the MAGNIMS approach. Positive CSF continues to be counted toward the diagnosis of PPMS.

The revised 2010 criteria continue to uphold the importance of objective evidence of at least one clinical attack in making a diagnosis of MS. The recently described entity of the radiologically isolated syndrome (RIS), in which an MRI picture characteristic of MS is discovered incidentally in an individual with no history of clinical attacks or significant neurological disability, does not qualify as MS under these criteria. The first, small longitudinal series of patients with RIS have suggested that about one-third will develop a CIS after 2–3 years of follow-up. The long-term probabilities of RIS evolving into CIS and MS are unknown.

Ancillary testing in the diagnosis of MS

Blood work should be sent to rule out conditions that can mimic MS. Serum vitamin B12 and TSH levels can be measured as deficiencies in vitamin B12 and thyroid hormone are reversible causes of focal neurologic symptoms. Serum NMO antibody testing should be performed where there are suspicious clinical or radiologic signs. ESR, C-reactive protein, ANA, anti-DNA, and ACE levels can serve as screening tests for inflammatory processes that may cause similar T2 multifocal lesions.

CSF studies have long been incorporated into the diagnostic workup of patients with suspected MS. CSF is probably most helpful in ruling out other differential diagnoses, particularly in PPMS. WBC count is usually normal or mildly elevated in MS, rarely >20. A WBC count >50 should lead one to question the diagnosis. Protein level should be within normal limits or mildly elevated <100 mg/dl. CSF opening pressure should likewise be normal. Oligoclonal banding and IgG index are measured as indicators of intrathecal antibody secretion. The gold standard for the detection of oligoclonal banding involves running CSF on agarose gel with isoelectric focusing followed by immunoblotting. The CSF banding is compared to the pattern from the patient's own serum with the presence of two or more oligoclonal bands *unique to the CSF* considered to be a positive finding. Quantification of the CSF IgG index is also predictive of MS where the index is increased. In general, it should be considered a complimentary procedure to oligoclonal banding using isoelectric focusing and immunofixation, as it has lower sensitivity and specificity. CSF oligoclonal banding or IgG index is positive in 85–90% of patients with MS. Presence of oligoclonal banding is associated with a greater probability of conversion to clinically definite MS in CIS cases but with somewhat lower sensitivity.

Oligoclonal banding is not specific for MS. The differential diagnosis of positive oligoclonal bands includes CNS infections (HIV, syphilis, Lyme disease, subacute sclerosing panencephalitis, chronic meningitis, measles, rubella), inflammatory diseases (SLE, neurosarcoidosis, NMO, ADEM), neoplastic processes (paraneoplastic disorders), and congenital disorders (adrenoleukodystrophy, CADASIL).

Evoked potentials can provide objective evidence of subclinical neurological deficits. A delay in the P100 response or asymmetry in responses between the eyes provides evidence of visual dysfunction. Visual evoked potentials are abnormal in over 80% of patients with MS. They are typically the most useful evoked potential and can be essential in identifying optic nerve lesions because the optic nerves are often not well visualized on conventional MRI. Somatosensory and brainstem auditory evoked potentials may also be helpful but are somewhat less sensitive.

Optical coherence tomography (OCT) is a new technique that allows for detection of optic nerve disease in MS through measurement of retinal nerve fiber layer thickness. Its sensitivity and specificity in determining optic nerve lesions remain to be defined.

Differential diagnosis of MS

Sound clinical reasoning continues to be a critical element in the diagnosis of MS. With lower lesion counts necessary to meet the 2010 McDonald diagnostic criteria, it is critical that these should only be applied where clinical history and MRI appearance are typical of MS. Several features on history and examination should give the clinician pause (Table 3.4 and Table 3.5).

There are various diseases that may mimic MS and should be considered during the diagnostic workup, depending on the patient's presenting features. One of the most frequently

Table 3.4 Historical Features Suggesting Against MS

Sudden or insidious onset (except of the latter in PPMS)
Onset before age 10 or after age 50
Constitutional symptoms
Involvement of other organ systems
Rash
Decreased LOC or encephalopathy
Cortical deficits (i.e., aphasia, neglect)

Table 3.5 Examination Findings Suggesting Against MS

Significant early cognitive deficits
Sensorineural hearing loss
Combination of UMN and LMN signs
Cranial neuropathies other than CN II, V, VII
Meningismus
Myopathy

concerning differentials is with other demyelinating diseases, mainly ADEM and NMO.

ADEM is a monophasic demyelinating process that is thought to follow infection or vaccination, although the infection may have been asymptomatic. Occasionally, a second relapse has been reported in cases of ADEM, although it is highly unusual. ADEM is much more common in children than in adults and is discussed in the chapter on pediatric MS. Presenting symptoms differ from MS in that encephalopathy is usually present and may be prominent. Seizures may occur. It typically takes patients weeks to months to recover, whereas the resolution of relapses is more rapid for the most part in MS. The classic MRI appearance is of larger, bilateral, diffusely enhancing white matter lesions. Gray matter involvement may be evident, which would be expected to be minimal on conventional MRI in MS. There may be up to 100 WBCs in the CSF, and there is often a modest elevation in CSF protein. The CSF is rarely positive for oligoclonal banding or an elevated IgG index. CSF studies are therefore often useful in predicting the likelihood of MS in first attacks that do not clearly conform with a diagnosis of ADEM or MS based on clinical features. The 2010 McDonald criteria need to be applied with caution in these instances, and sometimes, a final diagnostic decision must be postponed.

Acute hemorrhagic leukoencephalitis is a fulminant disease that is thought to be a form of ADEM. It presents with fever, meningismus, multifocal neurological signs, and decreased LOC and seizures following a URTI. Peripheral WBC and CSF WBC, RBC, protein, and opening pressure are elevated. Pathology on autopsy has revealed microvascular hemorrhagic lesions and necrotic venules with fibrinous exudates in these cases. Encephalitis, especially herpes simplex encephalitis, needs to be considered in the differential diagnosis and treated appropriately.

NMO is another demyelinating disease (covered in greater detail in another chapter) with a unique pathophysiology, involving antibodies against the aquaporin-4 water channel found in the foot processes of astrocytes at the blood–brain barrier. Clinically, NMO is defined by demyelinating lesions in the optic nerves and longitudinally extensive lesions (>3 vertebral segments) in the spinal cord. Brain MRI can be normal in NMO or there can be few lesions with a predominantly infratentorial distribution. There is predilection for disease in the region of the hypothalamus and around the third and fourth ventricles. Spinal cord MRI reveals longer lesions that are typically located in the central cord and often cause cord expansion. CSF may demonstrate a neutrophilic pleocytosis. NMO is more often seen in patients of Asian, African, and Latin origin; there should be a lower threshold to test for NMO in these populations. Patients with new complete transverse myelitis should also be tested. The diagnosis is made by meeting clinical criteria that include serum NMO antibody testing. Patients with NMO often do not have full recovery from relapses and may have more rapid progression. There are important implications for treatment, as NMO patients are often less responsive to routine corticosteroid treatment and may actually do worse with interferon therapy.

There are many other disorders that should be considered in the differential diagnosis of

MS, depending on the clinical circumstances (Table 3.3). A history of symptoms with sudden onset should lead one to consider a vascular process or mitochondrial disease. Onset at a young age should raise the possibility of a congenital disorder, infectious illness, or ADEM, and CSF studies may help in this differential. In patients with onset after age 50, leukoaraiosis and neoplastic disease in particular should be considered. Constitutional symptoms should prompt investigations into ADEM, other inflammatory disorders, CNS infection, and neoplastic disease.

Where there is encephalopathy, a broad differential, including all of the main etiologies listed in Table 3.3, should be entertained. Cortical deficits or lesions that affect both the white and gray matter should lead to evaluation for ADEM, a CNS vasculitis, a neoplastic process, Susac syndrome, or mitochondrial disease. Sensorineural hearing loss may rarely be seen in MS but should lead one to assess for Susac syndrome or mitochondrial disease. The coexistence of UMN and LMN findings is concerning for systemic autoimmune disease, HIV, Lyme disease, neurosyphilis, lymphoma, vasculitis, vitamin B12 deficiency, leukodystrophies, and mitochondrial disease.

If multiple cranial neuropathies occur, neurosarcoidosis, Lyme disease, neurosyphilis, vasculitis, and lymphoma and other neoplastic processes should be considered. Where there are progressive symptoms from onset, all of the diagnostic categories listed in Table 3.3 should be assessed for with serum and CSF studies, in addition to MRI. CSF studies and NMO testing should be pursued in cases of transverse myelitis, excluding a partial transverse myelitis with a lesion highly typical for MS. When no MRI lesions are found despite clinical attacks, psychiatric causes should be considered.

Conclusion

MS is a chronic demyelinating disease of the CNS involving multiple lesions separated in space and time. It may evolve according to several different clinical courses, of which relapsing–remitting is the most prevalent. Most patients eventually develop secondary disease progression with accumulating disability. The McDonald diagnostic criteria were revised in 2010 to allow for earlier diagnosis of the disease and simplification of the DIS and DIT requirements. These criteria should be applied only in typical clinical presentations and MRI appearances of MS. There are many illnesses that can mimic MS, and it is essential to evaluate for these where historical, examination, imaging, or laboratory findings do not meet with expectations.

Further Reading

Freedman, M.S., Thompson, E.J., Deisenhammer, F. et al. (2005) Recommended standard of cerebrospinal fluid analysis in the diagnosis of multiple sclerosis: a consensus statement. *Archives of Neurology*, **62**, 865–870.

Lublin, F.D. & Reingold, S.C. (1996) Defining the clinical course of multiple sclerosis: results of an international survey. *Neurology*, **46**, 907–911.

McDonald, W.I., Compston, A., Edan, G. et al. (2001) Recommended diagnostic criteria for multiple sclerosis: guidelines from the International Panel on the diagnosis of multiple sclerosis. *Annals of Neurology*, **50**, 121–127.

Miller, D.H., Weinshenker, B.G., Filippi, M. et al. (2008) Differential diagnosis of suspected multiple sclerosis: a consensus approach. *Multiple Sclerosis*, **14**, 1157–1174.

Montalban, X., Tintoré, M., Swanton, J. et al. (2010) MRI criteria for MS in patients with clinically isolated syndromes. *Neurology*, **74**, 427–434.

Polman, C.H., Reingold, S.C., Edan, G. et al. (2005) Diagnostic criteria for multiple sclerosis: 2005 revisions to the "McDonald Criteria". *Annals of Neurology*, **58**, 840–846.

Polman, C.H., Reingold, S.C., Banwell, B. et al. (2011) Diagnostic criteria for multiple sclerosis: 2010 revisions to the McDonald criteria. *Annals of Neurology*, **69**, 292–302.

Poser, C.M., Paty, D.W., Scheinberg, L.C. et al. (1983) New diagnostic criteria for multiple sclerosis: guidelines for research protocols. *Annals of Neurology*, **1**, 227–231.

Rovira, A., Swanton, J., Tintoré, M. et al. (2009) A single, early magnetic resonance imaging study in the diagnosis of multiple sclerosis. *Archives of Neurology*, **5**, 287–292.

Swanton, J.K., Rovira, A., Tintoré, M. *et al.* (2007) MRI criteria for multiple sclerosis in patients presenting with clinically isolated syndromes: a multicentre retrospective study. *Lancet Neurology*, **6**, 677–686.

Thompson, A.J., Montalban, X., Barkhof, F. *et al.* (2000) Diagnostic criteria for primary progressive multiple sclerosis: a position paper. *Annals of Neurology*, **6**, 831–835.

Tremlett, H., Paty, D. & Devonshire, V. (2006) Disability progression in multiple sclerosis is slower than previously reported. *Neurology*, **66**, 172–177.

4

MRI in Diagnosis and Disease Monitoring

María I. Gaitán[1,2] and Daniel S. Reich[1]

[1]National Institute of Neurological Disorders and Stroke, National Institutes of Health, Bethesda, MD, USA
[2]Dr. Raúl Carrea Institute for Neurological Research, FLENI, Buenos Aires, Argentina

Introduction

The introduction of magnetic resonance imaging (MRI) in multiple sclerosis (MS) has revolutionized our ability to diagnose the disease and monitor treatment response in the clinic and in clinical trials. It has, no less, deepened and transformed our understanding of the pathologic processes involved in the development and progression of the disease. On average, MRI is about 5–10 times more sensitive to ongoing inflammatory demyelination than clinical assessment (Harris *et al.* 1991) and is greatly superior to any other imaging method for lesion detection. McDonald and colleagues introduced MRI into the diagnostic criteria, emphasizing the presence of brain and spinal cord lesions and enabling earlier, more sensitive, and more specific diagnosis than considering clinical symptoms and signs alone. These MRI-based diagnostic criteria have twice been revised since they were first established in 2001, most recently in 2010 (Polman *et al.* 2011) (Table 4.1).

MRI has also provided new insights into the pathogenesis of the disease, particularly with respect to the blood–brain barrier. In this regard,

the key observation was that MRI performed after intravenous injection of chelates of gadolinium can detect blood–brain barrier opening occurring during lesion development (Grossman *et al.* 1986). MRI scanning also enabled the noninvasive and quantitative characterization of brain atrophy in MS, which occurs two to three times more rapidly than in the general population and which is generally thought to reflect the neurodegeneration that underlies the relentless accumulation of disability in progressive MS (De Stefano *et al.* 2010). MRI measurements such as T2 and T1 lesion volume, as well as the number of enhancing lesions, have also improved monitoring of the anti-inflammatory effects of disease-modifying therapies in clinical trials (Petkau *et al.* 2008).

This chapter has three main parts. First, we present the MRI findings that are useful to note on initial examination of a patient being worked up for MS. Second, we describe the use of MRI to monitor disease evolution over time, emphasizing insights from clinical trials that can be used in the clinic. Finally, we briefly present some of the most promising advanced MRI techniques.

Multiple Sclerosis and CNS Inflammatory Disorders, First Edition. Edited by Lawrence M. Samkoff and Andrew D. Goodman.

Table 4.1 2010 MRI Criteria for Multiple Sclerosis

Clinical Presentation	Additional Data Needed for MS Diagnosis
≥2 attacks[*]; objective clinical evidence of ≥2 lesions or objective clinical evidence of 1 lesion with reasonable historical evidence of a prior attack[†]	None[‡]
≥2 attacks[*]; objective clinical evidence of 1 lesion	Dissemination in space, demonstrated by: ≥1 T2 lesion in at least 2 of 4 MS-typical regions of the CNS (periventricular, juxtacortical, infratentorial, or spinal cord)[§]; or Await a further clinical attack[*] implicating a different CNS site
1 attack[*]; objective clinical evidence of ≥2 lesions	Dissemination in time, demonstrated by: Simultaneous presence of asymptomatic gadolinium-enhancing and nonenhancing lesions at any time; or A new T2 and/or gadolinium-enhancing lesion(s) on follow-up MRI, irrespective of its timing with reference to a baseline scan or Await a second clinical attack[*]
1 attack[*]; objective clinical evidence of 1 lesion (clinically isolated syndrome)	Dissemination in space and time, demonstrated by: For DIS: ≥1 T2 lesion in at least 2 of 4 MS-typical regions of the CNS (periventricular, juxtacortical, infratentorial, or spinal cord)[§]; or Await a second clinical attack[*] implicating a different CNS site; and For DIT: Simultaneous presence of asymptomatic gadolinium-enhancing and nonenhancing lesions at any time; or A new T2 and/or gadolinium-enhancing lesion(s) on follow-up MRI, irrespective of its timing with reference to a baseline scan; or Await a second clinical attack[*]

Insidious neurological progression suggestive of MS (PPMS)	1 year of disease progression (retrospectively or prospectively determined) plus 2 of 3 of the following criteria[§]: 1. Evidence for DIS in the brain based on ≥1 T2 lesions in the MS-characteristic (periventricular, juxtacortical, or infratentorial) regions 2. Evidence for DIS in the spinal cord based on ≥2 T2 lesions in the cord 3. Positive CSF (isoelectric focusing evidence of oligoclonal bands and/or elevated IgG index)

Source: Polman *et al.* (2011). Reproduced with permission of Wiley.

If the criteria are fulfilled and there is no better explanation for the clinical presentation, the diagnosis is "MS"; if suspicious, but the criteria are not completely met, the diagnosis is "possible MS"; if another diagnosis arises during the evaluation that better explains the clinical presentation, then the diagnosis is "not MS."

CNS, central nervous system; CSF, cerebrospinal fluid; DIS, dissemination in space; DIT, dissemination in time; IgG, immunoglobulin G; MRI, magnetic resonance imaging; MS, multiple sclerosis; PPMS, primary progressive multiple sclerosis.

*An attack (relapse; exacerbation) is defined as patient-reported or objectively observed events typical of an acute inflammatory demyelinating event in the CNS, current or historical, with duration of at least 24 h, in the absence of fever or infection. It should be documented by contemporaneous neurological examination, but some historical events with symptoms and evolution characteristic for MS, but for which no objective neurological findings are documented, can provide reasonable evidence of a prior demyelinating event. Reports of paroxysmal symptoms (historical or current) should, however, consist of multiple episodes occurring over not less than 24 h. Before a definite diagnosis of MS can be made, at least one attack must be corroborated by findings on neurological examination, visual evoked potential response in patients reporting prior visual disturbance, or MRI consistent with demyelination in the area of the CNS implicated in the historical report of neurological symptoms.

†Clinical diagnosis based on objective clinical findings for two attacks is most secure. Reasonable historical evidence for one past attack, in the absence of documented objective neurological findings, can include historical events with symptoms and evolution characteristic for a prior inflammatory demyelinating event; at least one attack, however, must be supported by objective findings.

‡No additional tests are required. However, it is desirable that any diagnosis of MS be made with access to imaging based on these criteria. If imaging or other tests (for instance, CSF) are undertaken and are negative, extreme caution needs to be taken before making a diagnosis of MS, and alternative diagnoses must be considered. There must be no better explanation for the clinical presentation, and objective evidence must be present to support a diagnosis of MS.

§Gadolinium-enhancing lesions are not required; symptomatic lesions are excluded from consideration in subjects with brainstem or spinal cord syndromes.

- *Conventional MRI*
  - The longitudinal (T1) and transverse (T2) relaxation of protons, when placed inside a strong magnetic field and irradiated with radiofrequency energy, can be used to generate images.
  - T2-FLAIR images are the standard for diagnosing MS. They differ from standard T2 images in that signal from free water, mostly cerebrospinal fluid, is suppressed by means of an *inversion pulse*.
  - STIR is another type of T2 image that is especially useful in evaluating the spinal cord and optic nerve.
  - Proton density images are useful for evaluating the brainstem and cerebellum, but newer T2-FLAIR protocols that acquire high-resolution data simultaneously from the whole brain (rather than slice by slice) may be equally good.
  - Intravenous gadolinium shortens T1 relaxation in blood vessels and areas of blood–brain barrier opening. This causes brightening (enhancement) in T1 images.
- *Nonconventional MRI*
  - Magnetization transfer images are indirectly sensitive to macromolecules, which in white matter are mostly contained in myelin.
  - Diffusion images measure the mobility of water molecules and provide indirect information about tissue orientation and microstructure.
  - In spectroscopy, the signal derives from brain metabolites including creatine, *N*-acetylaspartate (NAA) (found almost exclusively in neurons), choline, glutamate, lactate, and myoinositol.
  - Susceptibility (T2*) images are sensitive to small variations in the magnetic field induced by metals such as iron or gadolinium, certain types of tissue (notably myelin), and tissue orientation.

MRI at presentation

Lesions

On a gross anatomic level, MRI correlates well with pathology. Lesions visualized on MRI are usually small, round or oval in shape, asymmetrically distributed across the brain and spinal cord, and seen most readily in the white matter (Figure 4.1). Lesions are typically discrete at first and become more confluent as they accumulate. New lesions are usually clinically silent unless they substantially disrupt a clinically eloquent pathway, which happens most commonly in the optic nerve, brainstem, or spinal cord. However, even lesions in those locations can appear without accompanying symptoms. For differentiation of lesions due to MS from those due to other conditions, important features of lesions include morphology, signal intensity, location, and the presence and character of enhancement following gadolinium administration.

Signal intensity and morphology

Lesions in the acute phase are typically brighter than surrounding white matter (hyperintense) in proton density and T2 images, which most likely reflects a combination of inflammation, demyelination, and increased water content (edema), and they may have fuzzy borders. These same pathological characteristics, but particularly increased water content, cause acute lesions to be darker than surrounding white matter (hypointense) in T1 images. Enhancement (hyperintensity in T1 images) is due to opening of the blood–brain barrier. Older lesions are usually more sharply demarcated, persistently hyperintense in proton density and T2 images and isointense or hypointense in T1 images, and do not enhance with

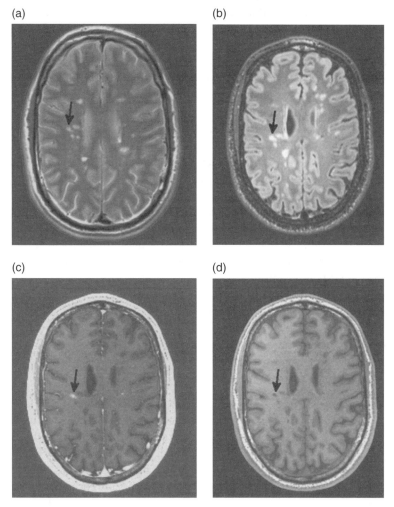

(a) (b) (c) (d)

Figure 4.1 Brain images of a 43-year-old man with active relapsing–remitting MS, performed on a 3 T scanner. (a) Proton density. (b) T2-FLAIR. (c) T1 without contrast. (d) T1 after injection of 0.1 mmol/kg gadobutrol. The arrows denote an enhancing lesion that was not present on the prior scan 1 month earlier. Note that the plane of section for the proton density image (a) is slightly different from that of the other images.

- Atrophy is profound in long-standing MS and begins early in the disease.
- Other diseases cause lesions in T2 images that may mimic MS. The presence of spinal cord lesions and veins in the center of most MS lesions (seen best on susceptibility or T2* images) makes MS much more likely.

gadolinium. These changes in signal intensity reflect resolution of edema, clearance of cellular debris, remyelination, and gliosis.

Lesion location

Brain lesions are commonly periventricular, juxtacortical (at the gray–white junction), and infratentorial (including brainstem and cerebellum), but they can occur anywhere. White matter lesions tend to have an ovoid configuration, to occur along the callososeptal interface, and to extend outward from the bodies of the lateral ventricles along the deep medullary veins (forming the so-called Dawson's fingers). White matter lesions may also extend into the gray matter, including both cortex and deep nuclei (particularly the thalamus). Lesions may also develop directly within the gray matter; these lesions have been classified as either intracortical or subpial. Intracortical lesions are quite small and represent only about 10% of all cortical lesions. Subpial cortical lesions, which may represent 50% of the total seen in pathology studies, are not apparent in conventional MRI and are exceedingly difficult to detect reliably even in nonconventional MRI, although consensus guidelines for lesion identification using a technique called double inversion recovery (DIR) have been published (Geurts *et al.* 2011). Major reasons for the poor MRI contrast between normal gray matter and cortical lesions include partial volume effects (inclusion of multiple tissue types within individual voxels), less extracellular water, and the relative paucity of myelin compared to white matter.

Black holes

Lesions that are hypointense on T1-weighted spin-echo images are called *black holes* if they persist longer than 6 months, because they are thought to reflect areas of substantial tissue destruction (van Waesberghe *et al.* 1999). In fact, most newly formed lesions are T1 hypointense due to the presence of edema, but roughly 80% of these lesions become isointense (revert to the signal intensity of normal white matter) within a few months as the edema resolves and the damaged tissue partially repairs itself. Only approximately 20% of lesions remain hypointense after 6 months and meet the *black hole* definition (Bagnato *et al.* 2003). It is important to realize, however, that not all T1 images are alike, and many more lesions appear persistently hypointense on contemporary scans for technical reasons alone.

Contrast enhancement

Enhancement within an MS lesion indicates the presence of active inflammation and is the imaging correlate of a clinical relapse (although, as mentioned earlier, contrast-enhancing lesions occur much more commonly than relapses) (Katz *et al.* 1993). Contrast enhancement is usually a transient phenomenon in MS lesions, usually disappearing over 2–6 weeks but occasionally lasting longer. Lesion enhancement is less common in primary and secondary progressive MS. Old lesions may re-enhance if they reactivate, but it is often difficult to distinguish a re-enhancing lesion from a new lesion that develops adjacent to the old one. Enhancement may appear homogeneous throughout the lesion (the so-called *nodular* pattern), or it may appear only on the periphery (*ring* pattern). These differences may depend on the size of the lesion and the time interval between gadolinium injection and scan acquisition, rather than true differences in lesion biology (Gaitan *et al.* 2011).

Brain atrophy

Brain atrophy occurs in MS at a rate of about 0.5% per year, about two to three times more rapidly than in healthy people of similar age (De Stefano *et al.* 2010). In clinical practice, an easy, practical, qualitative method for assessing brain atrophy is to use an ordinal scale based on global assessment of ventricular size and sulcal width. On this scale, atrophy is described as mild, moderate, or severe (Simon *et al.* 2006). With image-processing software, the brain volume can be normalized to the size of the cranial vault to generate the *brain parenchymal fraction*, a useful cross-sectional estimate of brain atrophy in MS (Fisher *et al.* 2008).

⚠ CAUTION!

Question your diagnosis when you observe the following:
- Normal MRI
- Substantial mass effect or displacement of nearby structures (rule out tumor)
- A lot of edema surrounding lesions (rule out tumor)
- Bleeding (rule out a vascular process)
- Symmetrically distributed lesions (rule out a toxic or metabolic process)
- Simultaneous enhancement of all lesions (rule out acute disseminated encephalomyelitis)

- Extensive leptomeningeal enhancement (rule out sarcoidosis and infections)
- Gray matter spinal lesions (rule out infarct)
- Long spinal cord lesions (rule out neuromyelitis optica)
- Enhancement lasting more than 3 months (rule out tumor)

Spinal cord

MS lesions are typically located in the posterior and lateral columns and, as in the brain, are for the most part multifocal and asymmetrically distributed. They develop in the periphery of the spinal white matter and are most frequently in the cervical spinal cord. They are usually less than one vertebral body in height and occupy less than half the cross-sectional area of the cord. By contrast, in neuromyelitis optica, lesions are usually much larger, typically more than three vertebral bodies in height. Spinal cord lesions are conventionally best detected in sagittal short-tau inversion recovery (STIR) images, but modern T1 and T2* imaging protocols show promise for improving detection of these often-hard-to-see lesions (Figure 4.2). As normal aging and small vessel disease do not typically cause spinal cord lesions, their presence is very useful for increasing diagnostic certainty. Thirty percent of patients with clinically isolated syndrome—often the initial presentation of MS—have asymptomatic spinal

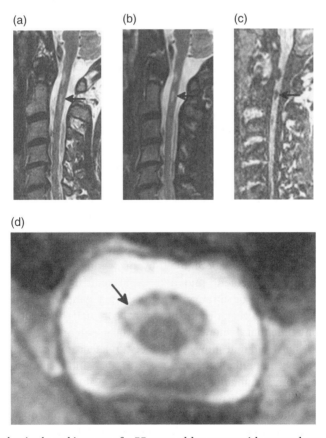

Figure 4.2 Cervical spinal cord images of a 55-year-old woman with secondary progressive MS, performed on a 3 T scanner. (a) Sagittal T2. (b) Sagittal STIR. (c) Sagittal T1. (d) Axial T2* at the C1–C2 disk level. The arrows denote a lesion in the right lateral column on all images.

cord lesions, and 90% of patients with definite MS have cord lesions (Lycklama à Nijeholt *et al.* 2003). Spinal cord atrophy can be detected in any disease subtype, but it appears to be most severe in progressive MS. New spinal cord lesions enhance with gadolinium, but for technical reasons, such enhancement is more difficult to observe than in the brain.

MRI diagnostic criteria

The diagnostic criteria for establishing the diagnosis of MS are based on three main principles: (1) evidence of dissemination in time (DIT), (2) evidence of dissemination in space (DIS), and (3) exclusion of alternative diagnoses. In 2001, the International Panel on the Diagnosis of Multiple Sclerosis presented new diagnostic criteria, the so-called McDonald criteria, which for the first time integrated brain and spinal cord lesions detected by MRI with traditional diagnostic approaches (history, physical exam, and laboratory test). This new set of criteria was designed to be a straightforward diagnostic scheme to enable practicing neurologists to more reliably and consistently diagnose MS. They also allowed earlier diagnosis with a higher degree of specificity and sensitivity. In 2005, the revisions to the McDonald criteria simplified things further while maintaining adequate sensitivity and specificity.

The most recent revisions, formulated in 2010 and published in 2011, for the first time enabled the diagnosis to be made, in the context of an appropriate clinical presentation, on the basis of a single scan. This is accomplished by integrating knowledge about the time course of lesion enhancement into a determination of the presence or absence of both DIT and DIS (Polman *et al.* 2011). Thus, an MRI performed at any time that demonstrates DIS (more than one lesion) and that shows the simultaneous presence of nonenhancing and asymptomatic gadolinium-enhancing lesions is sufficient to support a diagnosis of relapsing–remitting MS. For DIS, the requirement is that one or more T2 lesions be present in at least two of four cardinal locations (periventricular,

juxtacortical, infratentorial, and spinal cord). The appearance of a new T2 lesion on a follow-up scan, irrespective of the timing of the first scan, also fulfills criteria for DIT. The 2010 McDonald MRI criteria for both relapsing–remitting and primary progressive MS are reproduced in Table 4.1.

MRI consensus protocol

A standardized conventional MRI protocol has been proposed (Simon *et al.* 2006). In the brain, this protocol includes T1 images before and after contrast administration as well as proton density and T2 images (Table 4.2). For initial evaluation, a brain MRI study that mimics this standardized protocol should be acquired, and injection of contrast is strongly recommended. The standard dose of most gadolinium chelates, 0.1 mmol/kg, is based on a balance between safety, cost, and detection; however, in MS, it is clear that enhancement detection is higher with double and triple doses of contrast. The minimum delay for scanning is 5 min following the injection. Gadobutrol currently provides the best contrast between enhancing lesions and the background tissue (Lovblad *et al.* 2010). It is important to note that release of gadolinium ions from contrast agents appears to be relevant for the development of nephrogenic systemic fibrosis, a rare condition that occurs in patients with kidney failure and that is characterized by thickening and induration of the skin. Thus, contrast should only be administered in patients with potentially impaired kidney function when it is likely to affect clinical management, such as by uncovering an alternative diagnosis.

Spinal cord imaging may be useful if the main presenting symptoms can be localized to the spinal cord or if the results of the brain MRI are equivocal (Simon *et al.* 2006). However, artifacts related to cerebrospinal fluid flow and cardiac and respiratory motion may compromise evaluation of the spinal cord, and in practice, false positives and false negatives are quite common. The consensus recommendation for spinal cord MRI protocol is provided in Table 4.3.

Table 4.2 Consensus Brain MRI Protocol for Clinical Evaluation of MS

	Sequence	Diagnostic Scan for Clinically Isolated Syndrome	MS Baseline or Follow-up Scan	Comment
1	Three plane (or other) scout	Recommended	Recommended	Set up axial sections through subcallosal line*
2	Sagittal fast FLAIR	Recommended	Optional	Sagittal FLAIR sensitive to early MS pathology, such as in corpus callosum
3	Axial FSE PD/T2	Recommended	Recommended	TE_1 minimum (e.g., ≤30 ms) TE_2 (usually ≥80 ms) PD series sensitive to infratentorial lesions that may be missed by FLAIR series
4	Axial Fast FLAIR	Recommended	Recommended	Sensitive to white matter lesions and especially juxtacortical–cortical lesions
5	Axial pregadolinium T1	Optional	Optional	Considered routine for most neuroimaging studies
6	3D T1	Optional	Optional	Some centers use this for atrophy measure
7	Axial gadolinium-enhanced T1	Recommended	Optional	Standard dose of 0.1 mmol/kg injected over 30 s; scan starting minimum 5 min after start of injection

Source: Simon *et al*. (2006). Reproduced with permission of American Society of Neuroradiology. FSE indicates fast spin-echo (or turbo spin-echo); PD, proton density-weighted (long TR, short TE sequence); T1, T1-weighted (short TR, short TE sequence). Section thickness for sequences 3–6 is ≤3 mm with no intersection gaps when feasible. Partition thickness for 3D sequence 6 is ≤1.5 mm. In-plane resolution is approximately ≤1 × 1 mm.
*The subcallosal line joins the undersurface of the front (rostrum) and back (splenium) of the corpus callosum.

In general, the use of scanners with magnetic field strength equal to or higher than 1.5 T is strongly recommended in MS. Higher field strength increases the T1 relaxation time, providing better T1 images and better delineation of brain structures. Higher field strength also leads to improved image quality overall, with higher signal-to-noise ratio and the possibility of acquiring thinner sections in a reasonable scan time. At a minimum, we recommend acquiring 3 mm slices without gaps. When available, we prefer 3D sequences, in which data are acquired simultaneously from the whole brain rather than slice by slice, ideally using isotropic (cubic) voxels. T2-FLAIR images are generally acquired before gadolinium injection; however, in our experience, obtaining the T2-FLAIR images after gadolinium injection can improve the detection of enhancing lesions (Figure 4.3).

Table 4.3 Consensus Spinal Cord MRI Protocol for Clinical Evaluation of MS

	When Acquired Immediately Following an Enhanced Brain MRI		When Acquired without a Preceding Enhanced Brain MRI	
	Sequence	Recommendation	Sequence	Recommendation
1	Three plane (or other scout)	Recommended	Three plane (or other scout)	Recommended
2	Postcontrast sagittal T1	Recommended	Precontrast sagittal T1	Recommended
3	Postcontrast sagittal FSE PD/T2†	Recommended	Precontrast sagittal FSE PD/T2†	Recommended
4	Postcontrast axial T1	Through suspicious lesions	Precontrast axial FSE PD/T2*	Through suspicious lesions
5	Postcontrast axial FSE PD/T2*	Through suspicious lesions	3D T1$	Optional
6	Postcontrast 3D T1$	Optional	Postcontrast-enhanced sagittal T1¶	Recommended
7			Postcontrast-enhanced axial T1	Through suspicious lesion(s)

Source: Simon *et al.* (2006). Reproduced with permission of American Society of Neuroradiology.

FSE indicates fast spin-echo (or turbo spin-echo); PD, proton density-weighted (long TR, short TE sequence); T1, T1-weighted (short TR, short TE sequence); T2, T2-weighted (long TR, long TE sequence).

*Indications are (1) main presenting symptoms are at the level of the spinal cord, and these have not resolved; (2) if the brain MRI results are equivocal. No additional intravenous contrast is required if the spinal cord study immediately follows the contrast-enhanced brain MRI, as gain is very limited. The segment to be studied (cervical and/or thoracic) is based on clinical findings. Sagittal section thickness is 3 mm (no gap).

†PD series may depict lesions less apparent on heavily T2-weighted series.

*Increases confidence in the findings of sagittal series; may provide classic lesion characteristics.

$For volumetric analysis if desired.

¶Standard dose of 0.1 mmol/kg injected over 30 s; scan starting 5 min after start of injection.

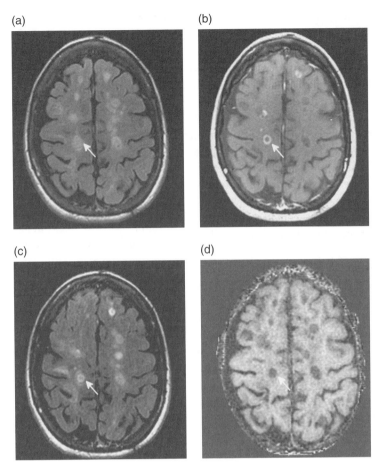

Figure 4.3 Brain images of a 51-year-old woman with active relapsing–remitting MS, performed on a 3 T scanner. (a) T2-FLAIR. (b) T1 after injection of 0.1 mmol/kg gadopentetate dimeglumine. Note the presence of four enhancing lesions, one of which is denoted by an arrow. (c) T2-FLAIR after contrast injection. Enhancing lesions are brighter than their nonenhancing counterparts. (d) MTR. Both enhancing and nonenhancing lesions are hypointense, probably due to a combination of demyelination and increased water content (edema).

MRI for monitoring disease and treatment

The primary goal of disease-modifying treatments in MS is to prevent the occurrence of new clinical relapses and ultimately disease progression. Since MRI is usually more sensitive to ongoing inflammation than clinical measures, MRI findings are often used as outcome measures to shorten phase I and II clinical trials of new MS therapies. Such outcome measures include the accumulation of new or enlarging T2 lesions, the presence of new contrast-enhancing lesions, change in the total lesion volume,

evolution of new lesions into *black holes*, and change in brain volume (Filippi & Rocca 2011). As discussed in the next section, advanced MRI techniques, such as magnetization transfer imaging, diffusion tensor imaging, and proton spectroscopy, can detect and quantify the extent of tissue damage inside and around lesions and can monitor how that damage changes over time.

In the clinic, follow-up MRI scanning is indicated when unexpected clinical worsening happens, for reassessment of disease burden prior to initiation of treatment, or when an alternative diagnosis is suspected (Simon *et al.* 2006).

Unfortunately, many of the changes detected by both conventional and advanced MRI are small and/or subtle, so it has been difficult to apply lessons learned from large populations in clinical trials, or in carefully controlled research settings, to the care of individual patients. Furthermore, interpretation of changes is difficult; an increase in lesion load in a patient under treatment may indeed reflect complete treatment failure, but it also could be the case that even more lesions would have accrued in the absence of treatment. Nevertheless, the standard of care in many centers is to acquire contrast-enhanced follow-up MRI scans to help in treatment decisions.

Since conventional MRI is highly sensitive to inflammation, if follow-up scans are performed carefully, meaning that imaging quality is high and patient positioning is similar, the radiological interpretation can provide very useful information about the evolution of the disease. The requirement for similar positioning will become less important as vendors integrate prospective scan alignment into their acquisition protocols and as registration techniques find their way into clinical image visualization software.

New lesion activity

Contrast is optional for follow-up studies, but it is exceedingly helpful as it allows determination of ongoing disease activity at the time of scanning. However, counting the number of contrast-enhancing lesions alone provides only a snapshot of disease activity. Although some new lesions may completely resolve, for the most part, new lesions permanently alter the local T2-weighted signal. Thus, detecting new or enlarging T2 lesions can provide information about ongoing disease activity over the interval since the previous scan. For this reason, a composite measure that integrates both contrast-enhancing lesions and new or enlarging T2 lesions has proved to be very useful in short- and long-term clinical trials for MS. Unfortunately, it is often difficult to find new T2 lesions, particularly if the lesions are small, data acquisition is not standardized, and the total lesion burden is

high. Subtraction imaging is a relatively new and highly promising tool that may alleviate this difficulty (Moraal *et al.* 2010).

Brain atrophy

Brain atrophy reflects tissue loss and represents a global measure of both demyelination and axonal loss in MS. The number and volume of T2 lesions, as well as more subtle MRI-detectable abnormalities in extralesional white matter and gray matter, affect brain atrophy. Quantitative atrophy estimation, involving postprocessing by automated or semiautomated methods, can detect progressive loss of brain volume and, in particular, the gray matter atrophy that appears to most strongly drive whole-brain atrophy (Fisher *et al.* 2008). Disease-modifying therapies can reduce brain atrophy, although after the initiation of treatment, care must be taken not to interpret an initial drop in brain volume (sometimes called *pseudoatrophy*) that is thought to be due to a reduction in inflammation. How to integrate brain volume measurement (which commonly varies substantially across scanners and scan acquisition parameters) into clinical practice is an ongoing area of research.

Limitations

The limitations of conventional MRI for disease monitoring include the weak associations with clinical status and the relatively poor sensitivity to some clinically relevant findings, such as gray matter disease and diffuse damage throughout the white matter. In addition, serial spinal MRI reveals only one-tenth as much activity as brain MRI in relapsing–remitting MS; whether this reflects differences in lesion accumulation or technical factors (poorer imaging) remains unclear.

Nonconventional MRI

The correlation between the lesion volume observed on conventional MRI and the clinical burden of disease is far from perfect. Possible explanations for this so-called clinical–radiological paradox include limited specificity for the pathological substrates of MS, difficulties in quantifying the extent of damage to extralesional white matter areas (the so-called normal-appearing white matter or NAWM), lack of sensitivity to gray matter lesions, variability of clinical expression of MS lesions in different areas of the brain, and the relative insensitivity of clinical disability scales, especially with respect to cognition. Advanced MRI techniques have begun to alleviate some of these issues because they can provide insight into the underlying pathology as well as the mechanisms of disease evolution and treatment response. However, the application and interpretation of these techniques in clinical practice and clinical trials remain a matter of intense research interest. See Science Revisited for information on specific techniques; their clinical relevance is discussed later.

Magnetization transfer imaging

This technique enables calculation of a semi-quantitative index, the *magnetization transfer ratio* (MTR). Low MTR can be caused by demyelination and axonal loss as well as edema and inflammation, particularly in newly forming lesions (Figure 4.3). Subtle decreases in MTR can be retrospectively detected in the weeks and months prior to lesion formation (Pike *et al.* 2000). A persistent increase of MTR following an initial decrease may indicate remyelination (Giacomini *et al.* 2009). Published experience with magnetization transfer imaging in clinical trials is so far limited, but it holds some promise in this regard.

Magnetic resonance spectroscopy

Spectroscopy is usually performed in single voxels but can also be acquired in entire slices via a technique known variously as chemical shift or spectroscopic imaging. Enhancing lesions may show elevated choline, which reflects ongoing synthesis and breakdown of membranes (in white matter, mostly myelin); the choline level returns to normal over a 4–6-month period. Transiently elevated lactate may reflect altered metabolism within enhancing lesions. The most prominent change in MS lesions, however, is a

decrease in the concentration of NAA, which may normalize after a few months or remain persistently low (Davie *et al.* 1994). Global NAA, measured across the whole brain, is also abnormally low in MS. Because NAA is detected almost exclusively in neurons and their processes, decreases in this metabolite can be interpreted as evidence of axonal injury. NAA levels correlates with axonal density and disability as measured with EDSS (Bjartmar *et al.* 2000).

Susceptibility-weighted imaging

Venous abnormalities and iron deposition in the MS brain are two topics of current interest. MS lesions develop around small parenchymal veins, and this can be directly demonstrated using T2* (or susceptibility) weighting (Figure 4.4b). Detection of veins is markedly improved at higher magnetic field strengths and can be accomplished at 3 and, even more effectively, at 7 T (Tallantyre *et al.* 2009). This type of imaging also demonstrates a hypointense peripheral rim around approximately 10% of MS lesions, which appears to correlate with iron accumulation in macrophages in the periphery of chronic active lesions (Pitt *et al.* 2010). As it is sensitive to some of the tissue changes that appear to be most relevant for the pathophysiology of MS, this technique may open a new window into the mechanisms of lesion development and evolution.

Diffusion-weighted imaging

Demyelination, remyelination, and neurodegeneration may produce abnormal water motion and thereby change measures of diffusion in tissue, to which MRI is sensitive. The total extent of diffusion, quantified as the mean diffusivity or apparent diffusion coefficient, is often especially high in contrast-enhancing and T1-hypointense lesions (Figure 4.4c) (Rovaris *et al.* 2005). However, transient decreases in mean diffusivity sometimes occur in acute MS lesions, especially in the optic nerve; this may reflect swelling of the myelin sheaths, cytotoxic edema, or intense inflammatory cell infiltration. Directional diffusion may also be measured using a technique known as diffusion tensor imaging. In addition to

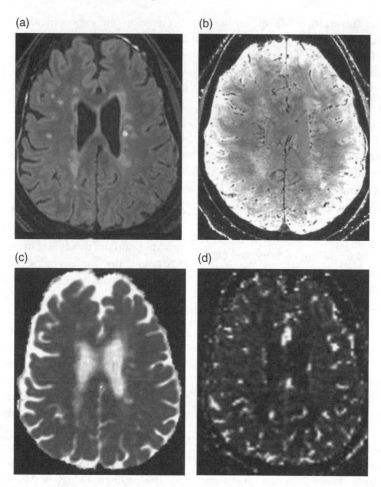

Figure 4.4 Brain images of a 64-year-old woman with primary progressive MS, performed on a 3 T scanner. (a) T2-FLAIR after injection of 0.1 mmol/kg gadobutrol showing an enhancing periventricular lesion. (b) T2* (susceptibility) image showing the presence of a vein (arrow) within the lesion. (c) Mean diffusivity map showing facilitated diffusion of water within the enhancing lesion. (d) Relative cerebral blood volume map showing elevated perfusion within the enhancing lesion.

allowing reconstruction of various white matter pathways, directional diffusion may in some situations help to distinguish axonal damage from other concurrent pathologies, although this is rarely the case in MS.

Perfusion-weighted imaging

Perfusion can be estimated by a variety of MRI techniques. Increased local perfusion can be detected in acute lesions (Figure 4.4d), and this finding may even precede lesion appearance on T2 images (Wuerfel *et al.* 2004). In chronic lesions and gray matter, perfusion is abnormally low, a finding that remains unexplained at present (Ge *et al.* 2005). Indeed, the overall relationship between blood flow and MS pathogenesis remains a topic of intense current interest.

Conclusions

In the three decades since it was introduced as a clinical tool, MRI has become the cornerstone diagnostic tool in MS and, as such, an indispensible part of patient care. Scientifically, it has opened up new avenues in MS research and enabled more rapid, precise testing of new drugs. With continued rapid evolution of the technology, some of the pathological and pathophysiological processes that were previously visible only under the microscope or in the test tube will become accessible to routine, noninvasive monitoring.

Acknowledgments

The authors thank Govind Nair for assistance with the figures; Irene Cortese for invaluable help with the exposition; the Neuroimmunology Clinic, National Institute of Neurological Disorders and Stroke (NINDS), and National Institutes of Health for patient care and scanning; and the Intramural Research Program of NINDS for financial support.

References

Bagnato, F., Jeffries, N., Richert, N.D. *et al.* (2003) Evolution of T1 black holes in patients with multiple sclerosis imaged monthly for 4 years. *Brain*, **126**, 1782–1789.

Bjartmar, C., Kidd, G., Mork, S. *et al.* (2000) Neurological disability correlates with spinal cord axonal loss and reduced N-acetyl aspartate in chronic multiple sclerosis patients. *Annals of Neurology*, **48**, 893–901.

Davie, C.A., Hawkins, C.P., Barker, G.J. *et al.* (1994) Serial proton magnetic resonance spectroscopy in acute multiple sclerosis lesions. *Brain*, **117** (Pt 1), 49–58.

De Stefano, N., Giorgio, A., Battaglini, M. *et al.* (2010) Assessing brain atrophy rates in a large population of untreated multiple sclerosis subtypes. *Neurology*, **74**, 1868–1876.

Filippi, M. & Rocca, M.A. (2011) MR imaging of multiple sclerosis. *Radiology*, **259**, 659–681.

Fisher, E., Lee, J.C., Nakamura, K. & Rudick, R.A. (2008) Gray matter atrophy in multiple sclerosis: a longitudinal study. *Annals of Neurology*, **64**, 255–265.

Gaitan, M.I., Shea, C.D., Evangelou, I.E. *et al.* (2011) Evolution of the blood-brain barrier in newly forming multiple sclerosis lesions. *Annals of Neurology*, **70**, 22–29.

Ge, Y., Law, M., Johnson, G. *et al.* (2005) Dynamic susceptibility contrast perfusion MR imaging of multiple sclerosis lesions: characterizing hemodynamic impairment and inflammatory activity. *AJNR–American Journal of Neuroradiology*, **26**, 1539–1547.

Geurts, J.J.G., Roosendaal, S.D., Calabrese, M. *et al.* (2011) Consensus recommendations for MS cortical lesion scoring using double inversion recovery MRI. *Neurology*, **76**, 418–424.

Giacomini, P.S., Levesque, I.R., Ribeiro, L. *et al.* (2009) Measuring demyelination and remyelination in acute multiple sclerosis lesion voxels. *Archives of Neurology*, **66**, 375–381.

Grossman, R.I., Gonzalez-Scarano, F., Atlas, S.W., Galetta, S. & Silberberg, D.H. (1986) Multiple sclerosis: gadolinium enhancement in MR imaging. *Radiology*, **161**, 721–725.

Harris, J.O., Frank, J.A., Patronas, N., McFarlin, D.E. & McFarland, H.F. (1991) Serial gadolinium-enhanced magnetic resonance imaging scans in patients with early, relapsing-remitting multiple sclerosis: implications for clinical trials and natural history. *Annals of Neurology*, **29**, 548–555.

Katz, D., Taubenberger, J.K., Cannella, B., McFarlin, D.E., Raine, C.S. & McFarland, H.F. (1993) Correlation between magnetic resonance imaging findings and lesion development in chronic, active multiple sclerosis. *Annals of Neurology*, **34**, 661–669.

Lovblad, K.O., Anzalone, N., Dorfler, A. *et al.* (2010) MR imaging in multiple sclerosis: review and recommendations for current practice. *AJNR—American Journal of Neuroradiology*, **31**, 983–989.

Lycklama à Nijeholt, G., Thompson, A., Filippi, M., Castelijns, J.A., Polman, C.H. & Barkhof, F. (2003) Spinal-cord MRI in multiple sclerosis. *Lancet Neurology*, **2**, 555–562.

Moraal, B., van den Elskamp, I.J., Knol, D.L. *et al.* (2010) Long-interval T2-weighted subtraction magnetic resonance imaging: a powerful new outcome measure in multiple sclerosis trials. *Annals of Neurology*, **67**, 667–675.

Petkau, J., Reingold, S.C., Held, U. *et al.* (2008) Magnetic resonance imaging as a surrogate outcome for multiple sclerosis relapses. *Multiple Sclerosis*, **14**, 770–778.

Pike, G.B., De Stefano, N., Narayanan, S. *et al.* (2000) Multiple sclerosis: magnetization transfer MR imaging of white matter before lesion appearance on T2-weighted images. *Radiology*, **215**, 824–830.

Pitt, D., Boster, A., Pei, W. *et al.* (2010) Imaging cortical lesions in multiple sclerosis with ultra-high-field magnetic resonance imaging. *Archives of Neurology*, **67**, 812–818.

Polman, C.H., Reingold, S.C., Banwell, B. *et al.* (2011) Diagnostic criteria for multiple sclerosis: 2010 revisions to the McDonald criteria. *Annals of Neurology*, **69**, 292–302.

Rovaris, M., Gass, A., Bammer, R. *et al.* (2005) Diffusion MRI in multiple sclerosis. *Neurology*, **65**, 1526–1532.

Simon, J.H., Li, D., Traboulsee, A. *et al.* (2006) Standardized MR imaging protocol for multiple sclerosis: consortium of MS Centers consensus guidelines. *AJNR—American Journal of Neuroradiology*, **27**, 455–461.

Tallantyre, E.C., Morgan, P.S., Dixon, J.E. *et al.* (2009) A comparison of 3T and 7T in the detection of small parenchymal veins within MS lesions. *Investigative Radiology*, **44**, 491–494.

van Waesberghe, J.H., Kamphorst, W., De Groot, C.J. *et al.* (1999) Axonal loss in multiple sclerosis lesions: magnetic resonance imaging insights into substrates of disability. *Annals of Neurology*, **46**, 747–754.

Wuerfel, J., Bellmann-Strobl, J., Brunecker, P. *et al.* (2004) Changes in cerebral perfusion precede plaque formation in multiple sclerosis: a longitudinal perfusion MRI study. *Brain*, **127**, 111–119.

5

Relapsing MS: Disease Staging and Therapeutic Algorithms

Mohsen Khoshnam and Mark Freedman

Multiple Sclerosis Research Unit, University of Ottawa, Ottawa, Ontario, Canada

Introduction

Multiple sclerosis (MS) starts out as a relapsing–remitting course in more than 80% of individuals and continues for almost two decades before yielding to secondary progressive (SP) MS. Most of the current disease-specific therapeutics in MS are approved for the relapsing phase with some modest but validated effects: they reduce attacks and MRI activity and slow the development of Expanded Disability Status Scale (EDSS) progression. Studies have shown that the earlier in the course of disease these agents are given, the better the chances of delaying disease progression. For nearly two decades, the mainstay of treatment was one of two therapies: interferon-β (IFN-β) or glatiramer acetate (GA). We are now moving into an era where additional choices exist, but choosing the best option for a given patient is the challenge. As data accumulate, we are beginning to see reasons for moving away from an empiric *one shoe fits all* approach to therapy to a more personalized patient-specific approach.

Disease-modifying drugs (DMD) started with the introduction of IFN-β-1b for the treatment of relapsing MS in 1993, followed by another IFN-β preparation IFN-β-1a (subcutaneous (SC) and IM) and by GA. These have been considered *first-line agents* in most countries. Mitoxantrone, a well-known chemotherapeutic agent, also attained a level of evidence that led to its approval for treating some MS patients showing signs of disease progression despite treatment with the first-line agents. Natalizumab was the first of a new wave of medications to be approved but was withdrawn from the market by the manufacturer because of emergence of PML and then reintroduced in 2006 with a *risk management* strategy. In 2010, fingolimod became the first oral DMD available, but there is inconsistency across the world as to whether it too should be considered second line, owing to a different toxicity profile, or first line, as is its current status in the USA—with a new safety recommendation from the FDA.

Although the exact mechanism(s) of action (MoA) of all the agents is not well understood, their role in MS disease control is believed to be primarily exerted by *immunomodulation* (though some may have inherent immunosuppressive capabilities), in that they affect immune system processes that are felt to contribute to the inflammatory events that cause damage to the CNS in MS as discussed in Chapter 2. Table 5.1 shows data on current DMD with their postulated MoA.

No single drug has proven yet to be universally efficacious in abrogating all measures of disease activity in MS and halting the disability progress. Furthermore, there are limited comparative data among current MS DMD to guide clinicians to choose the best option as an initial therapy. Nevertheless, data derived from a few active comparator studies evaluating the

Multiple Sclerosis and CNS Inflammatory Disorders, First Edition. Edited by Lawrence M. Samkoff and Andrew D. Goodman.

Table 5.1 Current DMD Administration, MoA, Adverse Reactions, and Pivotal Study

Drug	Route and Dosage	MoA	Risks and Adverse Reactions	Pivotal Study
IFN-β-1b	SC, IFN-β-1b 8 MIU every other day	Reduction in T-cell activation, induction of cytokine shift in favor of anti-inflammatory effect, prevention of T-cell adhesion and extravasation across the blood–brain barrier (BBB), induction of T-regulatory cells, apoptosis of autoreactive T cells, neurotrophic factor expression, antiviral effects; IFN-γ antagonism	Lymphopenia, injection site reaction, asthenia, elevated liver enzymes, flu-like symptoms, depression, suicidal ideation, and injection site necrosis	IFN-β MSSG 1993
IFN-β-1a	SC, 22 µg or 44 µg three times per week	Same as INF-β-1b	Same as INF-β-1b	PRISMS 1998
IFN-β-1a	IM, 30 µg weekly	Same as INF-β-1b	Same as INF-β-1b, flu-like symptoms more pronounced and lingering	MSCRG 1996
GA	SC, 20 mg daily	Induction of regulatory T cell by a shift from Th1 to Th2 and Th3 type; dose-dependent inhibition of MBP-specific T-cell responses; GA-specific Th2-type cell migration through the BBB; cross-reactivity of GA-induced T cells with MBP, MOG, and PLP; bystander suppression; neuroprotection due to increased production of brain-derived neurotrophic factor (BDNF) by GA-specific T cells	Approximately 15% of patients experience a self-limited, postinjection systemic reaction characterized by chest tightness, flushing, anxiety, dyspnea, and palpitations; minor skin site reactions; lipoatrophy	Cop 1 MSSG 1995

Drug	Dose	Mechanism	Side effects	Trial/Year
Natalizumab	IV, 300 mg every 4 weeks	Antagonist of VLA-4 inhibits the binding of leukocytes to vascular cell adhesion molecules (VCAM)-1 on the BBB and prevents trafficking into the CNS	Most commonly, headache, fatigue, arthralgia, urinary tract infection, lower respiratory tracts infections, gastroenteritis, vaginitis, extremity pain, diarrhea, and hypersensitivity reactions (mainly rash and urticaria); rare but serious adverse effects; cerebral lymphoma, liver toxicity, melanoma, and PML	AFFIRM 2006
Mitoxantrone	IV, 12 mg/m² body surface every 1–3 months to a maximum of 100–120 mg/m²	Intercalates with DNA, causing single- and double-stranded breaks, and inhibits DNA repair via inhibition of topoisomerase II, inducing immunosuppressive and immunomodulatory properties	Treatment-related leukemia, congestive heart failure due to cardiotoxicity, and infertility	MIMS 2002
Fingolimod	Oral, 0.5 mg daily	Modulation of sphingosine-1-phosphate (S1P) receptors in lymphoid tissues trapping autoimmune cells in lymph nodes	Nasopharyngitis, dyspnea, headache, diarrhea, nausea, and asymptomatic elevations of liver enzymes, rarely macular edema and treatment-induced bradycardia, most commonly seen with the first dose and cardiac arrythmia	FREEDOMS 2010

efficacy of DMD revealed that high-dose, high-frequency IFN-β preparations are superior to low-dose once weekly IFN-β, but were not shown to be superior to GA. Comparison of fingolimod to low-dose IFN-β-1a IM weekly injection demonstrated superiority of efficacy of fingolimod, albeit with a different and occasional serious side effect profile.

We use a classification of these agents into several groups based on risk benefit, yielding to the designation of *first line*, *second line*, or further. The first-line drugs are those with long postmarketing safety records and consist of the various IFN-β preparations and GA. In our practice, the second-line group currently consists of natalizumab, mitoxantrone, and fingolimod (though regulatory approval of fingolimod and natalizumab allows for first-line use in the USA), which are agents that might be more potent than first-line drugs but carry a higher risk of major side effects. All are associated with rare but life-threatening side effects.

Window

It is proposed that MS is essentially a two-stage disease: an early inflammatory stage, characterized by focal inflammation both in white and gray matter, and a later neurodegenerative stage, which is founded on the neuroaxonal damage caused by the inflammatory process

that has already attained a level that is irreversible and progressive and cannot be adequately repaired. In fact, recent evidence indicates that attacks in the first 1 or 2 years may have a major influence on later stage progression, while attacks occurring later may have less influence on disease progression. This suggests that an important early window of opportunity is present for initiation of disease-specific treatment that can minimize the inflammatory-induced damage, as is the goal of all DMD, accomplished through modulation of inflammatory events (manifest as clinical relapse and MRI activity). Effective early therapeutic intervention appears, therefore, key to diminishing the pathological process and preventing or slowing disability progression. Figure 5.1 depicts the window of opportunity.

Prognostic factors

Several studies have shown that a poorer prognosis can be anticipated in cases with some of the following characteristics: male gender; a later age at onset; motor, cerebellar, and sphincter involvement at onset; a progressive course at onset; a short interattack interval; a high number of early attacks; and a relevant early residual neurologic deficit. Some paraclinical measures might also confer prognostic considerations such as MRI, cerebrospinal fluid (CSF) analysis, and evoked potentials. These tend to not only predict

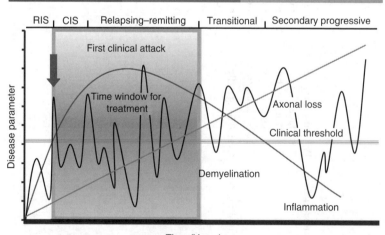

Figure 5.1 MS: Pathology versus clinical course of the disease.

the early conversion to a relapsing course in CIS patients but also indicate which patients may have an earlier progression (e.g., MRI).

EVIDENCE AT A GLANCE

CSF analysis is not commonly included in the measures for staging the disease activity, but abnormal white blood cell (WBC) count was shown to have a correlation with the severity of inflammatory reactions in the CNS and is cleared from CSF following effective anti-inflammatory and immunmodulatory treatments.

In addition to giving us a prognosis, some of these features might also help to place a particular patient into the *window* of therapy by indicating whether it is early, warranting a safe but mild treatment, or late, where more aggressive therapy may be more effective.

The pivotal studies that established current therapies, together with postmarketing monitoring of their efficacy in last two decades, have revealed that they are not curative but can offer partial efficacy in terms of disease control with a variable degree of response among patients. There is no indication as yet of an a priori profile in a patient's biologic or clinical characteristics to guide us to the best choice of therapy that will produce the optimal response in a given patient, but recently, researchers have suggested some biological markers that might predict treatment response or be used for monitoring treatment in MS patients in the future.

Overall, the research offers tantalizing data, and we anxiously await the results of larger studies on bigger cohorts of patients for maturation of the novel idea of biomarkers in MS treatment optimization, and until then, we must rely on common markers of disease activity (relapse, disability progression, and MRI activity) in our clinical practice.

SCIENCE REVISITED

Neutralizing antibodies (NAbs) have become commercially available for monitoring treatment with IFN-β and natalizumab. In the case of IFN-β, these can lead to a reduction in biological responsiveness to the drug, whereas with natalizumab, NAbs may be associated with severe allergic-type reactions as well as loss of treatment effect. In the case of IFN-β, it is not routine to monitor for their appearance unless there is a sense that patients have shown a poor response to therapy. With natalizumab, it is routine in our center to measure for the appearance of NAbs within the first 6 months of treatment.

Several studies have investigated the presence of antibodies against GA; in most studies, the majority or all patients were found to be seropositive. The biological meaning of these antibodies remains unknown, since the pathway leading to the clinical effect of this drug is still obscure.

Therapy

The major factors that affect our decision-making for choosing an option in MS treatment are:

1) Clinical course of MS: We do not have evidence-based medicine in treatment of PPMS, but CIS, RRMS, and early SPMS are our target patients for treatment.
2) The stage of patient in the window of opportunity for treatment: Estimated by considering prognostic factors, history, and physical examination (EDSS) and MRI.
3) The early aggressive course of disease: Especially if aggressive, warrants a different approach regardless of the patient's early status in time frame of window of opportunity.

After starting patients on DMD, we enter into a dynamic and sometimes challenging phase of treatment monitoring. The main purposes of this phase are to determine a patient's adherence to the regimen, which is a prerequisite for effectiveness, and to assess disease response.

Patient adherence involves the combination of patient interest and enthusiasm in maintaining therapy, tolerance to side effects, and the regimen schedule. Adherence can be maximized through educational discussion in a realistic discussion about the expected efficacy

Table 5.2 Pre- and Postmedication Laboratory Tests

Agent	IFN-β	GA	Natalizumab	Fingolimod	Mitoxantrone
Prior to initiation	CBC/diff., LFT, and TFT	N/A	Chest X-ray, HIV, CBC, serum electrolytes, urea, Cr, LFT, serum protein and albumin, beta-HCG in women of reproductive age, TFT, screening of immune deficiency by counting CD4/CD8 cells, anti-JCV Ab titer	CBC, LFT, serum cholesterol level, ECG and retinal examination in diabetics and those with history of uveitis, anti-VZV antibody titer to ensure the immunity	CBC/diff, cr, LFT, beta-HCG in women of reproductive age, LV gated scan or echocardiography for study of LV (LVEF must be >50%)
Monitoring post dosing	CBC/diff., LFT monthly for 6 months and then every 6 months plus TFT	N/A	CBC/diff., LFT, and serum proteins will be done 1 month after the first infusion and then every 3 months, antinatalizumab Ab titer after first or second infusion, anti- JCV Ab titer reanalysis if negative at baseline	CBC and LFT are done in 3 months time for the first year after initiation of therapy with a retinal exam for all treated patients in between 3 and 6 month; serum cholesterol level is done yearly	After each infusion, CBC/diff., Cr, LFT, and beta-HCG (in women) will be tested. After the sixth dose, another LV gated scan or echocardiography is done (LVEF must be >50%), and then yearly CBC/diff. is done for the rest of patient's life

CBC/diff., complete blood count and differential; Cr., creatinine; LFT, liver function tests; LVEF, left ventricular ejection fraction; TFT, thyroid function tests.

of treatment and its usual side effects. Furthermore, adherence is aided through methods and instruments to improve injection techniques and lower the rate of injection site problems. Systemic side effects of IFN-β, such as flu-like symptoms, can be diminished by proper timing for injection according to a patient's activity and premedication. Detecting drug side effects is partly based on a patient's knowledge of symptoms, and this in turn requires up-front education about the medication and how it should be used.

Table 5.2 summarizes some laboratory tests that should be considered, depending on the individual, before starting the relevant therapy as part of premedication evaluation and after starting medication for side effect monitoring.

Disease response monitoring is by far the more challenging part of management, as there is no standardized evidence-based protocol for this and we rely mostly on treatment recommendations by consensus opinion. Unlike clinical trials, there is no placebo group with which to compare a patient's response to therapy; thus, the best practice is to compare the patient's clinical state to the pretreatment period. This is even more challenging in CIS patients, since we do not have any pretreatment phase of activity. Typically, we would monitor three parameters: relapse, disease progression (EDSS), and MRI, in addition to insuring that each patient is tolerant of the medication and not showing any signs of toxicity.

Relapse parameters that concern us as to the level of disease activity are the rate, severity, and degree of recovery of neurological dysfunctions following each attack.

The Kurtzke EDSS is the most common measurement of disease progression assessment that has been used both in the clinic and in clinical trials with MS patients. Any increase from the baseline could indicate progression of disease or residual effects from relapses that should be interpreted based on the baseline score and time course of disability establishment. A significant and sustained increase in EDSS following a relapse developing in a short period of time could indicate a more severe inflammatory process. EDSS increments

sustained for more than 6 months are usually considered indicative of disability progression. MRI measures of disease activity such as contrast-enhancing lesion(s) (CEL), new or enlarging T_2-hyperintense lesion(s), T_1-hypointense lesion(s) (or black holes), and atrophy have all been examined, but new T_2 lesions +/− CEL are the most consistent and validated measures of disease activity. MRI has already been utilized as a surrogate marker of treatment efficacy in drug trials. A meta-analysis of 23 randomized placebo-controlled trials in RRMS, involving a total of 6591 patients, identified a strong correlation between the effect of treatment on relapses and number of MRI lesions measured. More than 80% of the variance in treatment effects on relapses was explained by the variance in MRI measures. Contrast enhancement and new or newly enlarging lesions identified with T_2 have greater utility in evaluating effectiveness of treatment, and MRI metrics (atrophy and T_1 black holes) have weak predictive value for future disability and correlate poorly with T_2 lesion burden in progressive disease.

None of the current *guidelines* for monitoring therapy have been standardized in large cohort of patients in long prospective studies but are based on clinical and MRI data that indicates inflammatory or degenerative activity of MS in patients, reflecting the temporary or permanent damage in myelin and neuroaxonal tissues. One practical recommendation is a simplified version of the Rio score instrument, a tool that uses the same clinical and MRI measures over the first year of treatment to predict response to therapy. The Rio scoring system was found to be useful for predicting response to SC IFN-β-1a among 373 patients with RRMS who were followed for 4 years in the PRISMS study. The patients were classified at 1 year using the Rio criteria, which determine response based on a score of 0 (responsive) or a score of 1–3 (unresponsive) when 1 point is assigned to each of the following:

- >2 active T2 lesions on MRI
- ≥1 relapse
- An EDSS score increase ≥1 (confirmed after 6 months)

After 1 year of treatment, the patients were classified using a simplified Rio scoring system (EDSS not included) in which 1 point is assigned to the presence of ≥2 active T2 lesions between months 6 and 12 and relapse is scored as follows:

- 0 relapses = 0
- 1 relapse = 1 and ≥2 relapses = 2

After 1 year, 29.9% of patients were Rio responders, and 37.3% were responders according to the simplified score. Both the Rio score and the simplified Rio score significantly predicted subsequent relapse frequency ($p < 0.001$ for each) as well as disease progression ($p = 0.03$ and $p = 0.002$, respectively).

Such a practical guideline can be applied in clinical practice to monitor the response to therapy and determine the status of patient as a responder or nonresponder for planning the future of management.

★ TIPS AND TRICKS

MRI is essential for diagnosis and *staging* of the disease prior to initiating treatment. In the treatment follow-up period, we obtain a single MRI performed at 1 year to help provide important information regarding subclinical response to treatment. MRI is indicated anytime unusual symptoms arise that suggest another condition (e.g., PML in the case of natalizumab treatment) or as a new *baseline* should a more aggressive treatment be considered. In some centers, annual MRIs are done during the first few years of first-line disease-modifying therapy and more frequently to monitor patients receiving natalizumab for early signs of PML.

More frequent visits are warranted in the first 2 years of treatment, to insure adherence and reaffirm with patients the goals of therapy and dispel misconceptions they may perceive regarding the aims of treatment. Usually three or four visits in the first year would be considered useful and then perhaps every 6 months. Specific precautions should be followed according to the established policies in respective countries regarding the administration of agents such as fingolimod, natalizumab, and mitoxantrone. Some examples include the first dose monitoring for fingolimod and NAb testing for natalizumab before administering the second or third dose, while anti-JCV antibody titer is checked as a premedication workup and suggested every 6 months in case of antibody negativity to detect seroconverters. In case of a stable treatment course in patients after 24 months of follow-up, the visits may be scheduled yearly (for first-line treatments), but patients should still be encouraged to report any unusual side effects as well as any sudden change in the course of disease.

☝ CAUTION!

NAbs against natalizumab occur less frequently (6%) than IFN-β but are associated with a clear loss of clinical and radiological efficacy and confer susceptibility to subsequent allergic reactions even anaphylaxis. We recommend that measurement of NAb to natalizumab be part of the routine management with that agent and in our center is tested up front after the first or second infusion.

Initiation

In considering which agent to choose for initiation of therapy, it is first important to place the patient in the *window of opportunity* for therapy.

Early window

CIS and early RRMS without characteristics of aggressive disease are *early* window patients. Our current practice is to start a first-line agent that may offer effective disease control without offering any significant toxicity (i.e., a high benefit: risk agent). First-line agents today are the IFN-β preparations, GA, or fingolimod in some countries. Patient follow-up should be regular in the first year to monitor for adherence, side effects, and drug efficacy.

Late window

Patients who present *late* in the window are those who have had a lot of prior subclinical disease activity determined by MRI and are felt to have a poorer prognosis with imminent advancing disease. For example, evidence of T_1 hypointensities (black holes) or obvious atrophy (of the brain or spinal cord) on MRI at presentation not only signifies the severity of disease but also tells us that such patients have acquired a significant amount of irreversible disease. For these patients, the perception is that there is little time to try and fail on a first-line option so perhaps a better strategy would be to reach for a more potent drug with a higher risk of adverse effects but a better chance of quickly abrogating the remaining inflammation in an effort to stave off permanent disability progression.

Options here could be fingolimod (in countries where it is not available first line), natalizumab, or mitoxantrone. In the case of the latter two agents, treatment could have a limited time or maximal dose exposure, and the goal would be to establish *control* and revert back to a safer first-line option. In this sense, choosing a second-line agent first for a period of time to *induce control* and then maintaining that control with a first-line agent have been referred to as *induction strategy*.

This strategy is also applied for those early window patients who present with aggressive MS and are treatment naïve. What might entail an *aggressive course* of disease is a patient who has already experienced several attacks in a relatively short period of time with involvement of different eloquent parts of CNS, which has led to early sustained EDSS changes. Other examples might be a slow and incomplete recovery from attacks despite the use of high-dose corticosteroid therapy. An early (often first) MRI showing a high T_2 lesion load, or follow-up studies showing new T2 or enhancing T_1 lesions, possibly with location in eloquent CNS areas such as the brainstem might also be poor prognostic factors indicative of a more aggressive disease.

Suboptimal response

Pivotal studies and postmarketing experience with all current treatments indicate that they control the inflammatory disease activity rather than induce complete remission. Nonetheless, one should strive for *optimal control* for any given patient. In spite of all advances in the neuroimmunology, the ideal treatment for patients with MS remains an unmet need. Current disease-specific treatments are only partially effective in preventing MS relapses and disability progression in all patients, but for some, they may well offer excellent long-term disease control.

Suboptimal response could entail poor adherence as well as the notion of *breakthrough disease* or the continued disease activity despite good adherence.

Intolerance: Lateral therapy

Both injection site reactions (in parenteral drugs) and systemic side effects may reach a level so that continuation of therapy is no longer tolerated by the patient or will be more detrimental than helpful. In such cases, switching to another drug with a different MoA but a similar safety and efficacy profile is a logical decision. Usually, GA is switched to one of IFN-β and vice versa. In case of needle phobia or needle fatigue as a cause of intolerance and poor adherence, one of current oral drugs will be the practical solution.

Mild breakthrough: Lateral therapy

Not all breakthrough disease activity indicates a *treatment failure*, but in case of mild disease activity such as new subclinical MRI lesions, mild EDSS change lasting more than 6 months, and occurrence of mild relapses in short duration with good recovery, the clinician could decide to switch among the first-line DMD. If patient is receiving low-dose IFN-β preparation, the common practice is to switch to a high-dose, high-frequency agent, or in the case of breakthrough on a high-dose, high-frequency IFN-β, one could consider a switch to GA and vice versa. If disease activity is not under control after a period of at least 6 months after switching, second-line drugs should be considered.

Major breakthrough

There is no standard definition for a *major* breakthrough in RRMS, but clinicians usually decide this based on the severity of a relapse (e.g., that causing significant change in the EDSS or that showing a poor recovery after high-dose pulse steroid therapy ± enhancing lesion(s) in new MRI). Depending on clinician experience, drug availability, costs and insurance coverage, and clarification of risk benefit for the patient, one of the following strategies is applied for patients in this category.

Combination therapy

The rationale behind combination therapy in MS is to target the early inflammatory disease process from different dimensions by using more than one drug with different MoA. In the last two decades, many combinations in various trials were tested without satisfactory results. In a randomized phase II trial, oral teriflunomide as add-on therapy to IFN-β showed acceptable safety and tolerability and reduced MRI disease activity compared with IFN-β alone. This study provides class II evidence that oral teriflunomide, 7 and 14 mg, added to IFN-β, is safe. T1 CEL burden was significantly reduced with both teriflunomide doses. In the near future, we expect more evidence to support such combinations with first- or second-line MS DMD for enhancing the efficacy.

Rescue therapy

The rationale behind this strategy is to use a stronger drug for a short course of therapy (usually 6–24 months) to subdue a disease that cannot be confined by the usual first-line drugs. Mitoxantrone has been used in this way, and there is data derived from several studies to support its application. Natalizumab might be much safer in terms of PML development, when it is used in the short term, for 1 or 2 years, regardless of JC virus Ab status, but the syndrome akin to the immune reconstitution inflammatory syndrome (IRIS) that typifies withdrawal from the agent might complicate its discontinuation. On the other hand, compassionate use of immunosuppressant or immunomodulatory drugs that are used in other diseases can also be considered as a form of rescue therapy.

Rituximab, alemtuzumab, daclizumab, and cyclophosphamide have been tried in this way, but only alemtuzumab now had level I evidence that it is effective in breakthrough patients.

Escalation

Switching to one of the second-line agents after first lines fail to adequately contain the disease is the usual strategy when patients are still considered to be *early* in the window. Typically, a switch among the first-line agents is tried, but if there is continued breakthrough, then escalation to second or higher agents is probably warranted. This switch can be for a defined period of time (e.g., 1–2 years for natalizumab or mitoxantrone) and then a return to first-line therapy once disease control appears to be evident. Escalation however might need to be maintained. Given that mitoxantrone has predefined dosing limits, that drug will almost certainly require a switch after maximal dosing is attained. Long-term treatment with natalizumab (>24 months) is the single greatest risk factor for developing the serious complication PML, especially in patients who have positive JCV serology.

Rapid advancement

Occasionally, clinicians may encounter RRMS patients who develop a rapidly progressive phase of disease despite treatment with first-line agents or following a severe relapse. Neither steroid treatment nor plasma exchange has been shown to alter anything but the duration of an attack, so a strategy needs to be adopted to counter rapidly advancing disease. For such cases, interval use of chemosuppressive agents such as cyclophosphamide has been used, or extreme treatments such as bone marrow transplantation could be considered.

Conclusion

The field of MS therapeutics has been rapidly evolving over the last two decades. With the advent of even newer agents with different MoA, we should be able to achieve good control for the majority of relapsing patients, especially if started early in the course of disease.

Furthermore, successful biomarker research might further enhance our ability to treat early disease by targeting populations that are likely to be *good responders* thereby saving the time lost on trial and failure of agents. Indeed, such approaches have already started to select out patients for particular therapies in the form of *personalized medicine.*

Clearly, the greatest unmet need in terms of treatment is that of regeneration or repair. Similarly, we have not really addressed a major component of disease, that of the cognitive decline. There are a vast array of new molecules and potentially therapeutic techniques that are currently under investigation in different pre-clinical and clinical phases with varied MoA and target pathways.

Although many of the strategies for the purpose of remyelination and repair may be several years away from clinical application, it is clear that we are entering to an era in which early disease control is possible and we may be closer to attaining a *disease activity-free* state for many individuals using a personalized approach.

Newer oral agents

As this chapter went to press, two new oral agents were approved for the treatment of RRMS, teriflunomide (TF) and dimethyl fumarate (DMF, also known as BG12). TF is a reversible inhibitor of dihydroorotate dehydrogenase, an enzyme involved in the de novo synthesis of endogenous pyrimidine for DNA metabolism. As such, TF is thought to modulate activation and proliferation of rapidly dividing cells, including activated T- and B-lymphocytes involved in MS pathology. DMF is an activator of the nuclear 1 factor (erythroid-derived 2)-like 2 (Nrf2) antioxidant response pathway that inhibits the cytotoxic effects of oxidative stress in experimental models of CNS neuroinflammation, resulting in demyelination and neurodegeneration seen in MS. DMF may also have direct anti-inflammatory properties.

In a 2-year placebo-controlled study, TF at doses of 7 and 14 mg daily both significantly reduced annualized relapse rates (by 31.2% and 31.5%, respectively) and cranial MRI disease activity compared with placebo. Beneficial effect on sustained disability was demonstrated by the 14 mg dose only. Adverse effects, seen equally at both the 7 and 14 mg doses, included hair thinning, nausea, and diarrhea. Elevations of alanine aminotransferase at levels ≥ 1 of the upper range of normal were seen more often in patients treated with either dose of TF compared with placebo. TF is a category X agent and is absolutely contraindicated in pregnancy.

DMF has been investigated as a treatment for RRMS at doses of 240 mg bid and 240 mg tid in two phase-3 placebo-controlled randomized studies. In both trials, DMF at 240 mg bid (the FDA-approved dosage) favorably reduced relapse rate by 44% and 53%, respectively. DMF also significantly reduced multiple measures of MRI disease activity. Beneficial effects of DMF on sustained disability progression were demonstrated in one study (38% with twice daily DMF and 34% with thrice daily DMF) but failed to reach significance in the other study. Adverse effects of DMF in both studies included flushing, nausea, diarrhea, and leukopenia/lymphopenia. Flushing and gastrointestinal effects appeared to diminish greatly after 1 month of treatment while leukopenia and lymphopenia plateaued after 12 months. However, grade-2 leukopenia ($<3.0 \times 10^9/l$) and grade-3 lymphopenia ($<0.5 \times 10^9/l$) were seen in 10% and 5%, respectively, of patients in the twice-daily DMF group. No malignancies or opportunistic infections attributed to DMF were seen in these trials.

The role of these therapies in the treatment of RRMS will almost certainly evolve as their use increases in clinical practice. Their place in the treatment algorithm of RRMS will depend upon the emergence of unanticipated toxicity with their long-term administration.

Further Reading

Clerico, M., Faggiano, F., Palace, J., Rice, G., Tintorè, M. & Durelli, L. (2008) Recombinant interferon beta or glatiramer acetate for delaying conversion of the first demyelinating event to multiple sclerosis. *Cochrane Database of Systematic Reviews,* CD005278.

Costello, F., Stuve, O., Weber, M.S., Zamvil, S.S. & Frohman, E. (2007) Combination therapies for multiple sclerosis: scientific rationale, clinical trials, and clinical practice. *Current Opinion in Neurology*, **20**, 281–285.

Fox, R.J., Miller, D.H., Phillips, J.T., *et al.* (2012) Placebo-controlled phase 3 study of oral BG-12 or glatiramer in multiple sclerosis. New England Journal of Medicine, **367** (12), 1087–1097.

Freedman, M.S. & Forrestal, F.G. (2008) Canadian treatment optimization recommendations (TOR) as a predictor of disease breakthrough in patients with multiple sclerosis treated with interferon b-1a: analysis of the PRISMS study. *Multiple Sclerosis*, **14**, 1234–1241.

Gajofatto, A., Bacchetti, P., Grimes, B., High, A. & Waubant, E. (2009) Switching first-line disease-modifying therapy after failure: impact on the course of relapsing–remitting multiple sclerosis. *Multiple Sclerosis*, **15**, 50–58.

Giovannoni, G., Comi, G., Cook, S. *et al.* (2010) A placebo-controlled trial of oral cladribine for relapsing multiple sclerosis. *The New England Journal of Medicine*, **362**, 416–426.

Hartung, H.P., Gonsett, R., Konig, N. *et al.* (2002) Mitoxantrone in progressive multiple sclerosis: a placebo-controlled, double-blind randomized multicenter trial. *Lancet*, **360**, 2018–2025.

Karussis, D., Biermann, L.D., Bohlega, S. *et al.* (2006) A recommended treatment algorithm in relapsing multiple sclerosis: report of an international consensus meeting. *European Journal of Neurology*, **13**, 61–71.

Le Page, E. & Edan, G. (2009) Long-term experience with induction treatment regimens in multiple sclerosis. *Journal of the Neurological Sciences*, **277** (Suppl. 1), S46–S49.

Malhotra, S., Bustamante, M.F., Pérez-Miralles, F. *et al.* (2011) Search for specific biomarkers of IFNβ bioactivity in patients with multiple sclerosis. *PLoS One*, **6** (8), e23634.

Multiple Sclerosis Therapy Consensus Group (MSTCG), Wiendl, H., Toyka, K.V. *et al.* (2008) Basic and escalating immunomodulatory treatments in multiple sclerosis: current therapeutic recommendations. *Journal of Neurology*, **255**, 1449–1463.

Nicholas, J., Morgan-Followell, B., Pitt, D., Racke, M.K. & Boster, A. (2012) New and emerging disease-modifying therapies for relapsing-remitting multiple sclerosis: what is new and what is to come. *Journal of Central Nervous System Disease*, **4**, 81–103.

O'Connor, P., Wolinsky, J.S., Confavreux, C., *et al.* (2011) Randomized trial of oral teriflunomide for relapsing multiple sclerosis. New England Journal of Medicine, **365** (14), 1293–1303.

Rio, J., Comabella, M. & Montalban, X. (2009) Predicting responders to therapies for multiple sclerosis. *Nature Reviews Neurology*, **5**, 553–560.

Rio, J., Castillo, J., Rovira, A. *et al.* (2009) Measures in the first year of therapy predict the response to interferon beta in MS. *Multiple Sclerosis*, **15**, 848–853.

Rio, J., Comabella, M. & Montalban, X. (2011) Multiple sclerosis: current treatment algorithms. *Current Opinion in Neurology*, **24**, 230–237.

Sormani, M.P., Rovaris, M., Comi, G. & Filippi, M. (2007) A composite score to predict short-term disease activity in patients with relapsing–remitting MS. *Neurology*, **69**, 1230–1235.

Valenzuela, R.M., Costello, K., Chen, M., Said, A., Johnson, K.P. & Dhib-Jalbut, S. (2007) Clinical response to glatiramer acetate correlates with modulation of IFN-gamma and IL-4 expression in multiple sclerosis. *Multiple Sclerosis*, **13** (6), 754–762.

6

Progressive MS Treatment Algorithms

Megan H. Hyland[1] and Jeffrey A. Cohen[2]

[1]Neuroimmunology Unit, Department of Neurology, University of Rochester School of Medicine and Dentistry, Rochester, NY, USA
[2]Mellen Center for Multiple Sclerosis Treatment and Research, Neurological Institute, Cleveland Clinic, Cleveland, OH, USA

Background

Progressive forms of multiple sclerosis (MS) differ from relapsing–remitting MS (RRMS) in their clinical course, imaging characteristics, and response to disease-modifying therapy, making it important to have distinct treatment approaches. Secondary progressive MS (SPMS) is defined by an initial relapsing–remitting (RR) course followed by gradual worsening with or without superimposed relapses or minor remissions. Primary progressive MS (PPMS) is characterized by gradual disease progression from the outset without distinct relapses. Approximately 50% of RRMS patients transition to SPMS after 10 years, and nearly 90% convert to SPMS after 25 years. Factors that contribute to a more rapid onset to progressive disease from a RR course include male gender, older age of disease onset, early motor symptoms, and a shorter time to second relapse. However, these factors have relatively modest predictive ability, and the absence of such factors does not guarantee a good prognosis. A primary progressive (PP) course is the initial presentation of 10–15% of all MS patients. PPMS affects a relatively higher percentage of men and has an older age of onset compared to RRMS, with a median age of onset similar to that of the typical transition from RRMS to SPMS.

Although the time from disease onset to progression is variable in SPMS, the time from the start of progression until attainment of distinct levels of disability is more uniform. Using the Disability Status Scale (DSS) to measure disability, a natural history cohort study demonstrated a median time from onset of progression to DSS score of 3 of 1.4 years; median times from onset of progression to DSS scores of 6 and 8 were 4.5 and 24.1 years, respectively. A comparable rate of disease progression is observed in PPMS, supporting the concept that the two forms of progression have similar underlying pathogenic mechanisms.

Clinical manifestations of progressive MS typically include worsening motor symptoms and spasticity with significant contribution to gait impairment and largely irreversible disability. Magnetic resonance imaging (MRI) studies demonstrate an overall greater T2 white matter lesion burden in SPMS patients compared to RRMS, but the development of new white matter lesions and gadolinium (Gd)-enhancing lesions generally occurs with decreasing frequency over time. PPMS shares some of the MRI characteristics seen in SPMS (fewer new or Gd-enhancing lesions) but typically has fewer focal lesions and an overall smaller lesion burden than SPMS. These MRI findings along with the relative paucity of relapses support the suggestion that decreased or more isolated inflammatory changes occur during the progressive disease phase.

Multiple Sclerosis and CNS Inflammatory Disorders, First Edition. Edited by Lawrence M. Samkoff and Andrew D. Goodman.
© 2014 John Wiley & Sons, Ltd. Published 2014 by John Wiley & Sons, Ltd.

The mechanisms for disease progression are still not fully understood. Wallerian degeneration and axonal injury resulting from chronic demyelination following relapses are one component of the proposed mechanism, but axonal loss has been seen in early disease, and white matter lesion burden and atrophy do not correlate strongly with disease progression. However, the concept of MS as a neurodegenerative disease with progression that may occur longitudinally is also becoming more widely recognized. MRI has become increasingly sensitive, and different techniques now allow measurement of gray matter demyelination and atrophy. Cortical lesions have been shown to increase at a greater rate in actively progressive disease, and gray matter atrophy also has a greater rate of increase during SPMS. The identification of different factors contributing to relapsing and progressive disease mechanisms aids in the understanding why medications effective in RRMS do not seem to work as well in progressive forms of MS. It also supports the notion that progressive forms with relapses or MRI lesion activity can be treated more like RRMS, while alternative strategies may be needed for progression without relapses.

Challenges to clinical trials in progressive MS

The data on efficacy of disease therapies in progressive forms of MS are limited. Some of this is the result of specific challenges to clinical trials in progressive disease. One challenge is to accurately categorize patients as they transition from RRMS to SPMS when they tend to have features of both forms of the disease. An additional challenge is the rather slow, insidious progression of disease, which often may be difficult to quantify. The Expanded Disability Status Scale (EDSS), a commonly used clinical trial metric, has several recognized limitations. These limitations may have less impact on trials in RRMS because additional informative metrics are available, such as relapse rate and MRI lesion activity. However, the far fewer relapses and MRI lesion changes seen in progressive MS require that trials depend much more heavily on the EDSS. Known EDSS issues include the inequality between score changes of the same magnitude at different points along the scale (i.e., an increase in 1 point from 1.0 to 2.0 has less clinical significance than an increase from 6.0 to 7.0) and insensitivity to detect important sources of disability (e.g., cognitive impairment, upper extremity dysfunction). Additionally, the optimal duration of time over which worsening of disability should be confirmed is unclear; a 3-month confirmation is often the standard but has been shown to revert on occasion and alter clinical trial results. A 6-month confirmation is more likely to detect sustained changes but results in fewer *events*. Finally, the slow progression of disability that may occur in progressive forms of MS and the relative insensitivity of the EDSS also are problematic because it may take several years to accrue detectable change in disability, and this may not be captured in the typical clinical trial duration of 2–3 years. This may be particularly difficult in PPMS in which relapses do not occur.

However, one advantage with clinical trials in progressive MS is that they generally can be performed without an active comparator. Placebo-controlled trials do not raise the same ethical and practical concerns as in RRMS due to the lack of therapy with proven efficacy in progressive MS.

Clinical trials in progressive MS

The disease-modifying therapies used to treat RRMS tend to be more effective in treating the inflammatory aspect of the disease. Of the eight medications that have been approved for treatment of RRMS by the US Food and Drug Administration (FDA) and European Medicines Agency (EMA), only one form of interferon (IFN)-beta is approved by the EMA for SPMS in patients who have demonstrated recent relapses. Mitoxantrone is the only medication specifically approved by the FDA for SPMS (or worsening RRMS), and its approval for SPMS varies from country to country within the region of the EMA. Glatiramer acetate is approved

Table 6.1 Summary of Disease-Modifying Therapy Clinical Trials

Treatment	Secondary Progressive Multiple Sclerosis	Primary Progressive Multiple Sclerosis
IFN-beta	No effect on sustained EDSS progression Statistically significant benefit on relapse rate, new T2 MRI lesions, Gd-enhancing lesions	No effect on sustained EDSS progression
Glatiramer acetate	Limited trial evidence	Trend toward decrease in sustained EDSS progression
Natalizumab	Ongoing placebo-controlled trial	No trial evidence
Fingolimod	Limited trial evidence	Ongoing placebo-controlled trial
Mitoxantrone	Improvement in composite outcome that included sustained EDSS progression and relapses	Limited trial evidence
MP	No effect on sustained disability measured by composite outcome. Secondary analysis showed high-dose benefit on time to sustained disability	
Methotrexate	No significant improvement in sustained EDSS progression. Statistically significant improvement in composite outcome including EDSS, Ambulation Index, 9-Hole Peg Test	
Cyclophosphamide	Variable evidence—overall showed disease stabilization in patients who were younger, had shorter disease duration, had secondary progressive disease	

EDSS, Expanded Disability Status Scale; Gd, gadolinium.

for RRMS. Natalizumab and fingolimod are approved for relapsing forms of MS by the FDA, allowing for use in SPMS with relapses, while approval is restricted to RRMS by the EMA. There are currently no medications approved for usage in PPMS. Clinical trial data are summarized later and in Table 6.1.

Interferon-beta

Of the four randomized placebo-controlled clinical trials of IFN-beta in SPMS, three failed to show significant benefit on time to confirm EDSS worsening. The trials did show benefit on reduction of relapse rate, new T2 lesions, and Gd-enhancing lesions. This finding supports the concept that IFN-beta may be beneficial in early SPMS or in SPMS with relapses where relapses and MRI lesion activity would have greater impact. The one trial that showed a positive effect of IFN-beta-1b on EDSS

progression (European Study Group) generally had a younger study population with shorter disease duration and more recent baseline relapses, again supporting the use of IFN-beta for *relapsing forms of MS* rather than purely progressive disease.

The intramuscular (IM) form of IFN-beta-1a was investigated in 50 PPMS patients who received either placebo or one of two IFN-beta-1a doses (30 or 60 μg weekly). The study demonstrated greater side effects with the higher IFN-beta-1a dose but no benefit on the primary endpoint, sustained EDSS progression. IFN-beta-1b was compared with placebo in 49 PPMS patients but showed no treatment effect on sustained EDSS progression over 2 years. There was a treatment effect observed on MS Functional Composite, but the study population was too small to demonstrate clinically meaningful outcomes.

IFNs may worsen spasticity, which is common in progressive MS; glatiramer acetate is a better first option when considering a therapy trial in a patient with significant spasticity.

Glatiramer acetate

Though not studied in SPMS, there was an investigation in a PPMS population of the effect of glatiramer acetate versus placebo on the time to a 3-month sustained disability progression using the EDSS. This large study enrolling 943 patients had the goal of 3-year follow-up but was terminated early due to projected lack of efficacy.

Mitoxantrone

In addition to IFN-beta, another medication that has been tested more extensively in SPMS is the chemotherapeutic agent mitoxantrone. A study of 194 patients with worsening RRMS or SPMS compared mitoxantrone (5 and 12 mg/m² doses) to placebo administered once every 3 months for 24 months. Patients receiving 12 mg/m² of mitoxantrone compared with placebo demonstrated statistically significant improvement in the primary outcome, a global analysis of five clinical measures that included EDSS change, number of relapses, time to first relapse, standardized neurological status change, and change in Ambulation Index. Similar to some of the IFN-beta trials, the patients involved in the study described previously were generally younger than typical SPMS patients with disease durations <10 years and average baseline EDSS <5.0. Rare but serious adverse events have been observed with mitoxantrone, most notably cardiotoxicity and acute myeloid leukemia (AML). Because of these concerns, mitoxantrone has a cumulative dose limit of 140 mg/m², and its use has decreased recently.

Cyclophosphamide

Another chemotherapeutic agent, cyclophosphamide, whose mechanism of action involves CD4+ T-cell depletion and a reduction in Th1 response, has been studied in several trials in progressive MS. Early individual and small group treatment success led to an initial randomized trial comparing adrenocorticotropic hormone (ACTH) alone with either ACTH combined with plasma exchange and oral cyclophosphamide or ACTH and intravenous (IV) cyclophosphamide in a total of 58 patients with progressive MS. The study was unblinded but showed improvement or stabilization in 80% of the IV cyclophosphamide group as compared with 20% of the ACTH group, and the effect was shown to last for an average of 18 months. These results prompted an additional single-blind trial, the Northeast Cooperative Treatment Group, which studied 261 progressive MS patients for possible prolonged disease stabilization with addition of booster treatments following initial induction. Different induction protocols were used without significant differences identified, but there was a relatively small but significant effect of booster dosing. It was also shown that younger patients, those with shorter duration of progression, and those with SPMS were more likely to benefit from booster therapy.

Although there have also been negative single-blind studies of cyclophosphamide in progressive MS, there has been debate about whether the results negate the positive findings because the studies were conducted in older patient populations with different treatment administration protocols.

In general, the recommended cyclophosphamide protocol treats patients with monthly pulses and allows for dose adjustment to attain a goal white blood cell (WBC) count nadir between 1500 and 2000/mm³. The common side effects seen with cyclophosphamide include alopecia, nausea, infertility, leukopenia, bladder toxicity, and malignancy (most commonly bladder). Aggressive hydration is recommended along with drug administration to prevent some of the urologic complications. There is a lifetime maximum dose of 80–100 g. Monitoring should include midmonthly WBC counts and yearly cystoscopy after 3 years of treatment.

Methotrexate

The immunosuppressant methotrexate inhibits dihydrofolate reductase and has also been studied as treatment of progressive MS. A study of 60 patients (30% PPMS, 70% SPMS) compared oral methotrexate 7.5 mg weekly to placebo over 36 months and showed a benefit of methotrexate on the primary endpoint, a composite outcome measure consisting of EDSS, Ambulation Index, 9-Hole Peg Test, and Box and Block Test. However, there was no difference between treatment and placebo groups for sustained EDSS progression. Overall, low-dose methotrexate is generally safe with the most common side effects including nausea, diarrhea, and infection. Complete blood counts and comprehensive metabolic profiles should be monitored at 1, 2, and 4 weeks and then every 1–3 months.

Methylprednisolone

Another medication studied in the treatment of progressive MS is IV methylprednisolone (MP), which was studied at high and low doses (500 and 10 mg/day) administered for three consecutive days in bimonthly pulses over 2 years in SPMS patients. The study of 108 patients showed no significant difference between the two treatment groups in the proportion of patients experiencing sustained disability progression as measured by a composite outcome. However, a planned secondary analysis demonstrated a significant increase in time to onset of disability in the high-dose IVMP group compared with the low-dose group. This suggests that there may be a role for the use of intermittent pulse-dose IVMP in SPMS patients, although the optimal dose and frequency are not well defined. The baseline patient and disease characteristics from the aforementioned study were not described in detail, so it is also difficult to know whether the IVMP treatment effect is more likely attributable to early SPMS patients and patients with more frequent baseline relapses. The potential utility of intermittent IVMP must be weighed against potential adverse effects. For example, effects of high-dose steroids on blood sugar levels may complicate use in patients with diabetes. The effects on bone density should be considered in patients with severe osteoporosis with high fall risks.

Other disease-modifying therapies

Several other immunosuppressive medications have been evaluated in progressive MS patients in small groups with some anecdotal success. In addition to those studies, PPMS patients ($n = 439$) were evaluated in a double-blind, placebo-controlled trial of rituximab over 96 weeks. Confirmed disease progression measured by EDSS showed a trend toward being delayed in the treated group, but statistically significant delay was only seen in subgroup analyses of patients who were younger and had baseline inflammatory lesions. Many of the other medications typically used in RRMS have not been adequately studied in progressive MS. Both natalizumab and fingolimod are FDA approved for *relapsing forms of MS*, but their effect on progressive disease has not been fully investigated. A randomized placebo-controlled clinical trial is currently underway to examine the effect of natalizumab on disability progression in SPMS patients (as measured by the EDSS and timed 25-Foot Walk) over 2 years. A placebo-controlled trial of fingolimod is being conducted in PPMS patients.

Monitoring progressive MS in clinical practice

RRMS patients are generally monitored clinically through history and physical exam for assessment of relapses; radiological monitoring with periodic brain MRI is also relatively straightforward and high yield for identifying new T2 or Gd-enhancing lesions. As noted previously, these are not particularly effective means of monitoring progressive MS due to the infrequency of relapses and new MRI lesions. Accumulation of disability is the primary clinical measure of progressive MS, but the most accepted standard of grading disability, the EDSS, is not widely used in practice due to limited time constraints for patient follow-up visits. An increasingly used measure of progressive MS through imaging is quantification of brain atrophy, but this is not yet a widespread or easily reproducible measure across different sites. Therefore, the typical way to monitor patients tends to encompass clinical history (i.e., patient descriptions of new difficulties with ambulation or activities of daily living). Additionally, shorter standardized physical exam measures, such as components of the MS Functional Composite, may be used. A common measure is the timed 25-Foot Walk, which can be tracked over time to indicate persistent disease progression.

Another important aspect of monitoring progressive MS patients is verification that disability progression is due to MS. For example, when RRMS patients first appear to be transitioning to progressive disease, MRI studies of the brain and/or cervical spine should be considered to rule out a structural abnormality, such as spondylotic myelopathy. Additionally, the same MS mimics that are investigated during the initial diagnosis of MS should be reconsidered as possible contributing factors to disease progression. Based on the clinical history, it may be reasonable to check TSH, vitamin B12, and other blood work to rule out other possible etiologies for clinical disease progression.

> **⚠ CAUTION!**
>
> When patients first appear to be transitioning to SPMS, it is important to consider structural or metabolic etiologies as an alternative to disease progression. Useful tests may include cervical spine MRI and blood work including a complete blood count, thyroid studies, and vitamin B12 level.

Treatment of progressive MS in clinical practice

The overall modest effectiveness of treatment options in progressive MS combined with a lack of evidence regarding other possible therapies has led to a treatment strategy involving substantial variability in opinion and practice. One possible treatment algorithm is outlined in Figure 6.1. As noted previously, the subset of progressive MS patients who tend to be most responsive to therapies includes those who are younger with shorter disease duration, recent disease activity on MRI (new or Gd-enhancing lesions), rapid disease progression, or (in the case of SPMS) recent relapses. This subset of patients can be treated with an algorithm similar to that used in RRMS patients. However, there are certain caveats and alternative considerations as outlined later.

> **⚠ CAUTION!**
>
> The potential risks of unproven disease-modifying therapy options in progressive MS need to be balanced with likelihood of benefit.

> **✶ TIPS AND TRICKS**
>
> Progressive MS patients who are younger with shorter disease duration, a recent relapse, recent MRI lesion activity, or response to IV steroids are more likely to respond to a trial of a disease-modifying therapy.

In treatment-naïve PPMS patients, the initial approach is often to try one of the more established treatments, such as glatiramer acetate or IFN-beta. The former is sometimes preferable as it is less likely to cause side effects or worsening of spasticity. If a patient does not tolerate these initial treatments or continues to worsen, another option is the use of pulse-dose IVMP administered every other month as long as the patient demonstrates benefit and treatment tolerance. There is no published evidence supporting the use of natalizumab or fingolimod in the treatment of PPMS. However, fingolimod has demonstrated an effect on slowing disability progression and reducing brain volume loss in RRMS patients, and it is

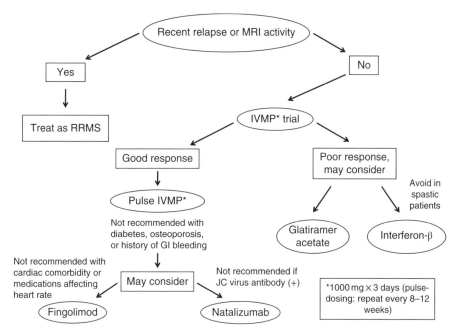

Figure 6.1 Approach to treatment of progressive MS.

currently being studied in PPMS patients. Its use may be considered in young patients without contraindications provided that the risks and potential benefits are weighed appropriately. Other more aggressive therapy options such as mitoxantrone or cyclophosphamide have greater potential for significant adverse events and, given their lack of clear efficacy, are typically only considered for very rapidly progressive disease.

In SPMS, one subset of patients to consider includes the relatively treatment-naïve patients—those initially opposed to treatment during the relapsing phase of the disease or who followed more of a *benign* course but who ultimately seek therapy due to accumulation of disability. There is again no evidence behind treatment guidelines, but similarly to treatment-naïve PPMS patients, trial of glatiramer acetate or IFN-beta is a reasonable first step with similar side effect considerations.

For SPMS patients who are already on treatment but continue to have worsening of disability, it becomes important to assess for evidence or likelihood of recent or ongoing inflammation. Without a clear history of recent

relapse, it makes sense to consider checking a brain MRI to evaluate for evidence of new interval lesions or active inflammation. A trial of IVMP may also give patients and providers insight as to the potential benefit of disease-modifying therapy. Since IVMP is thought to act largely through anti-inflammatory mechanisms in MS, the patients who notice improvement or stability of symptoms in response to IVMP are generally felt to be more likely to behave like patients with relapses and are most likely to potentially benefit from a change in their current treatment.

One option for patients who benefit from IVMP would be to continue its use in pulse doses every other month. However, other options for patients who are considered to have active inflammation, particularly those who clearly have superimposed relapses, would include natalizumab or fingolimod. There again is no evidence to support the use of either of these medications in SPMS, though a clinical trial of natalizumab in SPMS is currently recruiting patients. Nevertheless, if there is no contraindication, it may be reasonable to offer natalizumab or fingolimod on a trial basis

(6–12 months) to see if the disease appears to stabilize. There are patients who seem to symptomatically improve due to the anti-inflammatory effect of disease-modifying therapies such as natalizumab. Yet if patients continue to have disease progression, these therapies should generally be discontinued given that they are unapproved treatments that do not have long usage histories or safety profiles like those of IFN-beta or glatiramer acetate.

In patients with clear disease progression without relapses or other suggestion of inflammatory activity, it is even more important to assess patients for side effects of treatments and to carefully weigh the potential risk of more aggressive therapies with the likelihood of benefit. JC virus antibody testing is now commercially available and is recommended to help assess patient risk of progressive multifocal leukoencephalopathy with use of natalizumab. It may be argued that this stratification is particularly important when considering natalizumab in the treatment of SPMS patients where the benefit is not as well defined.

As natalizumab and fingolimod have become increasingly utilized treatment options, the roles of cyclophosphamide and mitoxantrone have diminished. The former is not approved for use in MS but may be considered for patients with active disease who are transitioning from RRMS to SPMS. Both medications are now reserved for rare patients with rapid progression who may not be candidates for or do not tolerate the other second-line agents. If selected, the recommendations for monitoring with cyclophosphamide have been mentioned previously and for mitoxantrone include a complete blood count and nuclear cardiac scan or echocardiogram at baseline, prior to each infusion, and for several years post treatment.

Stopping disease-modifying therapy

Another important issue that must be addressed in the treatment of progressive MS patients is: when should patients stop disease-modifying therapy? Although the natural history of MS demonstrates a diminishing frequency of relapses and decreasing inflammation, the exact timing of this decline varies from patient to patient. Occasionally, patients who have had a long-standing *quiet* disease course may abruptly suffer a severe relapse. There is no absolute way to predict a patient's disease course, and this has led to a lack of evidence regarding appropriate timing of disease-modifying therapy discontinuation.

A 2009 epidemiological study was conducted surveying both neurologists and patients with progressive MS to obtain information regarding patient and practitioner rationales for discontinuation of disease-modifying therapy. In addition to opinions, the investigators also observed the actual practices of practitioners. The study highlighted that many neurologists would prefer to stop disease-modifying therapies but do not always accomplish this plan. Patient reluctance to stop treatment was an often cited reason, but there are many factors that must be weighed in the decision to stop treatment. Factors that must be considered include duration of disease stability, patient comorbidities, treatment side effects, potential treatment adverse events, and, of course, the patient's wishes. It is not an issue that can be ignored as the number of patients on treatment who convert to SPMS will continue to increase, and the cost of treatment is substantial.

Neuroprotective strategies

There is great interest in potential neuroprotective or repair-promoting treatment strategies for progressive MS. Thus far, studies of possible neuroprotective treatments such as lamotrigine have not yielded positive results in MS. However, there is increasing evidence that vitamin D deficiency is correlated with MS activity, and recent studies suggest that MS patients with lower vitamin D levels may be at greater risk for relapses. Studies have also shown that patients are able to tolerate substantially higher levels and doses of vitamin D than previously recommended. A randomized placebo-controlled trial of vitamin D in MS patients is underway, but until more data are available, a relatively low-risk treatment to offer progressive MS patients is vitamin D supplementation to attain goal levels >30 ng/ml.

Other treatment considerations

The importance of symptomatic treatment to address issues such as spasticity, bowel and bladder symptoms, fatigue, and other manifestations in progressive MS cannot be overemphasized and is addressed at length in later chapters of this book. Similarly, the impact of MS on the social, emotional, and financial health of patients and their support networks, particularly later in the disease when physical and cognitive disability is greater, is another extremely important issue discussed later in the book in more detail.

However, there are other treatment-related considerations specific to progressive MS that should be noted. Progressive MS generally occurs in older patients who have other comorbidities that must be addressed. Routine use of IVMP is not an ideal treatment option for type II diabetics or those at risk of developing diabetes. Additionally, the concern for development of macular edema on fingolimod is higher in diabetic patients. Older age and decreased weight bearing due to disability also puts patients at greater risk of osteoporosis, so patients managed on IVMP should be carefully followed with bone density scans and appropriate pharmacologic therapy for osteoporosis prevention. Progressive MS patients are more likely to be on an antihypertensive medication, and there are new concerns being raised about the safety of fingolimod in patient taking beta-blockers or calcium channel blockers. In the case of more severely disabled patients with very limited mobility, routine immunizations such as a flu shot or pneumonia vaccine should be considered. In paraplegic patients, there is also a greater risk of deep vein thrombosis, and the potential risks and benefits of anticoagulation should be weighed carefully.

> ★ TIPS AND TRICKS
>
> Bone health is particularly important in progressive MS patients who are on recurrent steroid treatment and may have decreased weight-bearing activity. Bone density scans, calcium and vitamin D supplementation, and more aggressive therapies for osteoporosis should be utilized appropriately.

Further Reading

Cohen, J.A. & Rudick, R.A. (eds) (2011) *Multiple Sclerosis Therapeutics*, 4th edn. Cambridge University Press, Cambridge.

Goodkin, D.E., Rudick, R.A., Medendorp, S.V. *et al.* (1995) Low-dose (7.5 mg) oral methotrexate reduces the rate of progression in chronic progressive multiple sclerosis. *Annals of Neurology*, **37**, 30–40.

Goodkin, D.E., Kinkel, R.P., Weinstock-Guttman, B. *et al.* (1998) A phase II study of IV methylprednisolone in secondary-progressive multiple sclerosis. *Neurology*, **51**, 239–245.

Hartung, H.P., Gonsette, R., Konig, N. *et al.* (2002) Mitoxantrone in progressive multiple sclerosis: a placebo-controlled, double blind, randomised, multicentre trial. *Lancet*, **360**, 2018–2024.

Hauser, S.L., Dawson, D.M., Lehrich, J.R. *et al.* (1983) Intensive immunosuppression in progressive multiple sclerosis. *The New England Journal of Medicine*, **308**, 173–180.

Lonergan, R., Kinsella, K., Duggan, M., Jordan, S., Hutchinson, M. & Tubridy, N. (2009) Discontinuing disease-modifying therapy in progressive multiple sclerosis: can we stop what we have started? *Multiple Sclerosis*, **15**, 1528–1531.

Lublin, F.D. & Reingold, S.C. (1996) Defining the clinical course of multiple sclerosis: results of an international survey. *Neurology*, **46**, 907–911.

Reynolds, R., Roncaroli, F., Nicholas, R., Radotra, B., Gveric, D. & Howell, O. (2011) The neuropathological basis of clinical progression in multiple sclerosis. *Acta Neuropathologica*, **122**, 155–177.

Rio, J., Comabella, M. & Montalban, X. (2011) Multiple sclerosis: current treatment algorithms. *Current Opinion in Neurology*, **24**, 230–237.

Panitch, H., Miller, A., Paty, D. *et al.* (2004) Interferon beta-1b in secondary progressive MS. *Neurology*, **63**, 1788–1795.

Vukusic, S. & Confavreux, C. (2007) Natural history of multiple sclerosis: risk factors and prognostic indicators. *Current Opinion in Neurology*, **20**, 269–274.

Weinshenker, B.G., Bass, B., Rice, G.P.A. *et al.* (1989) The natural history of multiple sclerosis: a geographically based study. *Brain*, **112**, 1419–1428.

Whitaker, J.N., McFarland, H.F., Rudge, P. & Reingold, S.C. (1995) Outcomes assessment in multiple sclerosis clinical trials: a critical analysis. *Multiple Sclerosis*, **1**, 37–47.

Wolinsky, J.S., Narayana, P.A., O'Connor, P. *et al.* (2007) Glatiramer acetate in primary progressive multiple sclerosis: results of a multinational, multicenter, double-blind, placebo-controlled trial. *Annals of Neurology*, **61**, 14–24.

7

Sex-Determined Issues in Multiple Sclerosis

Callene Momtazee and Barbara Giesser

Department of Neurology, MS Division, UCLA School of Medicine, Los Angeles, CA, USA

Epidemiology of MS and gender

Most autoimmune diseases over the past century have developed a predilection for females. At the beginning of the 19th century, the ratio of women to men with multiple sclerosis (MS) was 1:1. Now, that ratio is approaching 3:1. There are many theories as to why MS, as well as other autoimmune conditions such as lupus and rheumatoid arthritis, is steadily increasing in women. Most of these theories center around the effect of male and female chromosomes, sex hormones, and their interaction with the environment.

One such theory is that the immune systems of women seem to be more active than men. Females show stronger responses to vaccination and can resist infections more effectively than males (Greer & McCombe 2011). Additionally, the composition of immune cells also seems to vary between women and men. Women have a higher percentage of T cells than men and a higher ratio of CD4:CD8. Interestingly, more estrogen receptors are seen on CD4+ helper T cells than on CD8+ suppressor T cells.

Sex hormone differences may also contribute to the gender inequality seen in the incidence of MS. Men are diagnosed with MS later in life than women, which coincides with the natural decline in testosterone in men as they age. This raises the question as to whether or not testosterone may be protective in those younger males who are genetically predisposed to develop MS. Although the traditional thinking is that MS disables male patients more rapidly than their female counterparts, it is unclear if this is true for relapsing–remitting MS (RRMS) patients. Some studies have shown that men transition to secondary progressive MS (SPMS) at a faster rate than women (5–10 years for men from RRMS diagnosis vs. 15 years for women) but that both sexes progress to SPMS usually around ages 40–45 (Voskuhl & Giesser 2011). Additionally, men have fewer enhancing lesions and relapses in the earlier stages of their disease. This suggests that men may be protected at earlier ages from the inflammatory stage of MS, even though both sexes transition to the more degenerative or progressive phase of MS at a similar chronological age. Once in the progressive stage, both sexes progress in disability at the same speed. Interestingly, primary progressive MS (PPMS), which is thought to be less inflammatory in nature than RRMS, continues to show an incidence ratio of 1:1 men and women (Voskuhl & Giesser 2011).

Lastly, males and females do experience different interactions between their bodies and their environment. As the possible link between low vitamin D levels and the incidence of MS is elucidated, studies have looked at gender differences. Overall, men have more sun exposure and use less sunscreen than women, which may provide another element of protection for their gender (Greer & McCombe 2011).

Multiple Sclerosis and CNS Inflammatory Disorders, First Edition. Edited by Lawrence M. Samkoff and Andrew D. Goodman.

EVIDENCE AT A GLANCE

Men develop RRMS at a lower rate than females at a ratio of roughly 3:1 female to male. They also tend to develop MS later in life, but transition to the progressive phase of the disease at the same age as women (40–45 years old). Younger men's protection in MS is speculated to be due to both sex hormone and chromosomal differences. PPMS, a less inflammatory condition than RRMS, continues to show a 1:1 female to male ratio.

Basic science of sex hormone and chromosome differences seen in MS

Actions of sex hormones

Sex hormones are lipophilic and easily cross the blood–brain barrier. The possible neuroprotective effect of sex hormones in MS was studied in the mouse model experimental autoimmune encephalomyelitis (EAE). In mice, as seen in humans, males appear less susceptible to the disease than females. Castration of the males increases their risk of disease, presumably because it decreases testosterone (Voskuhl & Giesser 2011). Additionally, male mice show lower levels of testosterone during EAE relapses. In humans, there is some evidence that male MS patients may have lower levels of testosterone than controls. Pilot studies involving supplemental exogenous testosterone showed some improvement on both cognition and brain atrophy measures (Voskuhl & Giesser 2011). Larger studies are needed to confirm this effect of treatment.

Female sex hormones are also being studied as possible neuroprotective agents in MS. There are three types of estrogen in women: estradiol, estriol, and estrone. Estrone is primarily produced in the body's fat cells and estriol by the fetal placental unit during pregnancy, and estradiol is the main form of estrogen, produced by the ovaries, which regulates menstruation.

As will be discussed in detail later in this chapter, women with MS experience a decrease in relapses during their third trimester of pregnancy. In a pilot study, patients treated with oral estriol that mimicked levels found during the sixth month of pregnancy experienced an 80% reduction in gadolinium-enhancing lesions on MRI (Voskuhl & Giesser 2011). A current, phase III, multicenter, double-blind randomized controlled trial is being conducted to further assess estriol's protective effects on relapses and new MRI lesions has just been completed;results are pending. Interestingly, in immune modulation, high doses of estrogen augment Th2 responses and low doses seem to augment Th1 responses (Greer & McCombe 2011). Given that Th2 immune shifts are thought to be protective in MS, this could be one putative mechanism of the protection provided by female hormones.

EVIDENCE AT A GLANCE

Effects of sex hormones on MS
Lipophilic sex hormones easily cross the blood brain barrier. Estrogen is an immunomodulator, and at higher doses augments the body's Th2 immune response which is thought to be beneficial in the course of MS. In mice, lower levels of testosterone exacerbate EAE.

Gender effects seen in genetics of MS

The genetics of MS transmission suggest a link to the HLA class II genes and specifically HLA-DRB1*15 (Chao et al. 2011). As stated earlier, there are roughly three female RRMS patients for every male with the disease. Although MS does not show a Mendelian inheritance pattern, offspring of parents with MS have a greatly elevated risk of developing MS as compared to the general population, with the bulk of this risk apparently transmitted through the mother. Also, in regard to vertical transmission, more mother–daughter affected pairs are seen than father–son duos (Chao et al. 2011).

The X chromosome itself may increase the susceptibility to MS. In transgenic mice, the presence of two X chromosomes (regardless of whether or not the mouse had ovaries or testes) showed an increase of susceptibility to EAE (Greer & McCombe 2011). Further, certain antigen targets in MS, such as myelin proteolipid protein, are encoded on the X chromosome itself (Greer & McCombe 2011). Lastly, in humans, there seems to be a *skewing* of X chromosome inactivation in women with autoimmune disease. In typical females, each cell shows an inactivation of one of her X chromosomes, and this ratio is usually around 1:1 so that half of the X chromosomes expressed are from either parent. But certain studies have shown that females with autoimmune disease present a preponderance of X chromosomes being active from only one parent or a skewed X inactivation (Greer & McCombe 2011).

Reproductive issues in MS

Menstrual cycle and menopause

Experiencing menarche at a younger age has been seen to increase the risk of MS. And for PPMS, there may be a delayed progression to EDSS when menarche begins later, at age 13 years or more (D'hooghe *et al.* 2012). While MS does not appear to have a particular effect on the regularity of the menstrual cycle or the onset of menopause, there is some evidence that women may experience an increase in their MS symptoms premenstrually (Voskuhl & Giesser 2011). In one study, MRI lesions were seen more frequently during the luteal phase of a woman's cycle (Greer & McCombe 2011). More studies are necessary to elucidate the cause of this phenomenon.

Interestingly, oral contraceptive pills (OCPs) do not seem to provide a protective effect in MS (D'hooghe *et al.* 2010). In fact, there is some evidence in one population study that users of OCPs experience progress to EDSS 6 faster, especially if they began using OCPs as a teen (D'hooghe *et al.* 2012). It is unknown why this type of synthetic estrogen is not beneficial in MS.

There is little data on the effect of menopause on MS. Although MS symptoms may be seen to increase perimenopausally, there has been no benefit seen from the use of hormone replacement therapy (HRT) in the progression of MS (Greer & McCombe 2011).

Effects on fertility

In general, MS does not seem to have any significant impact on fertility or reproductive health (Voskuhl & Giesser 2011). For patients who do happen to experience infertility, there is limited evidence to suggest that in vitro fertilization (IVF) may be associated with more frequent MS exacerbations if the IVF procedure fails or if GnRH agonists are used (Michel *et al.* 2012), although these studies had very few patients and other studies have found no difference with different fertility medications.

However, MS patients take many disease- and symptom-modifying medications that can affect both fertility and a developing fetus. Patients of both genders who require second-line therapy with chemotherapeutic or immunosuppressant agents such as mitoxantrone, azathioprine, methotrexate, and cyclophosphamide may experience a decrease in fertility and should be counseled about the option of sperm and egg banking if pregnancy is desired following cessation of treatment. The disease-modifying therapies (DMTs) and common symptom medications used in MS are listed in Table 7.1 and Table 7.2 along with their pregnancy safety categories for reference.

Contraceptive issues

Given the potential risk of certain DMTs to the developing fetus, female MS patients may wish to take contraceptive precautions against pregnancy if it is not immediately desired. If pregnancy is immediately desired, it is recommended that patients stop their interferon or glatiramer acetate therapy at least one to two cycles prior to trying to become pregnant (Voskuhl & Giesser 2011) and at least two cycles for the oral therapy fingolimod given its half-life. Natalizumab should be discontinued 3 months prior to conception (Hellwig *et al.* 2011). Dimethyl fumarate has a short half life and its metabolite does not accumulate, so theoretically no wash out period should be necessary

(Lu *et al.*, 2014). Conservative patients may wish to have one normal menstrual cycle off of dimethyl fumarate prior to conception.

Table 7.1 DMTs—Pregnancy Safety Categories*

Disease Modifying Therapy	Pregnancy Category
Beta-interferon-I-b	C
Beta-interferon-I-a	C
Fingolimod	C
Glatiramer acetate	B
Terflunomide	X
Dimethyl fumarate	C
Natalizumab	C
Mitoxantrone	D
Cyclophosphamide[†]	D
IVIG[†]	C
Azathioprine[†]	D
Methotrexate[†]	X

Source: Voskuhl and Giesser (2011). Adapted with permission of Oxford University Press. A, no evidence of fetal harm in human studies; B, no evidence of fetal harm in animal studies; C, evidence of fetal harm in animal studies or no data available; D, evidence of fetal harm in humans, use may be justified in some circumstances; X, evidence of fetal harm in humans, not indicated for use in pregnancy.
*FDA pregnancy risk category definitions.
[†]Not approved MS therapy by FDA or other regulatory agencies.

The teratogenic potential for terflunomide may be up to 2 years after cessation of administration. The minimum recommended wash out period is at least 8 months. Facilitated elimination may be accomplished with cholestyramine or activated charcoal (Lu *et al.*, 2014).

There are no official guidelines as to the pros and cons of the use of OCPs or HRT in MS patients. Although estrogens may have a protective effect in MS as described earlier, there is no current evidence to suggest that estradiol, in the amounts contained in OCPs, is helpful in treating or preventing MS (Voskuhl & Giesser 2011). It is recommended that individual patients decide what contraceptive method is best for them in consultation with their doctors.

Congenital effects

To date, there is no evidence that babies born to mothers with MS experience congenital malformations or stillbirths at a higher rate than the general population (Argyriou & Makris 2008). A national pregnancy registry of patients with MS, diabetes, and epilepsy showed that MS patients displayed a higher incidence of intrauterine growth restriction and cesarean delivery than controls (Kelly *et al.* 2009) but that overall patients with MS tend to have healthy, full-term pregnancies.

The main MS-related risk to the developing fetus is the fact that children born to parents with MS have an increased risk of developing

Table 7.2 Symptom Management Medications—Pregnancy Safety Categories

Agent	Symptom	Pregnancy Risk Category
Corticosteroid	Acute exacerbation*	C
Baclofen	Spasticity	C
Diazepam	Spasticity,* anxiety	D
Tizanidine	Spasticity	C
Gabapentin	Seizure, pain,* spasticity*	C
Amantadine	Fatigue*	C
Modafinil	Fatigue*	C
Oxybutynin	Overactive bladder	B
Tolterodine	Overactive bladder	C
Dalfampridine	Improve walking	C

Source: Voskuhl and Giesser (2011). Adapted with permission of Oxford University Press.
*No FDA indication for this use or no indication for use in MS.

MS, roughly 20–50 times that of the general population, depending upon the study cited (Voskuhl & Giesser 2011). A Danish population-based registry study of 8205 MS patients since 1968 found that the lifetime risk of a daughter developing MS born to an MS-affected parent was 2.9%. For sons, the risk was 2.8%. This is compared to the general population risk in Denmark of developing MS of 0.5% for females and 0.3% for males (Nielsen *et al.* 2005). This data will vary based upon the location and ethnicity of the patients being studied naturally and may be difficult to extrapolate to patients who are not of Northern European descent.

Pregnancy and the MS patient

Epidemiology

While pregnancy can be considered a *protected state* in MS, previously conducted population studies were unclear as to the long-term protective effects of pregnancy in women with MS. There is some evidence that women who have had children take longer to reach an EDSS of six than women who have not had children (Greer & McCombe 2011). But authors note that this may indicate that women who have greater amounts of disability, or perhaps more aggressive MS, may just choose not to get pregnant. Women with MS are more likely to never have children than the general population (Ponsonby *et al.* 2012). Other previous studies show that there is no effect of parity on disability progression outcome measures in MS (D'hooghe *et al.* 2010).

The Ausimmune study recently attempted to address this question by examining the age of onset of a first clinical demyelinating event (FCD). They found that per patient an increasing number of offspring was associated with a dose–response trend toward a later age of developing an FCD for women but not men. In fact, there was a 49% reduction in the risk of FCD for each birth. This trend persisted even after adjusting for sun index scores and vitamin D levels, smoking, body mass index, HLA-DR15 gene presence, and other potential risk factors for developing MS. Hence, the presumptive mechanism of this decreased MS risk is thought to be due to the pregnancies themselves

(Ponsonby *et al.* 2012). This study is also important because it studied FCD, not when women were diagnosed with MS. Therefore, these patients were not choosing to be childless because of their diagnosis. Interestingly, the age of first birth for women in Australia has increased to 31.9 years in 2008 as compared to 23.2 years in 1961. During this same time period, the female-to-male ratio of MS has increased significantly, prompting the study authors to wonder if these environmental factors are related (Ponsonby *et al.* 2012).

Although the 9 months of pregnancy is a protected state for exacerbations in MS patients, as discussed earlier, the effect of multiple pregnancies on the course of the disease and progression in disability had been unclear until now. There is some evidence that pregnancy may increase the time until reaching SPMS, but evidence on pregnancy and its effect on disability progression (EDSS score) is mixed (Voskuhl & Giesser 2011). Longer-term and prospective studies are required to address these specific questions.

Clinical concerns

Women with MS who wish to become pregnant should not be discouraged from doing so as they were in years past. Any patient with a chronic or potentially disabling medical condition is labeled as a high-risk pregnancy. But it is now well known that MS patients experience a decrease in relapses during pregnancy and a potential rebound in relapses in the postpartum time frame. The *Pregnancy and Multiple Sclerosis*, or PRIMS, study addressed this question by prospectively following 227 pregnancies in women with MS. They found that the mean relapse rate for the women was 0.7 per year before pregnancy, 0.2 during the third trimester of pregnancy, and an uptick to 1.2 during the *fourth trimester* or postpartum period (Vukusic *et al.* 2004; Figure 7.1). Even with this increase in relapse activity postpartum, it is important to note that most patients followed did not incur a relapse during this 3-month time period (72% remained relapse-free). Also, keep in mind that only 2.2% of patients

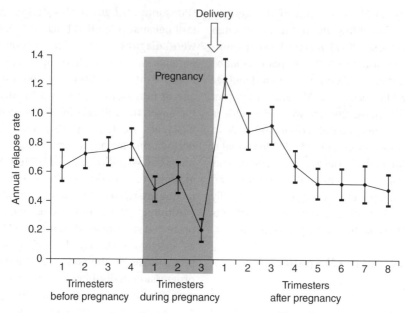

Figure 7.1 ARR in the year before pregnancy, during pregnancy, and in the 2 years after delivery among 227 women with MS (vertical bars represent means and 95% confidence intervals). Source: Vukusic *et al.* (2004). Reproduced with permission of Oxford University Press.

went on DMTs in the 6 months following delivery, meaning the majority of these women were medically unprotected against MS during the postpartum trimester. In this study, the predictors for women who would experience a relapse included women with more frequent relapses the year before and during pregnancy and women with higher levels of disability prepregnancy.

⚙ SCIENCE REVISITED

MS is thought to be primarily a cell-mediated type of autoimmune disease. During pregnancy, there is a shift from Th1 (cell-mediated) to Th2 (humoral) immune responses to protect the fetus from maternal rejection and provide for the passive transfer of maternal antibodies to protect against infectious disease. This immune system shift is thought to be a principle basis in the decrease in relapses seen in MS patients during pregnancy (Voskuhl & Giesser 2011).

During the PRIMS trial, no relation to postpartum relapse was seen between epidural use (18.9% of patients followed) and breastfeeding (54.6% of patients). Neither was the number of previous pregnancies, gender of fetus, age of MS onset, age of pregnancy onset, disease duration, nor total number of relapses prior to pregnancy related to the postpartum relapse rate (Vukusic *et al.* 2004).

As outlined earlier, MS is thought largely to be a cell-mediated autoimmune disease. During pregnancy, a woman's immune system tends to shift from a Th1 (cell-mediated) predominance to a Th2 (humoral-mediated) response. This prevents the fetus, which is technically a foreign body, from being rejected by the mother's immune system. Lupus (SLE) patients, in contrast, tend to experience exacerbations of their disease during pregnancy. This may be because SLE is a humoral-based autoimmune disease; hence, the shift from Th1 to Th2 responses during pregnancy is disadvantageous from a standpoint in SLE (Voskuhl & Giesser 2011).

Neuromyelitis optica (NMO), also a demyelinating disease of the central nervous system, is thought to be humorally based via the aquaporin-4 antibody. A recent study of 190 women looked at the influence of pregnancy on NMO disorder and found via retrospective questionnaires that the annualized relapse rate (ARR) for NMO was unchanged during pregnancy but quite raised during the postpartum period. It is unknown as to why this relapse pattern differs from SLE which is also humorally based. Perhaps there are other as yet unknown immune mechanisms at play in NMO disease. The T cells induce inflammation which then creates a favorable environment for the AQP4 antibodies to then go in and destroy astrocytes (Pohl *et al.* 2013). Only 26 women experienced a pregnancy after the diagnosis of NMO. Of the 40 pregnancies reported, 77% were associated with a postpartum relapse. The ARR was 5.3 in the first trimester after pregnancy and 3.7 in the second trimester after pregnancy regardless of prepregnancy relapse rates, type of delivery, epidural anesthesia, or breastfeeding status. Patients using immunosuppressant therapy had lower postpartum relapse rates 6–12 months after delivery. Hence it is recommended that NMO patients restart DMT as soon as possible after pregnancy (Kalluri *et al.* 2011; Kim *et al.* 2012).

Management of pregnant patient: Before, during, and after

Before pregnancy

Women with MS who wish to become pregnant should discuss this with their neurologist and should stop their DMT use before trying to become pregnant as discussed earlier. The protective effects of most DMTs will be gone a few months after discontinuation (Voskuhl & Giesser 2011). Therefore, women who have difficulty becoming pregnant, and are not on a DMT, are at an increased risk for relapse and should keep in close contact with their physicians should new neurologic symptoms arise.

⚠ CAUTION!

MS patients who wish to become pregnant should discontinue interferons and glatiramer acetate one to two menstrual cycles prior to conception if possible. Fingolimod should be discontinued at least two cycles prior to conception. Natalizumab should be discontinued three cycles prior to conception (Hellwig *et al.* 2011). The washout period for teriflunomide is 8 months to 2 years. No DMTs are approved for use during pregnancy or breastfeeding.

During pregnancy

As discussed earlier, DMTs are contraindicated for use during pregnancy. Additionally, most symptom management drugs used for MS complications are also contraindicated during pregnancy (see Table 7.2). Therefore, lifestyle changes and nonpharmacologic aids are encouraged as a substitute. For example, many pregnanat women have increased bladder frequency, therefore MS patients may require frequent timed voiding in order to help prevent sudden urgency or incontinence from spastic bladders instead of relying on medications. Fatigue is also an obvious concern, and energy conservation strategies should be discussed and put in place proactively (Voskuhl & Giesser 2011).

Acute relapses can occur during pregnancy, despite the protection that pregnancy can afford. Should an MS patient experience a new exacerbation, it is important to distinguish if it is a pseudoexacerbation (e.g., from a urinary tract infection, heat, etc.). If it is determined to be a true exacerbation, then a short course of IV methylprednisolone is considered safe as it is inactivated by the placenta but should be avoided during the first trimester if possible (Argyriou & Makris 2008). IVIG may also be used and may be preferable during the first trimester as it is safe throughout pregnancy (Achiron *et al.* 2004; Argyriou & Makris 2008).

MRIs are safe for both mother and fetus to be performed during pregnancy, preferably after the first trimester, but the use of gadolinium is discouraged as its fetal safety is unproven (Argyriou & Makris 2008). All other common tests used in MS patients, such as evoked potentials and lumbar punctures, are safe during pregnancy.

Just as there are no genetic or blood tests for MS, there are no prenatal tests to determine the likelihood of transmission of MS to the fetus (Argyriou & Makris 2008).

Management of labor and delivery

Unless an MS patient has been on chronic steroids for some reason, there is no need for pulse steroids during labor. Additionally, there is no increased risk for cesarean versus vaginal delivery in MS patients, nor are there differences seen in maternal or fetal outcomes in the different types of anesthesia (Argyriou & Makris 2008). Hence, an MS patient's labor should be managed by their obstetrician as is appropriate to the safety of the mother and baby.

After pregnancy

As discussed earlier, the PRIMS trial showed an increase in MS relapses during the postpartum period. Since some DMTs can take several months to reach their full protective effect, women who are not breastfeeding are encouraged to start DMTs as early as 2 weeks after delivery in order to help protect them from relapses as soon as possible. The number and frequency of relapses experienced by a patient prior to pregnancy are the best predictors for postpartum relapses. If a patient was poorly controlled before pregnancy, this can be an ideal time to change DMT choice.

Studies are ongoing to see if there is a way to counteract the rebound in inflammation and relapses seen in female MS patients after giving birth. One European multicenter phase III study, the POPART'MUS trial, is looking at treating patients proactively with a combination of high-dose progestin and estradiol. The investigators then will compare the percentage of patients who are relapse-free during the first 3 months after delivery as well as the number of new and enhancing lesions seen on MRI.

Breastfeeding is not allowed during this study, nor are other DMT agents. The goal is to enroll at least 300 patients (Vukusic *et al.* 2009).

IVIG has also been studied as a means to reduce relapses in the pregnancy and postpartum periods. Achiron *et al.* (2005) compared women retrospectively who received IVIG during the postpartum period as well as receiving IVIG during the pregnancy and postpartum period to controls and saw that there was a significant decrease in relapses in the IVIG-treated groups (Argyriou & Makris 2008). Double-blind, placebo-controlled trials are needed to confirm this finding.

> ★ **TIPS AND TRICKS**
>
> MS patients experience healthy pregnancies comparable to the general population and need not be managed differently obstetrically in regards to type of delivery or anesthesia.

Breastfeeding

Breastfeeding and MS remain a controversial topic. As discussed earlier, women are encouraged to restart DMT therapy after delivery in order to protect themselves from relapses as quickly as possible postpartum. But, the degree of transmission of DMT agents via breast milk is unclear, therefore, none of the DMTs are recommended for use while nursing. Studies that have looked at breastfeeding and relapses have been contradictory to date. Certain small studies show breastfeeding to be protective against MS relapses when done exclusively and not combined with or supplemented by formula feeding (Greer & McCombe 2011), but more investigation is needed.

Corticosteroids, often used for MS relapses, are transmitted into breast milk and therefore should be avoided (Argyriou & Makris 2008). Should a patient require steroids for a relapse postpartum, breastfeeding must be temporarily halted during treatment and shortly after. IVIG can be used instead for relapses however as it is considered safe for use while breastfeeding (Argyriou & Makris 2008).

MRI scans with gadolinium contrast are another concern for nursing mothers with MS. Although recent radiologic literature states that the amount of gadolinium expressed via breast milk and ingested by the infant is small, in practice, we recommend that our patients stop breastfeeding and *pump and dump* for 24 h after gadolinium administration in order to be as cautious as possible (Sungren & Leander 2011).

Female cancers

In past decades, MS patients have shown similar to or somewhat lower incidence rates of cancer as compared to the general population. Breast cancer rates appear to be similar, whereas non-breast-related cancers may be slightly reduced. This has been postulated to be an effect of probable enhanced immune surveillance for cancerous cells, perhaps because of the T-cell-mediated mechanisms involved in patients with this disease.

Yet, since the introduction of DMTs, including both immune modulators and immune suppressants, there is some evidence that the cancer protection previously seen in MS may now be counteracted by disease-modifying treatment. One Israeli study, where cancer reporting is mandatory, showed that in MS patients not taking DMT, the incidence rates of cancer were reduced. But in patients who were taking immunomodulatory therapy, the cancer incidence approached that of the general population and was even trending higher. In fact, there was some evidence that patients using glatiramer acetate may have a slightly higher incidence of breast cancer. Interestingly, the overall incidence rate of cancer in male patients on or off DMT was still similar to the general population (Achiron *et al.* 2005). A subsequent population-based study in Denmark suggested that women with MS may have a higher incidence of breast cancer overall, independent of timing and amount of parity (Nielsen *et al.* 2006). This question will need to be continually addressed in future population studies as more classes of DMTs are approved and used in MS patients.

Male sex hormones and concerns for the male patient

As discussed, males develop MS less often than females and at a later age, perhaps because of the difference in male versus female sex hormones and chromosomes. In one study performed by Safarinejad, lower circulating levels of testosterone, LH, and FSH have been seen in male MS patients compared to controls (Safarinejad 2008). Additionally, injecting GnRHa into these 68 male patients did not elicit the usual increase in LH or FSH levels compared to control patients, thus indicating possible hypothalamic–pituitary–testis axis dysfunction. No hypogonadism was seen in the MS patients, also indicating that the dysfunction was central rather than peripheral. This study also measured semen quality. Those with progressive disease were seen to have lower sperm counts than those with RRMS, who in turn had lower counts than normal controls. However, while there is some evidence that MS patients may have decreased sperm count and motility, this does not necessarily translate into lower fertility rates (Safarinejad 2008), although more research is needed.

Unfortunately, little has been studied on health concerns specifically relating to the male MS patient. Male patients with MS are known to suffer from erectile dysfunction (ED) more often than controls, and there are reports that find that up to 50% of men with MS suffer from ED (Safarinejad 2008). Therefore, it is important to screen male patients for sexual dysfunction. Decreased libido and arousal can also be a major issue. Again, this may or may not be attributable to lower levels of testosterone. An examination by a urologist is recommended for male MS patients complaining of sexual dysfunction as this can be multifactorial and exacerbated by other conditions (such as heart disease, diabetes, or medication side effects). Treatment for ED in MS should mirror that of non-MS patients in that both medication and lifestyle changes may help.

Acknowledgments

Callene Momtazee has no supporting research grants at this time.

References

Achiron, A., Kishner, I., Dolev, M., *et al.* (2004) Effect of intravenous immunoglobulin treatment on pregnancy and postpartum-related relapses in multiple sclerosis. *Journal of Neurology*, **251** (9), 1133–1137.

Achiron, A., Barak, Y., Gail, M. *et al.* (2005) Cancer incidence in multiple sclerosis and effects of immunomodulatory treatments. *Breast Cancer Research and Treatment*, **89**, 265–270.

Argyriou, A. & Makris, N. (2008) Multiple sclerosis and reproductive risks in women. *Reproductive Sciences*, **15**, 755–764.

Chao, M.J., Ramagopalan, S.V., Herrera, B.M. *et al.* (2011) MHC transmission insights into gender bias in MS susceptibility. *Neurology*, **76**, 242–246.

D'hooghe, M.B., Nagels, G., Bissay, V. & De Keyser, J. (2010) Modifiable factors influencing relapses and disability in multiple sclerosis. *Multiple Sclerosis*, **16** (7), 773–785.

D'hooghe, M.B., Haentjens, P., Nagels, G., D'hooghe, T. & De Keyser, J. (2012) Menarche, oral contraceptives, pregnancy and progression of disability in relapsing onset and progressive onset multiple sclerosis. *Journal of Neurology*, **259** (5), 855–861.

Greer, J. & McCombe, P. (2011) Role of gender in multiple sclerosis: clinical effects and potential molecular mechanisms. *Journal of Neuro-immunology*, **234**, 7–18.

Hellwig, K., Haghikia, A. & Gold, R. (2011) Pregnancy and natalizumab: results of an observational study in 35 accidental pregnancies during natalizumab treatment. *Multiple Sclerosis Journal*, **17** (8), 958–963.

Kalluri, S.R., Rothhammer, V., Staszewski, O., *et al.* (2011) Functional characterization of aquaporin-4 specific T cells: towards a model for neuromyelitis optica. *PLoS One*, **6**, e16083.

Kelly, V.M., Nelson, L.M. & Chakravarty, E.F. (2009) Obstetric outcomes in women with multiple sclerosis and epilepsy. *Neurology*, **73**, 1831–1836.

Kim, W., Kim, S.H., Nakashima, I. *et al.* (2012) Influence of pregnancy on neuromyelitis optica spectrum disorder. *Neurology*, **78**, 1264–1267.

Lu, E., Wang, B.W., Alwan, S. *et al.* (2014) A review of safety-related pregnancy data surrounding the oral disease modifying drugs for MS. *CNS Drugs*, **28**, 89–94.

Michel, L., Foucher, Y., Vukusic, S. *et al.* (2012) Increased risk of multiple sclerosis relapse after in vitro fertilization. *Journal of Neurology Neurosurgery & Psychiatry*, **83**, 796–802.

Nielsen, N.M., Westergaard, T., Rostgaard, K. *et al.* (2005) Familial risk of multiple sclerosis: a nationwide cohort study. *American Journal of Epidemiology*, **162** (8), 774–778.

Nielsen, N.M., Rostgaard, K., Rasmusseum, S. *et al.* (2006) Cancer risk among patients with multiple sclerosis: a population based register study. *International Journal of Cancer*, **118**, 979–984.

Pohl, M., Kawakami, N., Kitic, M., *et al.* (2013) T cell-activation in neuromyelitis optica lesions plays a role in their formation. *Acta Neuropathologica Communications*, **1**, 85.

Ponsonby, A.L., Lucas, R.M., van der Mei, I.A. *et al.* (2012) Offspring number, pregnancy, and risk of a first clinical demyelinating event: the Ausimmune study. *Neurology*, **78**, 867–874.

Safarinejad, M.R. (2008) Evaluation of endocrine profile hypothalamic-pituitary-testis axis and semen quality in multiple sclerosis. *Journal of Neuroendocrinology*, **20**, 1368–1375.

Sungren, P.C. & Leander, P. (2011) Is administration of gadolinium based contrast media to pregnant women and small children justified? *Journal of Magnetic Resonance Imaging*, **34**, 750–757.

Voskuhl, R. & Giesser, B. (2011) Gender and reproductive issues in multiple sclerosis. In: B. Giesser (ed), Multiple Sclerosis, pp. 221–240. Oxford University Press, Oxford.

Vukusic, S., Hutchinson, M., Hours, M. *et al.* (2004) Pregnancy and multiple sclerosis (the PRIMS study): clinical predictors of post-partum relapse. *Brain*, **127**, 1353–1360.

Vukusic, S., Ionescu, I., El-Etr, M. *et al.* (2009) The prevention of post-partum relapses with progestin and estradiol in multiple sclerosis (POPART'MUS) trial: rationale, objectives and state of advancement. *Journal of the Neurological Sciences*, **286**, 114–118.

8

Pediatric Multiple Sclerosis

Robert Thompson Stone[1] and Brenda Banwell[2]

[1]Department of Neurology, University of Rochester Medical Center, Rochester, NY, USA
[2]Department of Pediatrics (Neurology), The Hospital for Sick Children, Toronto, Ontario, Canada

Introduction

Once felt to be extremely rare, awareness of pediatric-onset multiple sclerosis (MS) has grown substantially over the last two decades. Over this time, a myriad of studies have emerged evaluating natural history data, diagnostic considerations, treatment safety, and effect on cognition. The condition differs from adult-onset disease in that the brain is actively myelinating and the immune system is actively maturing concurrent with the disease process. Children with an initial demyelinating event are more likely than adults to ultimately have a monophasic course. Thus, differentiation between events that will be relapsing versus monophasic can be challenging. There is also a more variable spectrum of clinical presentation in children, especially under age 12. This chapter emphasizes the clinical, neuroimaging, epidemiologic, and treatment aspects of pediatric-onset MS and summarizes current means to distinguish MS from other forms of acquired demyelinating disease.

Definitions

In 2013, the International Pediatric Multiple Sclerosis Study Group (IPMSSG) revised consensus definitions for acquired demyelinating syndromes (i.e., acute disseminated encephalomyelitis (ADEM), clinically isolated syndrome (CIS), neuromyelitis optica (NMO), and pediatric MS).

ADEM, and multiphasic ADEM

ADEM

ADEM is defined by polyfocal neurological deficits accompanied by encephalopathy (profound irritability, impaired level of consciousness, or coma). Patients may experience concurrent optic nerve and spinal cord involvement. Acute central nervous system (CNS) infection, metabolic disease, and other etiologies for acute CNS decompensation must be excluded. The diagnosis of ADEM also rests on the clinical and radiologic improvement (albeit not necessarily complete) following the inciting event. As the time course of improvement is variable, the current definition of ADEM permits a period of 3 months during which clinical and radiologic findings may evolve. Radiologic features typical of ADEM are described in section "Diagnostic Considerations". Over 85% of children with ADEM will experience a monophasic illness with complete or near-complete neurological recovery. Children with spinal cord lesions and children requiring intense care are more likely to experience residual deficits.

Multiple Sclerosis and CNS Inflammatory Disorders, First Edition. Edited by Lawrence M. Samkoff and Andrew D. Goodman.
© 2014 John Wiley & Sons, Ltd. Published 2014 by John Wiley & Sons, Ltd.

Multiphasic ADEM

Multiphasic ADEM is defined as a second episode of ADEM, occurring more than 3 months from the initial illness, but not followed by any further events. If more than two demyelinating events occur, it would be considered a chronic disorder (most typically MS or neuromyelitis optica).

Distinguishing multiphasic ADEM from MS rests on the presence of polyfocal neurological deficits and encephalopathy during both attacks and on the absence of clinically silent new lesions detected on MRI scans performed between events. Approximately 5–15% of children with an initial attack meeting criteria for ADEM will ultimately be diagnosed with MS. The diagnosis of MS in a child with an initial ADEM event could be made if a new demyelinating event occurs in the absence of encephalopathy, 3 or more months after the initial event, and is associated with new radiologic findings that meet the 2010 Revised McDonald criteria for dissemination in space.

Clinically isolated syndromes (CIS)

CIS is defined as an initial acquired demyelinating syndrome with mono- or multifocal neurological deficits in the absence of encephalopathy. It should not meet the criteria for a diagnosis of MS based on baseline radiologic features.

Pediatric multiple sclerosis

Pediatric MS is defined by onset (first attack) prior to 18 years of age. Over 95% of pediatric MS patients experience a relapsing–remitting disease onset with multiple episodes of CNS demyelination separated in time (more than 30 days between attacks) and involving multiple areas of the CNS. An initial single nonencephalopathic episode with radiologic findings consistent with the 2010 Revised McDonald criteria for dissemination in space and time could also lead to the diagnosis.

Clinical outcome following a first demyelinating attack

The majority of adult patients with an acquired demyelinating event will ultimately be diagnosed with relapsing–remitting MS. The proportion of children diagnosed with MS after an initial attack may be lower relative to adults, likely owing to the higher frequency of ADEM in childhood.

In one pediatric cohort, after 3 years of follow-up, 57% were diagnosed with pediatric MS, monophasic ADEM was diagnosed in 29%, and 14% experienced monophasic CIS. A more recent study followed a cohort of children with acute demyelinating syndrome (ADS) for 3 years and utilized the IPMSSG definitions for classification. After the follow-up period, the patients were diagnosed with pediatric MS in 21%, monophasic disease in 76%, and relapsing demyelination other than MS (i.e., recurrent optic neuritis (ON), transverse myelitis (TM), or NMO) in 3%. Only 5% of children initially diagnosed with ADEM were subsequently diagnosed with MS. The risk of developing MS after an episode of childhood ON appears to be about 10–35%, with MS more likely to be diagnosed in children who have demyelinating lesions outside the optic pathways. Longitudinally extensive TM as an initial episode of ADS is less likely than the other forms of CIS to represent the first attack of MS.

Epidemiology and risk factors

Overall, the incidence of ADS appears to be between 0.5 and 1.5 cases per 100,000 children per year, while the incidence of pediatric MS is approximately 0.3–0.5 per 100,000 children per year. Prevalence data for pediatric MS is limited. It is commonly cited that 3–5% of all patients with MS present with their first attack during childhood, the majority of whom manifest between ages 10 and 18 years. Onset of MS prior to age 10 years is rare, occurring in only 20% of all pediatric MS patients. The mean age of onset for pediatric MS is 12–13 years, whereas for monophasic ADS the mean age of onset is younger, that is, at 8–9 years.

The female/male ratio in adolescent-onset MS patients is approximately 2–3:1, while male and female patients are equally represented when MS onset occurs prior to age 11 years. Hormonal influences on immune cell behavior or sex-specific expression of MS-relevant genes are postulated but as yet unproven explanations. In North America, pediatric-onset disease appears overrepresented in Black- or Asian-descent individuals. It has been observed that a high proportion of pediatric-onset MS patients are first-generation North Americans (a world region of high MS prevalence), while their parents often emigrated from world areas where MS is rare. These observations support a strong contribution of childhood environment on MS risk.

The pediatric MS population is a useful cohort in which to study environmental risk factors given that children experience MS onset in close proximity to the pathobiological factors relevant to disease etiology. Remote infection with Epstein–Barr virus (EBV) is associated with MS in both pediatric and adult cohorts. Remote infection with EBV (as evidenced by seropositivity for anti-EBNA-1 antibodies) can be detected in 75–90% of children with MS. However, EBV infection cannot be obligatory given that 10–25% of patients have no evidence of exposure to EBV. Given that MS prevalence is highest in world regions with low ambient sunlight exposure, decreased exposure to sunlight and consequent low serum vitamin D concentrations are potential environmental risk factors for the development of MS. Children with MS have lower vitamin D concentrations compared to healthy children, and lower serum vitamin D concentrations detected at the time of a first demyelinating attack are predictive of subsequent MS diagnosis.

Clinical presentation

There are many similarities between the clinical manifestations of pediatric and adult MS; however, the two populations are inherently different in that the pediatric brain is undergoing myelination and development concurrent with the MS disease process. Pediatric MS is relapsing–remitting in over 95% of cases, and thus, the discussion will focus on this form of disease. In very young children, an *ADEM-like* presentation occurs more commonly than in older children and adolescents. Ataxia, motor dysfunction, and brainstem deficits are the most common presenting signs and symptoms. Sensory disturbances as initial manifestations are far less common, which may be a function of the difficulty a younger child has in describing them. In older children, the presentation is most commonly monosymptomatic without encephalopathy, and sensorimotor symptoms as well as ON are the most common initial presentations. Cognitive impairment, fatigue, mood alterations, spasticity, bladder dysfunction, and tremor are features that may persist distinct from relapses.

There are several rare tumefactive MS variants that can occur in the pediatric population including Marburg variant, Balo concentric sclerosis, and Schilder myelinoclastic diffuse sclerosis. Only the latter entity is more common in children. It typically presents with subacute onset of headache, encephalopathy, and motor or cerebellar dysfunction in the latter half of the first decade. MRI shows extensive bilateral lesions that may have a tumefactive appearance. The symptoms and brain lesions are characteristically exquisitely sensitive to corticosteroids, but disease activity can recur and progress over time.

Disease course

The interval between the initial demyelinating event and subsequent relapse is variable, with a range from 1 month (the minimum time interval delineated by diagnostic criteria) to over 30 years. There is some evidence that younger onset disease is associated with a longer interval to second attack. However, there is conflicting evidence to suggest that the interval between attacks in pediatric-onset disease is shorter than in adults. Overall, the mean annualized relapse rate in the first 2 years is 2–3, and about half to two-thirds of patients diagnosed with pediatric MS will relapse within 1 year. Once the diagnosis is established, longitudinal studies have cited annualized relapse rates of 0.3–0.9.

Earlier onset in childhood is more likely than adolescent onset to be associated with polysymptomatic presentations accompanied by encephalopathy; however, most young patients have full recovery or only mild sequelae. There is intense interest in establishing predictors of disease course severity. This information is not only important for clinical decision-making but also critical for families struggling with the psychosocial consequences of such a diagnosis. Factors associated with relapses or with a risk of early disability include female sex, shorter interval between the first and second attack (less than 1 year), absence of encephalopathy at onset, characteristic MRI (see *MRI* discussion in the later text), less than full recovery after the first attack, and progressive disease at onset.

Regarding time to secondary progression, a good general estimate is provided by using *10-year epochs*. Patients with pediatric MS tend to reach secondary progression 10 years longer into their illness than those with adult MS but at an age 10 years younger. Pediatric-onset MS patients tend to enter into secondary disease progression (defined by progressive disability in the absence of clear relapses) 15–30 years after onset of disease, and this occurs at 30–40 years of age. In a large cohort study, the median time to reach Disability Status Scale (DSS) scores of 4, 6, and 7 occurred after 20, 28.9, and 37 years and at biological ages of 34.6, 42.2, and 50.5 years, respectively. This study also found that although the interval to secondary progression was longer in pediatric MS, once this phase was reached, the rate of disability accumulation was similar to that in adult patients.

Diagnostic considerations

MRI

There are no universally accepted MRI criteria for pediatric MS, and many studies are based on adult criteria. However, it is clear that pediatric patients, especially those under age 10, can have different MRI characteristics. In fact, the 2001 McDonald criteria for lesion dissemination using baseline scans alone were found to be only 50% sensitive in a cohort of pediatric MS patients and were even less sensitive in the youngest patients. Children have a higher percentage of enhancing lesions on initial MRI (70% vs. 20% in adult MS) and a greater proportion of infratentorial lesions (70% vs. 30% in adult MS). There is also an increased incidence of larger, tumefactive lesions in younger patients. Table 8.1 summarizes the MRI criteria that have been proposed to aid in differentiating ADEM from pediatric MS. Pediatric MS patients are more likely to have T1-weighted hypointense lesions (*black holes*) and T2 hyperintense lesions with periventricular predominance. Initial MRI in pediatric MS tends to have smaller lesion loads and more distinct lesion borders (Figure 8.1 and Figure 8.2). Lesions secondary to ADEM are more likely to either completely or partially resolve over time, whereas children with MS accrue new, clinically silent lesions.

Table 8.1 MRI Features on Baseline Scan That Predict Subsequent MS Diagnosis in Children

KIDMUS criteria	White matter lesions located perpendicular to the long axis of the corpus callosum	100% specificity
	Sole presence of well-defined lesions	11% sensitivity
Callen diagnostic criteria	At least two out of three of the following: 1. ≥5 lesions on T2-weighted images	52% specificity
	2. ≥2 periventricular lesions 3. ≥1 brainstem lesion(s)	82% sensitivity
Callen MS versus ADEM criteria	At least two out of three of the following: 1. Absence of diffuse, bilateral lesion pattern	95% specificity
	2. Presence of black holes 3. ≥2 periventricular lesions	75% sensitivity
Verhey *et al.* criteria	1. ≥1 T1 hypointense lesion(s) (black hole)	93% specificity
	2. ≥1 periventricular lesion(s)	84% sensitivity

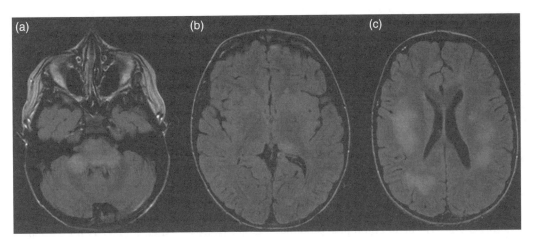

Figure 8.1 MRI in ADEM. (a) Axial FLAIR image showing bilateral cerebellar and brainstem lesions with patchy, indistinct borders. (b) Axial FLAIR image showing left thalamic and occipital lesions. (c) Axial FLAIR image showing large hyperintense lesions that are patchy and without periventricular predominance.

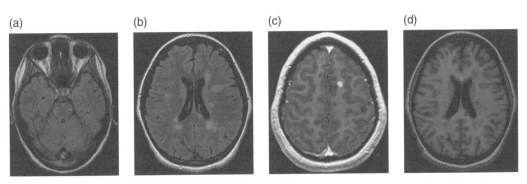

Figure 8.2 MRI in pediatric MS. (a) Axial FLAIR image with distinct, small brainstem hyperintense lesions. (b) Axial FLAIR image with numerous hyperintense lesions that have a periventricular predominance and distinct borders. (c) Axial T1 contrast-enhanced image showing a small left juxtacortical contrast-enhancing lesion. (d) Axial T1 imaging with several periventricular T1 hypointense lesions (*black holes*) that correlate with image (b).

Spinal fluid

The cerebrospinal fluid (CSF) characteristics of pediatric-onset disease are much like those in adults. There is frequently a mild lymphocytic pleocytosis with normal or slightly elevated protein. Children may be less likely than adults to have oligoclonal bands (OCBs), although the available data is limited by variable techniques for OCB measurement. One study using rigorous methods demonstrated that 92% of pediatric MS patients have CSF OCBs, a finding very similar to the prevalence of OCBs in adult-onset MS. Children with ADEM or NMO are typically negative for OCBs, although this is not absolute.

Evoked potentials

Similar to adult-onset disease, visual evoked potentials are more helpful than somatosensory and brainstem auditory potentials in aiding diagnosis. Around 50% of patients will have abnormal visual evoked potentials at the time of first attack, and nearly two-thirds of those patients will have no clinical evidence of ON.

Differential diagnosis

Other inflammatory, infectious, toxic, and neoplastic conditions should be considered when evaluating a child with acute neurological deficits. Inflammatory conditions (including systemic lupus erythematosus, Behçet syndrome, Sjögren syndrome, and sarcoidosis), although rare in the pediatric age group, can mimic features of MS. Headache, encephalopathy, cranial neuropathy, spinal inflammation, ON, and seizures can occur. Systemic involvement such as uveitis, oral and/or genital ulceration, dry eyes and mouth, arthralgia or arthritis, and rash should prompt appropriate investigations. Infections such as tuberculosis, human immunodeficiency virus (HIV), human T-lymphotropic virus (HTLV), and neuroborreliosis can mimic demyelination. CNS lymphoma can mimic the radiological appearance of MS but is rare in childhood. Vascular entities such as migraine, moyamoya syndrome, and primary CNS angiitis should be considered. While neurological deficits referable to vascular territories distinguish vasculopathy from MS, children with isolated small-vessel vasculitis typically have both clinical features and MRI findings that can be very difficult to distinguish from demyelination. Brain biopsy is required for diagnosis. Metabolic disorders, including leukodystrophies; mitochondrial diseases; amino and organic acid disorders; and peroxisomal disorders should be evaluated in children with symmetric MRI lesions, multisystem abnormalities, developmental disability, and progressive symptoms. Primary progressive MS is extremely rare in children. Table 8.2 highlights several conditions more common in pediatric patients.

☆ TIPS AND TRICKS

Consider alternate diagnoses in patients with a prominent history of constitutional symptoms, progressive course, multisystem abnormalities (i.e., skin, joint, kidney, and/or liver involvement), prominent lymphadenopathy, mucosal ulcers, uveitis, hearing loss, short stature, progressive visual loss or dementia, neuroimaging features of calcifications, or symmetric lesions.

Treatment of acute demyelinating attacks

The first line of therapy for acute attacks is corticosteroids, provided that the neurological deficits are of sufficient severity as to warrant treatment. Children typically receive a 3–5-day course of intravenous methylprednisolone at a dose of 20–30 mg/kg/day up to a maximum dose of 1000 mg/day. It is currently unknown whether high-dose oral corticosteroid is as effective as intravenous corticosteroid. There is also no consensus on the utility of an oral prednisone taper. However, when a taper is prescribed, a typical regimen would be 1–2 mg/kg/day of oral prednisone given in a single daily dose and tapered every 2–3 days over about 2 weeks. The side effect profile in pediatric patients is similar to that in adults.

Level 1A evidence exists for the use of plasmapheresis for adult MS patients who do not improve after a course of intravenous methylprednisolone. Pediatric MS data is limited, but at least one report showed complete or partial recovery in two-thirds of patients with plasmapheresis after failing intravenous corticosteroid therapy. Many pediatric MS experts follow the PLEX protocol published for adults. Intravenous immunoglobulin (IVIG) is considered possibly helpful in patients who do not respond to corticosteroids. When used, it is common practice to give 2 g/kg divided over 2–5 days.

Disease-modifying therapy

There are no formal trials of disease-modifying therapies (DMTs) in pediatric MS, although there is an accumulating body of data regarding safety and tolerability of DMT administration in pediatric MS populations. Care of pediatric MS patients is enhanced by a multidisciplinary team, with particular attention to assisting children and their families deal with the inherent anxiety and stress of a serious disease. Anxiety regarding injectable therapies also requires management. Adolescents should be encouraged to take responsibility for their treatment and potentially administer their own injections.

Table 8.2 Description of Pediatric-Specific Diagnoses That Can Mimic Pediatric MS

Category	Disease	Clinical Features	Diagnostic Clues
Systemic inflammatory disorders	Langerhans cell histiocytosis	Onset in childhood of macrophage attack on multiple organs (skin, bone, muscle, liver, lung, spleen, bone marrow). Progressive course with headache and malaise	Hypothalamic–pituitary dysfunction or cerebellar dysfunction. MRI shows bilateral, symmetric lesions in the dentate nucleus or basal ganglia
Leukodystrophies	Adrenoleukodystrophy (childhood cerebral form)	X-linked disorder with onset 5–8 years. Leads to progressive behavioral disturbance, motoric dysfunction, ataxia, intellectual deterioration, optic atrophy, and adrenal insufficiency	MRI shows bilateral, symmetric periventricular T2 hyperintensity with posterior predominance. Elevated plasma very long-chain fatty acids (VLCFA)
	Metachromatic leukodystrophy	Onset in first decade of progressive motoric dysfunction, ataxia, intellectual deterioration or behavioral changes, optic atrophy, and peripheral neuropathy	MRI shows bilateral, symmetric periventricular T2 hyperintensity with sparing of subcortical white matter. Abnormal nerve conduction studies. Elevated urine sulfatides
Inherited metabolic disorders	Mitochondrial disorders	Multiple systems affected, progressive (but fluctuating) course. Stroke-like episodes, seizures, headaches, progressive ophthalmoplegia, pigmentary retinal degeneration	MRI lesions nonspecific and occur in white matter and/or basal ganglia. Elevated serum and CSF lactate. Abnormal muscle biopsy

Sexually active adolescents should receive contraceptive counseling. Figure 8.3 illustrates an algorithm for initiation of treatment, monitoring, and escalation of therapy.

Interferon-beta

Treatments with interferon-beta-1a weekly intramuscular injection (Avonex) and the subcutaneous interferon-beta preparations (Rebif and Betaseron) are commonly prescribed as first-line therapy for pediatric MS patients. Full adult doses are used, although many clinicians will commence therapy at one-quarter or one-half of the final dose in order to enhance tolerability and to avoid elevation in liver transaminases. Monitoring of liver transaminases and blood counts should occur monthly or at least every 3 months for the first year. The risk of elevated liver transaminases may be higher in those under age 10, and thus, younger patients

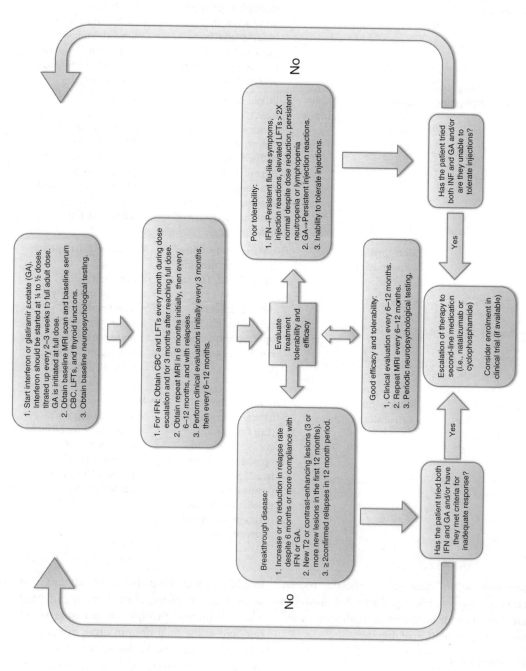

Figure 8.3 Treatment algorithm.

may need to be monitored more closely. Thyroid function tests should be checked at baseline and annually.

The most common clinical side effects of interferon therapy include flu-like symptoms (25–85%) and injection site reactions (5–10%). Pretreatment with acetaminophen (15 mg/kg/dose) or ibuprofen (10 mg/kg/dose) can be helpful to attenuate the flu-like symptoms. Overall, about 20–50% of pediatric MS patients discontinue interferon after a few years of treatment. While retrospective analyses of treated cohorts report reduction of relapse rate on therapy, such data can only be viewed as preliminary evidence of efficacy. There are no studies looking at neutralizing antibody production in pediatric patients, but as in adults, neutralizing antibodies could be checked with breakthrough disease.

Glatiramer acetate

Several studies have evaluated the safety and tolerability of glatiramer acetate given as once daily subcutaneous injection (Copaxone). Treatment is commenced at the full dose of 20 mg daily. The most common side effects were injection site reactions, occurring in 15–60% of patients, and transient systemic reactions (i.e., chest discomfort, palpitations, and flushing), occurring in 7–15%.

Escalation of care for severe MS

There is no consensus among experts as to what defines an inadequate treatment response, nor clear metrics to identify children at risk for aggressive disease. In one report, 16–44% of pediatric patients were defined as having an inadequate treatment response and ultimately switched therapy. In 2011, the IPMSSG published a document that reviewed the current state of therapies for pediatric MS and listed proposed criteria for inadequate treatment response. They stipulated that before determining inadequate response to any particular agent, the treatment should be prescribed for at least 6 months. Furthermore, the practitioner should be reasonably satisfied that the patient

was compliant with the medication (which can be particularly challenging in the adolescent population). In that setting, an inadequate response to treatment would be defined by at least one of the following: (1) increase or no reduction in relapse rate or new T2 or contrast-enhancing lesions on MRI from pretreatment period and (2) ≥2 confirmed relapses within a 12-month period or less. Children with poor recovery from relapses may need to be treated more aggressively than those who fully improve, and certain lesion localizations cause more functionally disabling deficits.

Natalizumab

Experience is limited with natalizumab in pediatric patients; however, there are several published reports that comment on the safety and tolerability. No patients in these reports developed any severe adverse events in up to 24 months of follow-up, and no pediatric MS patients have been reported with progressive multifocal leukoencephalopathy (PML). One study followed 19 patients with an age range of 6–16 years who had a pretreatment mean of five attacks over 28 months. They were treated with the full adult dose at initiation of therapy, and all patients remained relapse-free during follow-up. Reported side effects were minor and included headache, vertigo, pharyngitis, nausea, diarrhea, and fatigue. There is evidence that concurrent JC virus infection is less common in the pediatric age group, and growing evidence indicates that individuals seronegative for JC virus are at lower risk for PML. However, pediatric patients may be at increased risk for primary JC virus infection during treatment, and the effect of this is not known.

Other agents

Cyclophosphamide has been shown to reduce disease activity in patients refractory to first-line medications. One report cited a beneficial effect in 17 children with 80% showing stabilization or improvement in EDSS status. The treatment was overall well tolerated, although nausea was common, and adverse reactions included bladder transitional cell carcinoma, leukopenia, anemia, transient alopecia, osteoporosis, and amenorrhea. Furthermore, the suppression of disease did not seem to last beyond the time when the treatment was withdrawn. Oral contraceptives or leuprolide may help prevent gonadal failure in females, and males should consider sperm banking. Additionally, patients on cyclophosphamide need to be provided mesna therapy to reduce risk of hemorrhagic cystitis.

Rituximab has shown some promise in attenuating MS in adult studies, but the evidence in pediatric patients is lacking. Mitoxantrone is indicated for progressive disease in adults but carries a significant risk for cardiotoxicity and leukemia and is not endorsed for pediatric MS. There are several new therapies emerging for treatment of MS that are currently in phase II or III trials or have just recently been approved for use in adults. Future application of these therapies in the pediatric MS population would ideally be guided by clinical trials in pediatric MS and should at a minimum be supported by careful registry-based documentation of short- and long-term safety data.

Symptomatic therapy

Treatment of persistent symptoms is essential in maximizing quality of life. The most common symptoms in children include fatigue, spasticity, tremor, paroxysmal symptoms, bladder and bowel dysfunction, and cognitive impairment. The medications used to treat these symptoms are identical to those used in adults. Nonpharmacologic interventions should always be considered in any treatment regimen (e.g., physical and occupational therapy). Table 8.3 summarizes pediatric dosing regimens for commonly used medications.

Cognitive dysfunction and quality of life considerations

The burden of cognitive dysfunction is particularly significant in pediatric patients and differs from adult-onset MS likely owing to the impact of MS on the developing central nervous system. Other factors such as disruption of academics and the underlying neurodegenerative processes may contribute as well. In adult MS patients, the domains of cognition that are most significantly affected include visual–spatial function, memory, processing speed, and executive function (i.e., planning and sequencing and complex attention). In pediatric MS, these domains are also frequently impaired, but in addition, language (verbal fluency, naming, and comprehension) and intelligence can be affected. In one study, 25% of patients exhibited an intelligence quotient (IQ) between 70 and 89 versus 3.5% of control patients. Significant cognitive impairment (i.e., impairment on at least 2–3 cognitive tasks) occurs in one-third of pediatric MS patients. Over half show mild cognitive impairment. Two-thirds of patients show deteriorating cognitive performance over time as compared to initial performance on neuropsychological testing. The clearest risk factors for declining performance are increased age and duration of disease. The influence of EDSS score, number of relapses, and age at onset is unclear. Given the aforementioned findings, it is currently recommended that all patients with pediatric MS undergo a baseline neuropsychological evaluation, and cognitive status should be followed carefully. Some children will need school-based interventions and/or modification of curricula. It is important that educators be aware of the diagnosis and have a basic understanding of the physical, cognitive, and psychosocial consequences. The National MS Society published an excellent primer on pediatric MS for educators, and it is available on their website.

Similar to any chronic disease affecting children, pediatric MS has a significant impact on psychosocial functioning and quality of life. Physical symptoms can impact social functioning (e.g., fatigue and school absences limiting socialization and gait impairment limiting mobility) and cause embarrassment (e.g., bladder dysfunction). The disease can interfere with an adolescent's gaining of independence,

Table 8.3 Pediatric Dosing Regimens for Commonly Used Symptomatic Medications in Patients Weighing Less Than 40 kg

Medication	Indication	Formulation	Dosing Regimen
Amantadine	Fatigue	Capsule: 100 mg Liquid: 50 mg/5 ml	5 mg/kg/day given daily to BID. Max dose 150 mg/day
Amitriptyline	Headache, neuropathic pain	Tablet: 10, 25, 50, 75, 100, 150 mg	Start 10 mg QHS and titrate up by 10 mg q week as needed. Max dose 150–200 mg/day
Baclofen	Spasticity	Tablets: 10, 20 mg	Start 5 mg QHS and titrate up to 2–3 times daily. Typical maintenance dose 20–40 mg/day, max dose 60–80 mg/day
Carbamazepine	Paroxysmal symptoms, neuropathic pain	Tablet: 100, 200 mg Extended release tablet: 100, 200, 300, 400 mg Liquid: 100 mg/5 ml	Start 10 mg/kg/day divided BID. Typical maintenance dose 15–25 mg/kg/day divided BID–TID
Clonazepam	Spasticity, tremor	Tablets: 0.5, 1, 2 mg Oral dissolving tablets: 0.125, 0.25, 0.5, 1, 2 mg	Start 0.125 mg QHS and then titrate up to BID. Increase as needed by 0.125–0.25 mg/day
Diazepam	Spasticity, tremor	Tablets: 2, 5, 10 mg Liquid: 5 mg/ml	Start 0.5–1 mg given 2–4 times daily. Typical maintenance dose 0.1–0.8 mg/kg/day, max dose 30 mg/day
Docusate sodium	Constipation	Capsules: 50, 100, 250 mg Liquid: 50 mg/5 ml	5 mg/kg/day in 1–4 divided doses
Fluoxetine	Depression, anxiety	Tablet: 10, 20, 40 mg Liquid 4 mg/ml	Start 5–10 mg daily and titrate up as needed to average maintenance dose of 10–40 mg daily
Gabapentin	Neuropathic pain, paroxysmal symptoms	Tablet: 100, 300, 400, 600, 800 mg Liquid: 50 mg/ml	Start 10–15 mg/kg/day divided BID. Typical maintenance dose 25–35 mg/kg/day divided TID

(Continued)

Table 8.3 (*Continued*)

Medication	Indication	Formulation	Dosing Regimen
Oxybutynin	Neurogenic bladder	Tablet: 5 mg Extended release tablet: 5, 10, 15 mg Liquid: 5 mg/5 ml	Start 5 mg daily and titrate up as needed to a max dose of 5 mg TID
Polyethylene glycol	Constipation	Powder: 17 g per capful, mix in 4–8 oz of liquid	Start ¼ to ½ capful per day and titrate up as needed to 1 capful per day
Propranolol	Tremor, headache	Tablet: 10, 20, 40, 60, 80 mg Extended release: 60, 80, 120, 160 mg Liquid: 4–8 mg/ml	Start 1 mg/kg/day divided BID to TID. Typical maintenance dose 2–6 mg/kg/day divided BID to TID
Tizanidine	Spasticity	Capsule or tablet: 2, 4, 6 mg	Start 1–2 mg QHS (0.05 mg/kg) and then increase to twice daily. Typical maintenance dose 0.3 mg/kg/day divided BID
Tolterodine	Neurogenic bladder	Tablet: 1, 2 mg Long acting: 2, 4 mg	Start 0.1 mg/kg/day divided BID for age <5 years, 2 mg/day divided BID for age >5 years. Max dose 4 mg/day
Topiramate	Headache, neuropathic pain	Sprinkle: 15, 25 mg Tablet: 25, 50, 100, 200 mg	Start 1–2 mg/kg/day divided BID. Typical maintenance dose 5–10 mg/kg/day divided BID

which is an important developmental achievement. It can negatively impact a teenager's body image and interfere with the formation of mature peer relationships. Depression and anxiety are more common among the pediatric MS population and can significantly impact quality of life.

Patients with pediatric MS may show decreased health-related quality of life compared to siblings, and psychosocial functioning is most significantly affected. Practitioners need to be cognizant of these issues and screen patients frequently for mood or psychosocial difficulties. Signs of distress include somatic medical complaints, increased school absences, poor compliance with treatment, or risk-taking behaviors. The treating physician should coordinate the patient's care utilizing a multidisciplinary team including the patient's primary pediatrician; a neuropsychologist; physical, occupational, and speech therapists; and a psychological counselor. They should provide the patient and family with adequate information and support, help educate school staff, and help facilitate community support.

Conclusions and future directions

MS presents under the age of 18 years in 3–5% of cases. The majority of these patients are over age 10. There has been an increased awareness of pediatric MS over the last two decades, and this has prompted a surge in research. Children represent a unique population to study the pathobiology of MS and will help give incite to the complex interactions between genetic and environmental etiologic factors. An area of intense interest is the development of specific biomarkers to help distinguish pediatric MS from monophasic demyelinating disease, as well as predict course severity in relapsing disease. A challenge in the upcoming years will be to rigorously study the safety and efficacy of new treatments in pediatric patients. This would ideally be done through robust, multi-center clinical trials, and as the pediatric MS population is small, the treatment studies will have to be prioritized. Essential to the design of these trials will be the creation of a standardized outcome measure specific for pediatric patients that would ideally incorporate physical and cognitive disability along with psychosocial considerations.

Further Reading

Amato, M.P., Goretti, B., Ghezzi, A. *et al.* (2008) Cognitive and psychosocial features of childhood and juvenile MS. *Neurology*, **70**, 1891–1897.

Banwell, B., Ghezzi, A., Bar-Or, A., Mikaeloff, Y. & Tardieu, M. (2007) Multiple sclerosis in children: clinical diagnosis, therapeutic strategies, and future directions. *Lancet Neurology*, **6**, 887–902.

Banwell, B., Krupp, L., Kennedy, J. *et al.* (2007) Clinical features and viral serologies in children with multiple sclerosis: a multinational observational study. *Lancet Neurology*, **6**, 773–781.

Banwell, B., Shroff, M., Ness, J.M. *et al.* (2007) MRI features of pediatric multiple sclerosis. *Neurology*, **68** (Suppl 2), S46–S53.

Banwell, B., Kennedy, J., Sadovnick, D. *et al.* (2009) Incidence of acquired demyelination of the CNS in Canadian children. *Neurology*, **72**, 232–239.

Banwell, B., Bar-Or, A., Arnold, D. *et al.* (2011) Clinical, environmental, and genetic determinants of multiple sclerosis in children with acute demyelination: a prospective national cohort study. *Lancet Neurology*, **10**, 436–445.

Banwell, B., Bar-Or, A., Giovannoni, G., Dale, R.C. & Tardieu, M. (2011) Therapies for multiple sclerosis: considerations in the pediatric patient. *Nature Reviews Neurology*, **7**, 109–122.

Boiko, A., Vorobeychik, G., Paty, D., Devonshire, V., Sadovnick, D. & University of British Columbia MS Clinic Neurologists (2002) Early onset multiple sclerosis: a longitudinal study. *Neurology*, **59**, 1006–1010.

Chitnis, T., Tenembaum, S., Banwell, B. *et al.* (2012) Consensus statement: evaluation of new and existing therapeutics for pediatric multiple sclerosis. *Multiple Sclerosis*, **18**, 116–117.

Hahn, J.S., Pohl, D., Rensel, M., Rao, S. & International Pediatric MS Study Group (2007) Differential diagnosis and evaluation in pediatric multiple sclerosis. *Neurology*, **68** (Suppl 2), S13–S22.

Krupp, L.B., Banwell, B., Tenembaum, S. & International Pediatric MS Study Group (2007) Consensus definitions proposed for pediatric multiple sclerosis and related disorders. *Neurology*, **68** (Suppl 2), S7–S12.

MacAllister, W.S., Belman, A.L., Milazzo, M. *et al.* (2005) Cognitive functioning in children and adolescents with multiple sclerosis. *Neurology*, **64**, 1422–1425.

Ness, J.M., Chabas, D., Sadovnick, A.D. *et al.* (2007) Clinical features of children and adolescents with multiple sclerosis. *Neurology*, **68** (Suppl 2), S37–S45.

Renoux, C., Vukusic, S., Mikaeloff, Y. *et al.* (2007) Natural history of multiple sclerosis with childhood onset. *New England Journal of Medicine*, **356**, 2603–2613.

Verhey, L.H., Branson, H.M., Shroff, M.M. *et al.* (2011) MRI parameters for prediction of multiple sclerosis diagnosis in children with acute CNS demyelination: a prospective national cohort study. *Lancet Neurology*, **10**, 1065–1073.

9

Complementary and Alternative Medicine: Risks and Benefits

Allen C. Bowling

Colorado Neurological Institute, Englewood, CO, USA

Introduction

Clinicians who care for those with multiple sclerosis (MS) may find themselves in awkward situations related to *alternative medicine*. Many MS patients may ask questions about alternative therapies or provide lists of supplements that they are taking, yet clinicians with conventional medical training may feel that they lack the knowledge or experience to address these issues. However, there is a significant amount of evidence-based information about the safety and efficacy of these *alternative* therapies, and clinicians with conventional training may actually be in a position to improve the quality of MS care by providing objective information and guidance about these therapies.

Terminology

A variety of terms and definitions are used in the area of *alternative medicine*. In fact, the term *alternative medicine* is often used incorrectly. A more general, and often more appropriate, term is *unconventional medicine*, which refers to forms of medicine that are not widely taught in medical schools or generally available in hospitals. *Complementary* and *alternative* refer to the ways in which these unconventional therapies are practiced. *Complementary* indicates that these therapies

are used *in conjunction with* conventional medicine, while *alternative* indicates that they are used *instead of* conventional medicine. *Complementary and alternative medicine*, often indicated by the acronym *CAM*, refers to both approaches. The combined use of conventional and unconventional medicine is known as *integrative medicine*.

The National Institutes of Health (NIH) has developed a classification scheme for CAM therapies. In this scheme, there are several major categories of CAM therapies (Table 9.1). One specific therapy may fit into more than a single category. For example, acupuncture could be categorized as an *alternative medical system* and also an *energy therapy*.

Unconventional medicine use

Over the past two decades, there have been remarkable breakthroughs in the field of MS. Significant advances have been made in the diagnosis, treatment, and pathologic understanding of the disease. There are now many effective disease-modifying as well as symptomatic therapies. Despite these developments, however, conventional MS therapies have limitations. Both symptomatic and disease-modifying treatments may cause side effects or may be partially effective or ineffective in some patients. Furthermore, there may be

Multiple Sclerosis and CNS Inflammatory Disorders, First Edition. Edited by Lawrence M. Samkoff and Andrew D. Goodman.
© 2014 John Wiley & Sons, Ltd. Published 2014 by John Wiley & Sons, Ltd.

Table 9.1 NIH Classification of CAM Therapies with Representative Examples

Natural products
Herbs, vitamin, and mineral supplements

Mind and body medicine
Guided imagery, meditation

Manipulative and body-based practices
Massage, reflexology

Movement therapies
Pilates, Alexander technique

Traditional healing
Native American medicine

Energy medicine
Healing touch, magnet therapy

Alternative medical systems
TCM, Ayurveda

limited treatment options for some forms of MS, such as progressive disease, and for some MS symptoms, such as weakness, tremor, and incoordination.

The limitations of conventional MS therapy, as well as other factors, may lead many MS patients to become interested in, and use, CAM. Multiple studies indicate that one-half to three-fourths of those with MS in the USA and other Western countries use some form of CAM. Among MS patients, the vast majority who use unconventional medicine do so in a *complementary* manner. In other words, they use unconventional medicine in combination with conventional medicine and thus are using an *integrative medicine* approach.

Table 9.2 Risk–Benefit Profiles of MS-Relevant CAM Therapies

CAM Therapy	Risk–Benefit Profile
Acupuncture, Chinese herbal medicine, and traditional Chinese medicine	Low risk and possible symptomatic effects for acupuncture, theoretical risks and no known efficacy for Chinese herbal medicine
Antioxidants	Theoretical risks, no known efficacy
BVT	Rare risks, no known efficacy
Cooling therapy	Low risk, multiple possible symptomatic effects
Cranberry	Low risk, possible preventive effect on UTIs
Diets: the Swank diet and related diets	Low risk, possible disease-modifying effect
Echinacea and other *immune-stimulating* supplements	Theoretical risks, no known efficacy
Ginkgo biloba	Low risk, possible symptomatic effects on fatigue and cognition
Guided imagery	Low risk, multiple possible symptomatic effects
LDN	Low risk, multiple possible symptomatic effects
Marijuana (cannabis)	Moderate risk, possible disease-modifying and symptomatic effects
Massage	Low risk, multiple possible symptomatic effects
Reflexology	Low risk, multiple possible symptomatic effects
Tai chi	Low risk, multiple possible symptomatic effects
Vitamin B12	Low risk, therapeutic effects in those who are vitamin B12 deficient
Vitamin D	Low risk, definite effect on bone health and possible disease-modifying and symptomatic effects in MS
Yoga	Low risk, possible symptomatic effect on fatigue

> ### ✋ CAUTION!
>
> In clinical practice, there may be little or no discussion or consideration of CAM use. However, the majority of MS patients, sometimes unknown to their treating clinician, use some form of CAM.

The remainder of this chapter is a user-friendly guide to MS-relevant CAM therapies for clinicians. Therapies are listed in alphabetical order, and the emphasis is on concise presentation of safety and efficacy information that can be quickly conveyed to MS patients who are using, or considering, these therapies. A brief summary in bolded italics is included at the end of each section. Table 9.2 provides a listing and risk–benefit summary for the specific CAM therapies that are covered in this section.

CAM therapies

Acupuncture, Chinese herbal medicine, and traditional Chinese medicine

Traditional Chinese medicine (TCM) is an ancient, multimodal healing method. One component of this broad-based therapeutic approach is acupuncture. There are multiple other components, including herbs, nutrition, tai chi, exercise, stress reduction, and massage.

There are remarkably few studies of TCM in MS. Clinical trials of acupuncture for alleviating MS symptoms are too limited to be conclusive. In other conditions, acupuncture appears to relieve pain as well as nausea and vomiting. Although Chinese herbal medicine is sometimes touted as being effective for MS, there are actually no rigorous studies of this therapy in MS.

Acupuncture is usually well tolerated when done by a well-trained acupuncturist. In contrast, it is not known if Chinese herbal medicine interacts with conventional MS medication or if it is safe to use in those with specific medical conditions, including MS. Of concern, activation of immune cells, especially T cells and macrophages, may be caused by several commonly used Chinese herbs, including Asian ginseng, astragalus, and maitake and reishi mushrooms. This raises the theoretical risk that these herbs could worsen the disease course of MS or antagonize the therapeutic effects of immune-modulating and immune-suppressing medications.

In summary, acupuncture is generally safe and, though not well studied in MS, may alleviate pain. In contrast, Chinese herbal medicine, another component of TCM, has theoretical risks and is of unknown efficacy in MS.

> ### ✋ CAUTION!
>
> When considering MS and TCM, it is important to be aware of exactly what TCM therapies a patient is receiving. Acupuncture is low risk and may be reasonable for some patients to use, while Chinese herbal medicine poses theoretical risks, has no known efficacy in MS, and should probably be avoided. It is important to be aware that after an acupuncture session, patients may be given Chinese herbal therapy to take home with them.

Antioxidants

Free radicals cause cellular injury through oxidative damage. This oxidative damage may be decreased by antioxidant compounds. In MS, oxidative damage may play an important role in myelin and axonal injury, and thus, it is sometimes claimed that antioxidants should be used to treat MS.

In the animal model of MS (experimental allergic encephalomyelitis (*EAE*)), multiple antioxidant compounds have produced therapeutic effects. Small, short-term MS clinical trials with various antioxidants suggest that these approaches are well tolerated. However, these studies have not generally been powered adequately to assess efficacy.

Many antioxidants activate immune cells, including T cells and macrophages. As a result, antioxidant compounds carry theoretical risks of worsening MS or antagonizing the effects of disease-modifying medications. However, as noted, the limited clinical trials to date indicate that antioxidants are generally well tolerated in MS.

On the basis of theoretical and animal model studies, antioxidants could produce therapeutic effects in MS. However, there is no definitive evidence for their efficacy in MS, and there are theoretical risks associated with their use in MS.

> ★ TIPS AND TRICKS
>
> Expensive antioxidant compounds are sometimes marketed specifically to patients with MS and other neurological diseases. At this time, there is not rigorous information about the safety or effectiveness of any antioxidant compound in MS. This information should be conveyed to patients who are considering these therapies.

Bee venom therapy

Apitherapy is a term used for various unconventional treatments that utilize bees and bee products. One form of apitherapy that is sometimes claimed to be beneficial for MS is bee venom therapy (BVT), which involves the regular use of bee stings that are produced by placing bees on specific body parts with tweezers.

The highest quality study of BVT in MS is a randomized, crossover study of 26 patients with secondary progressive or relapsing–remitting MS. In this clinical trial, BVT did not produce any significant treatment effect with multiple outcome measures, including attack frequency, neurological disability, MRI activity, fatigue, and overall quality of life.

Although BVT is generally safe, there are rare adverse effects. Bee stings may rarely cause anaphylaxis, and thus, EpiPen devices should be available when this therapy is being used. In addition, some information on the use BVT for MS recommends bee stings around the eye as a treatment for optic neuritis. However, periorbital bee stings may actually *cause* optic neuritis and thus should be avoided.

In conclusion, BVT has not been shown to produce any significant therapeutic effects in MS. It is generally well tolerated but may rarely cause serious side effects.

> ★ TIPS AND TRICKS
>
> Many CAM therapies have not undergone formal clinical trial testing in MS and thus there is no information about safety or efficacy in MS. In contrast, BVT has actually undergone clinical trial testing and did not show any therapeutic effect in multiple outcome measures.

Cooling therapy

Cooling is an unconventional treatment that utilizes the known temperature sensitivity that occurs in MS. For more than 100 years, it has been recognized that small increases in body temperature (0.5°C) may provoke MS symptoms and, likewise, that small decreases in body temperature may relieve symptoms. On the basis of this observation, various cooling methods have been developed. These methods range from simple, commonsense strategies, such as drinking cold beverages and staying in air-conditioned areas, to more complex approaches, such as wearing specially designed cooling garments.

Several studies of variable size and quality have reported that cooling garments alleviate multiple MS symptoms. To rigorously follow up on these findings, a randomized, controlled, blinded trial of cooling in MS was conducted. This study found that cooling was associated with objective improvement in walking and visual function. Subjectively, there was improvement in strength, fatigue, and cognition. The therapeutic effects of cooling may be greater in those who are known to experience heat sensitivity.

Cooling strategies are generally well tolerated. Cooling may provoke worsening in a small subset of MS patients who are cold sensitive. Cooling garments may be awkward and cumbersome. At the onset of cooling, some people may experience mild discomfort.

Cooling is low risk and may relieve multiple MS symptoms.

Although cooling therapy is generally safe and may provide symptomatic relief, it may be underutilized in MS, especially during the summer months. Providing information about this therapy to MS patients during the springtime may give them time to proactively develop a cooling plan to use during the summer.

Cranberry

MS patients may experience recurrent urinary tract infections (UTIs) due to MS-associated bladder dysfunction. The fruit of the cranberry plant may prevent UTIs, presumably through a mechanism of action that is different from any conventional medication. Specifically, chemical constituents of the herb inhibit the adhesion of bacteria to the uroepithelium.

Herbal therapies that may be the most useful in clinical practice are those that contain active constituents with a mechanism of action that is different from that of any conventional medication. This appears to be the case with cranberry. Fructose and another molecule (proanthocyanidin) in cranberry exert inhibitory effects on bacterial adhesion that are not mimicked by any conventional medication. Interestingly, fingolimod (Gilenya), the MS disease-modifying medication, was developed through scientific studies that were designed to determine whether mushrooms used in traditional Chinese medicine contained any compounds with unique immunological mechanisms of action.

Multiple clinical studies indicate that cranberry may *prevent* UTIs. However, there is not evidence that cranberry effectively *treats* UTIs. Since UTIs may cause neurological decline (*pseudoexacerbations*) in those with MS, clinicians should monitor closely for UTIs in MS patients. Those who have definite UTIs should be treated promptly with antibiotics, *not* cranberry.

Reasonable doses of cranberry are usually well tolerated. There are case reports indicating that cranberry may increase the anticoagulant effect of warfarin. Chronic cranberry use may increase the risk of developing kidney stones.

Cranberry is a low-risk herbal therapy. It may prevent UTIs, but it should not be used to treat UTIs.

Diets: The Swank diet and related diets

Diets are among the most popular CAM therapies that are advocated for, and used by, MS patients. Many different diets have been claimed to be effective for MS. The diet that has undergone the most extensive study at this time is one that is low in saturated fats and high in polyunsaturated fatty acids (PUFAs), which include omega-3 and omega-6 fatty acids. A possible disease-modifying effect of this diet has been suggested by epidemiologic, in vitro, animal model, and clinical trial studies.

A dietary strategy that is low in saturated fat and high in PUFAs was originally developed by Swank and Dugan. This approach, known as the *Swank diet*, was claimed to have disease-modifying effects in MS. However, the clinical trial of this diet was not controlled, blinded, or randomized.

After the original Swank study, more rigorous trials were conducted with supplementation of specific PUFAs. Three randomized controlled trials of omega-6 supplements were conducted. Two of these trials reported a significant decrease in attack severity and duration. A reanalysis of the pooled data that was available from all three trials found therapeutic effects on disability progression in those with mild MS at the start of the trial.

The clinical trials of omega-3 supplements in MS have been more limited than those with omega-6 supplements. The most rigorous omega-3 trial was a large, randomized, double-blind, controlled trial of fish oil supplements. This study did not find a statistically significant disease-modifying effect. However, there was a trend that favored the treatment group ($p < 0.07$) for disability progression. A smaller randomized and controlled study of omega-3 fatty acid supplements in combination with conventional disease-modifying medications (glatiramer acetate or interferons) found trends favoring omega-3 supplements for emotional and physical function.

With regard to safety, omega-3 and omega-6 supplements are usually well tolerated in reasonable doses. Fish oil, a rich source of omega-3 fatty acids, has been classified as *generally regarded as safe (GRAS)* by the Food and Drug Administration (FDA). The safety of long-term use of other omega-3 fatty acid supplements and all omega-6 fatty acid supplements is not known. Omega-6 fatty acids may increase triglyceride levels and rarely have been associated with seizures. Mild anticoagulant effects may be produced by some omega-3 and omega-6 fatty acids. PUFA supplements (omega-3 or omega-6) may lead to vitamin E deficiency. As a result, supplementation with modest doses of vitamin E (such as 100 international units (IU) daily) may be indicated.

PUFA-enriched diets are usually well tolerated and have produced suggestive results in MS clinical trials of variable quality. The safety and efficacy of these diets in combination with disease-modifying medications have not been well studied. These diets should not be used instead of conventional disease-modifying medications.

☆ TIPS AND TRICKS

At this time, the two general dietary strategies for which there is the most suggestive evidence for a disease-modifying effect in MS are PUFA-enriched diets and vitamin D. Over the past several years, emerging studies actually provide stronger evidence for vitamin D and weaker evidence for PUFAs (see Vitamin D section). In terms of PUFA-enriched diets, the evidence for MS is certainly not definitive but patients who choose to pursue reasonable dietary strategies in this area may at least obtain cardiac benefits from the diet. Also, the observation that the best current dietary evidence in MS is for vitamin D and PUFAs

should be helpful for clinicians talking with MS patients about diets. Specifically, if patients ask about *any* dietary approach to MS, they can be told that, from an evidence-based approach, the best evidence at this point is for vitamin D and PUFAs.

Echinacea and other *immune-stimulating* supplements

Some lay publications on alternative medicine make the claim that *immune-stimulating* dietary supplements should be used by MS patients because MS is an *immune disease*. For MS, these publications actually recommend supplements that are known to activate T cells and macrophages. This type of information is erroneous and potentially dangerous.

Many different dietary supplements are associated with *immune stimulation*. This categorization is usually based on in vitro or animal model studies and therefore represents a theoretical risk. Popular herbs that activate T cells or macrophages include echinacea, alfalfa, ashwagandha (*Withania somnifera*), Asian ginseng, astragalus, cat's claw, garlic, maitake mushroom, mistletoe, shiitake mushroom, Siberian ginseng, and stinging nettle. Nonherbal *immune-stimulating* supplements include antioxidants (see Antioxidants section), melatonin, and zinc.

There are no documented therapeutic effects for echinacea and other immune-stimulating supplements in MS. In addition, these supplements pose theoretical risks in MS and should be avoided or used in limited amounts.

Ginkgo biloba

Ginkgo biloba is an herbal therapy that is derived from the leaf of the *ginkgo biloba* tree. The chemical compounds in ginkgo exert anti-inflammatory as well as antioxidant effects. Ginkgo could have symptom-relieving and disease-modifying actions in MS.

In the animal model of MS, some studies have shown that ginkgo decreases disease severity.

In a large study of MS patients, ginkgo was *not* effective for treating MS attacks. In small clinical trials, ginkgo has improved MS-associated cognitive dysfunction and fatigue.

Ginkgo is generally safe. However, it may produce anticoagulant effects and it may rarely provoke seizures. It should be avoided or used with caution by those with a history of seizures and those who take anticoagulant medications and antiplatelet agents, are undergoing surgery, or have coagulopathies. Ginkgo use has also been associated with dizziness, headaches, rashes, nausea, vomiting, diarrhea, and flatulence.

Ginkgo is a generally well-tolerated therapy that, in limited clinical trials, improved fatigue and cognitive dysfunction in MS patients. It does not appear to be effective for MS attacks.

Guided imagery

Guided imagery is a form of mind–body medicine in which one creates relaxing mental images. Guided imagery may be used on its own or combined with other relaxation methods, such as meditation or progressive muscle relaxation.

In a small MS study, guided imagery improved anxiety but had no effect on depression or multiple other MS symptoms. In other medical conditions, limited clinical trials have found possible therapeutic effects on anxiety, depression, pain, and insomnia.

Guided imagery is usually well tolerated. Guided imagery may cause anxiety, disturbing thoughts, and fear of losing control, especially in those with psychiatric conditions. Spasticity may sometimes be provoked by relaxation.

Guided imagery is generally well tolerated and may relieve anxiety and possibly other MS-associated symptoms.

✭ TIPS AND TRICKS

Guided imagery is one relaxation strategy that may be helpful for MS patients. Other relaxation methods that may be readily available but underutilized include various forms of meditation and mindfulness-based stress reduction.

Low-dose naltrexone (LDN)

It is sometimes claimed that low oral doses of naltrexone, an opiate antagonist, may be therapeutic in MS and many other diseases. In MS, low-dose naltrexone (LDN) has been claimed to relieve symptoms, prevent attacks, and slow disability progression.

Anecdotal accounts of the benefits of LDN in MS led to several formal clinical trials. One 8-week study of 80 patients with relapsing or progressive MS found that LDN had no effect on physical functioning but did improve pain and mental health. Another similarly designed study *did not* find any therapeutic effects of LDN. A 6-month, open-label study of LDN in 40 people with primary progressive MS found that LDN improved spasticity, *worsened* pain, and had no effect on depression, fatigue, or overall quality of life.

In the limited studies of LDN in MS, this therapy has usually been well tolerated. LDN may cause opiate withdrawal if given to patients who are being treated with opiates. In the study of primary progressive MS, one patient experienced neurological worsening.

LDN is generally well tolerated. Some, but not all, of the limited studies of LDN in MS indicate that it may produce therapeutic effects. Additional research is needed to determine if LDN is safe or effective in MS.

⚙ SCIENCE REVISITED

It has been proposed the LDN could produce a partial opiate agonist effect by increasing endogenous production of endorphins and also by increasing the affinity of the opiate receptor. If that is the case, then it is conceivable that LDN could be a non-exercise way to produce an "endorphin high" and thereby alleviate multiple subjective symptoms in a variety of medical conditions.

Marijuana (cannabis)

Marijuana, also known as cannabis, contains tetrahydrocannabinol (THC) and other related chemicals known as cannabinoids (CBs).

CBs have a variety of actions that could possibly be therapeutic in MS. CBs have immune-modulating and neuroprotective actions and thus could modify the disease course. Also, CBs are known to inhibit excessive neuronal activity and could thereby relieve some MS symptoms, such as spasticity and pain.

In the animal model of MS, CBs exert disease-modifying and symptomatic effects. In a large, well-designed clinical trial of marijuana in MS, CBs produced subjective, but not objective, evidence for symptomatic relief. A 12-month extension of this study found that THC produced a small improvement in spasticity and a possible effect on disability. *Sativex* is an orally administered form of cannabis. In multiple studies of variable quality, *Sativex* alleviated some MS symptoms, including pain, spasticity, and sleeping difficulties. Additional clinical studies of CBs in MS are needed and are currently underway in the UK.

Marijuana may produce many side effects. Its use has been associated with sedation, seizures, nausea, vomiting, impaired driving, incoordination, and poor pregnancy outcomes. Smoked marijuana may impair lung function and increase the risk of cancer of the head, neck, and lung.

Scientific and clinical studies suggest that marijuana may produce disease-modifying and symptomatic effects in MS. However, these efficacy findings are not definitive, marijuana may produce significant side effects, and marijuana use is illegal in many states and countries.

⚠ CAUTION!

In the USA, many states have made "medical marijuana" legal. Marijuana use is still illegal at the federal level. It is important for patients who are considering marijuana to understand that, even though medical marijuana may be legal for use in MS, its safety and efficacy in MS have actually not been established.

Massage

Massage is an ancient form of *bodywork*. Massage therapists manipulate, press, and rub muscles and other soft tissues of the body.

Although massage is widely available and popular, there are remarkably few formal studies of this therapy in MS. In a clinical trial, 24 MS patients were treated over 5 weeks with either *standard medical care* or standard medical care in conjunction with twice weekly massage therapy. Those who received massage showed improvement in multiple areas, including self-esteem, anxiety, depression, social functioning, body image, and *image of disease progression*. A randomized, controlled clinical trial of 30 MS patients found that abdominal massage relieved constipation.

Massage is usually well tolerated. Mild side effects include lethargy, headaches, and myalgias. Rarely, massage causes severe adverse effects, including hepatic bleeding and bone fractures. Massage should be used with caution or avoided by pregnant women and by patients with bone fractures, osteoporosis, skin infections, burns, open wounds, thrombosis, cancer, and heart disease.

Massage is a generally well-tolerated therapy that has produced suggestive therapeutic effects in limited MS studies.

Reflexology

Like massage, reflexology is a type of bodywork. Reflexologists apply manual pressure to specific sites, most of which are on the feet. These sites are claimed to correspond to specific organs or organ systems.

There are two controlled studies of reflexology in MS. Both studies included about 70 patients. In one study, subjects were treated with either reflexology or nonspecific calf massage. The treated group had significant reductions in spasticity, paresthesias, and urinary symptoms. In the other study, MS patients with pain were treated with reflexology or nonspecific foot massage. Both reflexology and sham massage were associated with improvement in pain, the primary outcome measure. There was also improvement in other symptoms, including fatigue and overall quality of life.

Reflexology is generally safe. It may produce mild side effects such as foot pain, fatigue, and changes in bowel and bladder function. Reflexology should be used with caution or avoided by those with significant foot conditions, such as bone or joint disorders, gout, ulcers, and vascular disease.

Reflexology is a low-risk therapy that has produced promising symptom-relieving results in two controlled MS studies. However, in one of these studies, similar beneficial effects occurred with reflexology and sham foot massage, which raises the possibility of a placebo response.

Tai chi

Tai chi has been practiced for centuries in China. Tai chi, like acupuncture, is a component of TCM. There are limited clinical studies of tai chi in MS.

There are two small, nonblinded trials of tai chi in MS. In these studies, tai chi produced suggestive therapeutic effects on walking, spasticity, and social and emotional functioning.

Tai chi is usually well tolerated. Mild side effects of tai chi include strained muscles and joints. There is a risk of falling with tai chi. Tai chi may be modified for those with disabilities. Tai chi should be used cautiously or avoided by those with fractures, significant joint injuries, severe osteoporosis, acute low-back pain, and significant joint injuries.

Tai chi is a low-risk therapy that has produced improvement in multiple MS symptoms in limited clinical trial testing.

Vitamin B12

It is sometimes claimed that MS patients generally may get multiple therapeutic effects by taking vitamin B12 supplements.

There are no clinical studies that demonstrate that vitamin B12 supplements produce significant therapeutic effects in MS patients generally. Importantly, however, there is a small subgroup of MS patients who are deficient in vitamin B12. For these patients, vitamin B12 supplementation is necessary.

Vitamin B12 supplements are generally well tolerated. Rare side effects include diarrhea, itching, and rashes.

Vitamin B12 supplements are generally safe. If vitamin B12 levels are normal, there is no evidence that vitamin B12 supplements provide therapeutic effects. If vitamin B12 levels are low, then vitamin B12 supplements (intramuscular or oral) are recommended.

Vitamin D

Vitamin D is relevant to MS for multiple reasons. Since MS patients are at risk for developing osteopenia and osteoporosis, vitamin D may play an important role in maintaining bone density in those with MS. Also, through its immune-regulating effects, vitamin D could produce disease-modifying effects in MS. Finally, vitamin D supplementation has possible neurological benefits, including improved gait stability and leg function, which could produce improvement in some MS symptoms.

Both low blood levels and low intake of vitamin D have been associated with increased risk for developing MS. In addition, low blood levels have been associated with increased risk for conversion of clinically isolated syndrome (CIS) to MS and also with increased risk for MRI activity, attacks, and progression of disability in those with MS. Large, well-designed intervention studies with vitamin D for MS prevention or disease-modifying or symptomatic effects have not been reported.

Vitamin D is generally well tolerated. The recommended daily amount (RDA) of vitamin D is 600–800 IU daily. High doses of vitamin D may cause multiple side effects, including nausea, vomiting, fatigue, hypertension, and renal damage. There is emerging evidence that high doses or high blood levels of vitamin D could *increase* the risk of fractures, falls, cardiovascular disease, all-cause mortality, and some cancers, including pancreatic. The tolerable upper intake level (UL) of vitamin D is 4000 IU daily.

In reasonable doses, vitamin D is a generally safe therapy that should be considered in MS patients who have low vitamin D levels. Vitamin D could have preventive, disease-modifying, and symptomatic effects in MS.

Yoga

Yoga is a component of Ayurveda, an ancient, multimodal healing method that was developed in India thousands of years ago. In spite of the widespread popularity of yoga, there have been limited studies in MS.

In MS, there is one well-designed clinical study of yoga. In this controlled trial, there were three arms: a control group that received standard medical care and two intervention groups that received standard medical care along with either yoga or conventional exercise. It was found that those who were treated with yoga or conventional exercise experienced significantly less fatigue than those in the control group.

When done appropriately, yoga is generally safe. Yoga may be modified for those with disabilities. There are some yoga groups and instructional programs specifically designed for people with disabilities. Vigorous physical activity and challenging positions should be done with caution or avoided by pregnant women and those with fatigue, heat sensitivity, gait instability, and significant cardiac, pulmonary, or bone conditions.

Yoga is generally well tolerated when it is practiced appropriately. In one rigorous clinical trial, yoga decreased MS-associated fatigue.

☆ TIPS AND TRICKS

Clinical trials of yoga as well as tai chi in MS are limited. Based on current evidence, both of those approaches are low risk and possibly therapeutic in MS. In contrast to some conventional exercise programs, yoga and tai chi have balance, stretching, and relaxation as integral components. These components may be beneficial to those with MS.

Conclusion

Most MS patients use some form of CAM. Likewise, most clinicians who provide care for these patients may be unfamiliar with CAM. This may create challenging patient–clinician situations in which CAM therapies are not being openly discussed and considered even though these therapies may produce beneficial or adverse effects on MS or interact with conventional MS medications. To improve this situation and improve overall quality of medical care for MS, clinicians may provide objective risk–benefit information about CAM therapies.

Further Reading

Ascherio, A., Munger, K.L. & Simon, K.C. (2010) Vitamin D and multiple sclerosis. *Lancet Neurology*, **9**, 599–612.

Bowling, A.C. (2007) Complementary and Alternative Medicine and Multiple Sclerosis. Demos Medical Publishing, New York.

Bowling, A.C. (2011) Complementary and alternative medicine and multiple sclerosis. *Neurologic Clinics of North America*, **29**, 465–480.

Bowling, A.C. & Stewart, T.M. (2003) Current complementary and alternative therapies of multiple sclerosis. *Current Treatment Options in Neurology*, **5**, 55–68.

Bowling, A.C. & Stewart, T.M. (2004) Dietary Supplements and Multiple Sclerosis: A Health Professional's Guide. Demos Medical Publishing, New York.

Bowling, A.C., Ibrahim, R. & Stewart, T.M. (2000) Alternative medicine and multiple sclerosis: an objective review from an American perspective. *International Journal of MS Care*, **2**, 14–21.

Jellin, J.M., Gregory, P.J., Batz, F. *et al.* (2012) Pharmacist's Letter/Prescriber's Letter Natural Medicines Comprehensive Database. Therapeutic Research Faculty, Stockton.

McClurg, D., Hagen, S., Hawkins, S. & Lowe-Strong, A. (2102) Abdominal massage for the alleviation of constipation symptoms in people with multiple sclerosis: a randomized, controlled feasibility study. *Multiple Sclerosis*, **17**, 223–233.

van Meeteren, M.E., Teunissen, C.E., Dijkstra, A. & van Tol, E.A. (2005) Antioxidants and polyunsaturated fatty acids in multiple sclerosis. *European Journal of Clinical Nutrition*, **59**, 1347–1361.

Oken, B.S., Kishiyama, S., Zajdel, D. *et al.* (2004) Randomized controlled trial of yoga and exercise in multiple sclerosis. *Neurology*, **62**, 2058–2064.

Polman, C.H., Thompson, A.J., Murray, T.J., Bowling, A.C. & Noseworthy, J.H. (2006) Multiple Sclerosis: The Guide to Treatment and Management, pp. 117–179. Demos Medical Publishing, New York.

Shinto, L., Yadav, V., Morris, C., Lapidus, J.A., Senders, A. & Bourdette, D. (2006) Demographic and health-related factors associated with complementary and alternative medicine (CAM) use in multiple sclerosis. *Multiple Sclerosis*, **12**, 94–100.

Stein, M.S., Liu, Y., Baker, J.E. *et al.* (2011) A randomized trial of high-dose vitamin D2 in relapsing-remitting multiple sclerosis. *Neurology*, **77**, 1611–1618.

Stewart, T.M. & Bowling, A.C. (2005) Polyunsaturated fatty acid supplementation in MS. *International MS Journal*, **12**, 88–93.

10

Symptomatic Management of MS

Jessica Robb, Lawrence M. Samkoff, and Andrew D. Goodman

Neuroimmunology Unit, Department of Neurology, University of Rochester School of Medicine and Dentistry, Rochester, NY, USA

Despite the introduction of disease-modifying agents for multiple sclerosis (MS), most individuals with MS continue to experience symptoms that interfere with their daily activities. This chapter will review the management of bladder, bowel, and sexual dysfunction (SD), pain, tremor, spasticity, and gait impairment related to MS.

Bladder dysfunction

Neurogenic bladder affects up to 70% of patients with MS at some time during the course of illness and may be present in up to 10% of patients at their initial presentation. Physiologic micturition requires storage of urine in the bladder and coordinated contraction of detrusor muscle and relaxation of the external sphincter to expel urine. This complex process depends upon integration of neuronal centers in the cerebral hemispheres, pons, and sacral spinal cord and their interconnecting fibers, which are frequently affected by demyelinating lesions of MS. Interruption of these pathways results in different patterns of bladder dysfunction.

Subtypes of bladder impairment in MS are classified as failure-to-store, failure-to-empty, and combined failure-to-empty-and-store, each produced by lesions in discrete anatomic loci. Although urinary symptoms are similar among these subtypes, it is important to distinguish them, as their management differs.

Suprasacral spinal cord lesions and suprapontine cerebral lesions are commonly associated with detrusor hyperreflexia, resulting in a small, poorly compliant bladder and a failure-to-store abnormality. Such patients present with urinary urgency, frequency, with or without urge incontinence. Detrusor-sphincter dyssynergia (DSD) may also occur with suprasacral cord lesions, resulting in inadequate relaxation of the external urinary sphincter during detrusor contraction. In DSD, the bladder fails to empty due to cocontraction of the detrusor and external sphincter muscles, leading to overall urinary retention. Patients with DSD may also complain of urinary urgency, frequency, and incontinence, as well as urinary hesitancy and a sensation of bladder fullness after voiding. Less commonly, sacral cord demyelinating lesions produce a hypotonic, overly compliant bladder that fails to empty. Patients may present with urinary frequency, overflow incontinence, and signs of incomplete emptying.

Patients with urinary complaints should often be evaluated first for a urinary tract infection (UTI) with urinalysis and urine culture, since treatment with antibiotics may reverse symptoms. However, most patients will have

Multiple Sclerosis and CNS Inflammatory Disorders, First Edition. Edited by Lawrence M. Samkoff and Andrew D. Goodman.

persistent problems regardless of presence or absence of UTI.

> ★ TIPS AND TRICKS
>
> Urinary symptoms in patients with MS are similar among different patterns of neurogenic bladder dysfunction. Patients should be evaluated for UTI before proceeding with further intervention.

Once UTI is excluded, postvoid residual urine volume (PVR) should be measured, either by ultrasound or sterile straight catheterization. PVR less than 100 mL^3 is indicative of detrusor hyperreflexia and failure-to-store neurogenic bladder; PVR greater than 100 mL^3 is found in failure-to-empty bladder dysfunction and can occur with either detrusor hyporeflexia or DSD.

> ★ TIPS AND TRICKS
>
> Bladder dysfunction in MS can be initially assessed with measurement of post-void residual volume using ultrasound. Urinary tract infection should be excluded, and treated as necessary, prior to intervention.

The mainstay treatments of failure-to-store bladder are the muscarinic anticholinergic agents (Table 10.1), which can be given in either short-acting or long-acting formulations. Nonselective antimuscarinics include oxybutynin, tolterodine, trospium, and fesoterodine. The M2- or M3-antimuscarinics, darifenacin and solifenacin, are more selective for cholinergic receptors in the bladder, thereby reducing systemic toxicity. Adverse effects of antimuscarinics include dry mouth, constipation, and delirium. These medications should be avoided in patients with cognitive dysfunction, narrow-angle glaucoma, and structural bladder output obstruction.

Patients who are intolerant of anticholinergic agents may benefit from detrusor muscle botulinum toxin (BTX)-A injections. Intranasal desmopressin (DDAVP) may be helpful to control nocturia but can produce hyponatremia, requiring monitoring of serum sodium and osmolality.

Patients with failure-to-empty bladder are at increased risk for UTI, renal dysfunction, and nephrolithiasis due to stagnation of urinary flow. This is usually best managed with sterile intermittent straight catheterization (ISC), performed several times daily. If urinary urgency and urge incontinence persist in the interval between ISCs, then an anticholinergic agent can be added. Low-dose antibiotics (nitrofurantoin) or urinary-acidifying agents (vitamin C) are often recommended in conjunction with ISC to reduce the incidence of UTI. Patients who cannot perform ISC due to difficulty with manual dexterity or lower extremity spasticity, or who are uncomfortable performing ISC, may benefit from an α-2-adrenergic blocking agent such as tamsulosin, which relaxes the external urinary sphincter, allowing for more effective bladder emptying. An algorithm demonstrating the management of patients with bladder dysfunction in MS is presented in Figure 10.1.

Table 10.1 Anticholinergic Agents for Detrusor Hyperreflexia

Agent	Dosage
Oxybutynin (Ditropan@, Ditropan XL@)	5 mg BID–TID (extended release: 5–30 mg qd)
Tolterodine (Detrol@, Detrol LA@)	1–2 mg BID (extended release: 2–4 mg qd)
Trospium (Sanctura@, Sanctura XR@)	20 mg BID (extended release: 60 mg qd)
Fesoterodine (Toviaz@)	4–8 mg qd
Darifenacin (Enablex@)	7.5–15 mg qd
Solifenacin (VeSIcare@)	5–10 mg qd

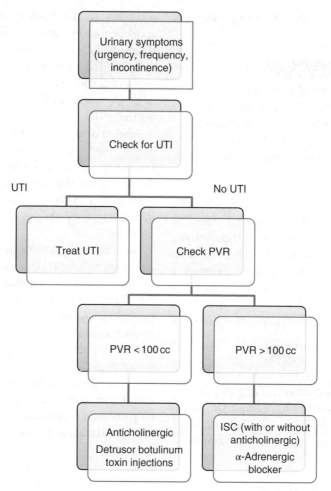

Figure 10.1 Algorithm for management of bladder symptoms in MS. ISC, intermittent straight catheterization.

Bowel dysfunction

Bowel disorders are common in MS. Constipation, fecal incontinence, or both occur in 29% to over 50% of individuals with MS. In one survey of 155 patients with MS, 34% spent more than 30 min daily managing their bowel symptoms, and bowel dysfunction was rated as equally disabling as mobility impairment.

The pathophysiology of bowel dysfunction in MS is primarily due to disruption of cerebral and spinal cord pathways that modulate gastrointestinal transit, pelvic floor muscle tone, anorectal autonomic and sensory function, and volitional motor control of the external anal sphincter. Constipation in MS is further exacerbated by physical immobility and the use of anticholinergic agents for concomitant neurogenic bladder.

Management of MS-associated constipation typically relies on conservative strategies, such as timed bowel elimination, maintenance of physical activity and hydration, and use of stool-bulking agents and dietary fiber. Medical therapies include stool softeners, rectal stimulants (polyethylene glycol or bisacodyl suppositories), laxatives, and enemas. Lubiprostone, a bowel-motility agent, is currently under investigation as a potential treatment for MS-associated constipation.

Fecal incontinence may occur as a result of stool impaction, which can be corrected with manual disimpaction and anticonstipation measures. Fecal incontinence associated with urgency is best addressed with anticholinergic agents. In addition, biofeedback has also been reported to ameliorate both constipation and fecal incontinence in patients with MS.

> ★ **TIPS AND TRICKS**
>
> Constipation in MS can be addressed by conservative measures, such as timed bowel evacuation, enhancing physical activity, maintaining adequate hydration, dietary fiber, and stool bulk-forming agents.

Sexual dysfunction

SD in patients with MS is common, affecting up to 50–73% of men and 40–70% of women with MS. The causes of SD in MS are multifactorial, including neuroanatomic disruption due to demyelinating lesions in the spinal cord, pons, and cerebral hemispheres (primary or neurogenic SD); interference of sexual activity due to MS-associated disability, such as spasticity, fatigue, cognitive dysfunction, neurogenic bladder, and pain (secondary SD); and disturbances due to psychologic and emotional complications of MS (tertiary SD). Finally, many agents used to manage MS symptoms, such as anticholinergics for bladder dysfunction, antispasticity medications, and selective serotonin reuptake inhibitors (SSRIs) for depression, may produce SD.

Symptoms of SD in men with MS include reduced libido, erectile dysfunction (ED), and ejaculatory–orgasmic disturbances. Women with MS also complain of reduced libido, as well as decreased vaginal lubrication, abnormal vaginal sensation, anorgasmia, and dyspareunia. SD can occur early in the MS disease course and impacts adversely on quality of life. Unfortunately, many patients are reluctant to discuss sexual complaints with their neurologist, and the physician may also be uncomfortable in discussing symptoms of SD.

Thus, SD may be underreported in the MS population. Screening for SD is recommended at the initial patient visit and during follow-up examinations. Validated self-administered tools, such as the MS Intimacy and Sexuality Questionnaire-19 (MSISQ-19), may be useful for this purpose.

Neurogenic ED in men with MS may be effectively treated with phosphodiesterase-5 (PDE-5) inhibitors, including sildenafil, vardenafil, and tadalafil (Table 10.1). PDE-5 inhibition produces smooth muscle relaxation, resulting in reduced penile venous return and sustained erection. In a randomized, placebo-controlled study of 217 men with MS and ED, sildenafil citrate in doses from 25 to 100 mg significantly improved both ED (89% vs. 24%, $p < 0.001$) and quality of life compared with placebo. Adverse effects of sildenafil were mild and consisted of headache, flushing, and dyspepsia, none of which resulted in drug discontinuation. In another controlled study of sildenafil in 203 men with MS and ED, the overall benefit of sildenafil on ED compared with placebo was less robust (32.8% vs. 17.6%, $p < 0.04$). Cardiovascular events occurred in three patients. Although vardenafil and tadalafil have not been specifically studied in MS, anecdotal evidence supports their effectiveness. It is important to emphasize the PDE-5 inhibitors are contraindicated in patients using nitrates for coronary artery disease (Table 10.2).

Nonpharmacologic approaches for ED can be considered for patients whose symptoms are refractory to PDE-5 inhibitors or for whom adverse drug effects are intolerable. These include intracavernous vasodilator agents

Table 10.2 PDE-5 Inhibitors for ED

Agent	Dosage
Sildenafil (Viagra®)	50–100 mg prior to sexual activity (start 25 mg if age >65)
Vardenafil (Levitra®)	10–20 mg prior to sexual activity (start 5 mg if age >65)
Tadalafil (Cialis®)	5–20 mg prior to sexual activity (alternative 2.5–5 mg daily)

(e.g., papaverine, alprostadil) and vacuum-based penile prostheses.

There is no established medical therapy for SD in women with MS. In one double-blind, placebo-controlled, crossover study of 19 females with MS-associated SD, sildenafil failed to demonstrate significant benefit, although there was some improvement in vaginal lubrication in the sildenafil group. Treatment of SD in women with MS relies mostly on nonpharmacologic modalities. Vaginal lubricants may be useful to enhance perineal sensation and ameliorate vaginal dryness. Topical estrogen may be helpful for vaginal dryness and dyspareunia in women who are postmenopausal. External vibratory stimulation of the vagina and clitoris may augment physiologic vasocongestion and orgasm.

Treatment of secondary SD in both men and women with MS is directed at ameliorating MS-related symptoms impairing sexual function, such as spasticity, pain, and fatigue. Premedication with agents directed at these specific symptoms before sexual activity may reduce their impact on sexual function.

Tertiary SD in both men and women with MS, typically manifested by reduced libido, is associated with the psychosocial consequences of chronic illness, including mood dysfunction, negative self-image, and fear of rejection. Clinical depression is present in over 50% of MS patients during the course of their disorder. Treatment of depression, which is discussed in another chapter of this book, whether pharmacologically or with cognitive behavioral therapy, can improve tertiary SD. Unfortunately, the commonly used SSRIs for depression may themselves produce adverse effects on sexual function; bupropion produces less SD and may be more useful in patients whose SD is thought to be in part due to SSRI therapy.

It is important to emphasize that effective treatment of SD in patients with MS requires a multidisciplinary approach, involving the neurologist, MS nurse specialist, and mental health therapist. These resources may be best provided by a tertiary MS clinic.

☆ TIPS AND TRICKS

Sexual dysfunction (SD) in patients with MS is underreported due to reluctance of both the patient and neurologist to discuss. A self-administered screening questionnaire can be helpful to select patient who require evaluation for MS-associated SD.

Pain

Not only is pain common among MS patients, but it is a particularly troublesome symptom. Several studies estimate that 50% of MS patients experience MS-related pain during the course of the disease. The chance of an MS patient experiencing pain increases with age, worsening disease severity, and increased disease duration. One study found that one-third of MS patients ranked pain as one of their worst MS symptoms. Pain affects many aspects of patients' lives. Patients with higher levels of pain report reduced quality of life and decreased level of function. Another study found that greater than 41% of MS patients report that pain interferes with daily life most of the time. MS patients with pain have higher utilization of healthcare, as compared with those without pain. Increased levels of pain in MS patients were also correlated with decreased satisfaction with their care from healthcare providers.

The mechanism for pain caused by MS lesions of the central nervous system (CNS) is not fully understood. Ectopic impulses produced at demyelinated lesions likely play a role. There are also likely contributions from central sensitization and lack of inhibition of central pain pathways.

More research has been conducted on symptomatic management of pain from peripheral neurologic origin, such as diabetic neuropathy, than pain of central neurologic origin. However, many of the symptomatic treatments of peripheral pain have been successfully adapted to treat pain of central neurologic origin.

Overall, there a few principles to consider when treating pain of CNS origin. Finding an effective treatment in any given patient often involves a trial-and-error process. In addition, while mood and sleep disorders are not the underlying cause of the pain experienced by MS patients, treating these disorders often lessens the perception of pain. As is true of the treatment of other disorders, monotherapy is ideal. If polytherapy is needed, it is useful to combine medications with different mechanisms to maximize benefit and minimize side effects.

Pain directly caused by MS can be further divided into two categories, paroxysmal and constant pain. Paroxysmal pain is most commonly experienced as trigeminal neuralgia (TN) and Lhermitte's phenomenon. Constant pain is typically experienced as limb dysesthesias. These two categories will be addressed in turn.

Paroxysmal pain

TN is a severe lancinating facial pain that lasts for seconds to minutes and can occur multiple times per day. It is often triggered by activities such as chewing or toothbrushing. The reported prevalence is 1–2% in MS patients, which is considerably higher than in the general population. Up to one-third of TN in MS patients is bilateral, which is rare in idiopathic TN. TN in MS is attributed to intrapontine demyelinating lesions involving the trigeminal entry zone.

Carbamazepine is typically the first-line treatment for TN in both MS and non-MS patients. Oxcarbazepine is an effective alternative. Both of these medications reduce the frequency of attacks of TN by 50%. Hyponatremia occurs more often with oxcarbazepine than carbamazepine but is otherwise relatively well tolerated. Gabapentin and pregabalin may also be useful alternatives. Second-line agents include baclofen, lamotrigine, topiramate, valproic acid, and phenytoin. For rapid control of severe, frequent TN attacks, rapid dose escalation can be used despite the potential for the side effects of dizziness, fatigue, and gait instability. For these severe cases, one can also use the IV form of valproic acid or phenytoin.

Both conventional surgical approaches, such as microvascular decompression and balloon rhizotomy, and stereotactic radiosurgery can be used to treat TN in MS patients with pain refractory to medical therapy (Table 10.3; Figure 10.2).

Paroxysmal dystonic spasms of the limbs, most commonly affecting the upper extremity, are not uncommon in MS and are attributed to demyelinating lesions in the spinal cord. Although brief in duration (usually lasting less

Table 10.3 TN Treatments

	Medication	Starting Dose	Typical Dose	Notes
First-line agents	Carbamazepine	100 mg BID	200–400 mg BID	Extended-release dosing described
	Oxcarbazepine	300 mg QHS	300–900 mg BID	Can cause hyponatremia
Second-line agents	Baclofen	10 mg daily	10–30 mg TID	
	Gabapentin	100–300 mg TID	300–600 mg TID	
	Lamotrigine	25 mg daily	200–400 mg daily	Titrate slowly due to risk of Stevens–Johnson syndrome
	Phenytoin	100 mg TID	100–300 mg TID	
	Pregabalin	75 mg BID	150–300 mg BID	
	Topiramate	25 mg QHS	100–200 mg BID	Can cause cognitive slowing
	Valproic acid	250 mg BID	250–500 mg BID	

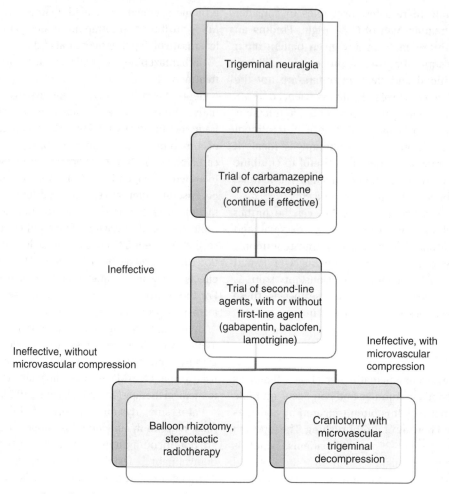

Figure 10.2 Algorithm for management of TN in MS.

than 1 min), they may occur in clusters and are often painful. Other paroxysmal symptoms seen in MS include dysarthria, ataxia, and itching. Paroxysmal events in MS can be controlled with carbamazepine, although other anticonvulsants or baclofen may be used if necessary.

Lhermitte's phenomenon is a brief electrical sensation shooting down the spine that occurs during neck flexion. Stretching of demyelinated sensory pathways in the cervical spinal cord is thought to be the mechanism. Up to 40% of MS patients experience this symptom during the course of their disease. This is often seen in the setting of an exacerbation and will improve considerably over time or with corticosteroid treatment. Typically, medication is not used;

instead, patients avoid neck flexion. However, if this symptom is persistent and very bothersome, it may be treated with carbamazepine or gabapentin.

Optic neuritis is painful in more than 90% of cases. This is often described as a sharp retro-orbital pain that is worse with eye movement. It is usually responsive to treatment with corticosteroids. Glossopharyngeal and occipital neuralgia are relatively uncommon in MS but are treated with the same medications as are used for TN.

Constant pain

Dysesthetic limb pain (DLP) is the most common form of constant MS-induced pain.

This is typically a burning sensation more commonly experienced in the lower limbs than the arms or trunk. Twenty-three percent of MS patients experience DLP at some point during the disease course, frequently in the setting of a spinal cord lesion. Physical exertion or heat can exacerbate this pain. Unfortunately, the pain is typically most bothersome when patients are trying to sleep, which significantly impacts quality of life.

First-line therapies for DLP include amitriptyline and gabapentin. Amitriptyline is typically started at 25 mg QHS and titrated as needed and tolerated up to 150 mg QHS. When using amitriptyline, one must be aware of the anticholinergic side effects, including urinary retention and constipation, as well as the possibility for cardiac conduction abnormalities in patients with cardiac comorbidities. Other effects of amitriptyline can be beneficial, including improvement in mood and sleep. Gabapentin has also been used successfully used to treat limb dysesthesias. Typically, a slow titration is used until symptom relief is achieved with a daily maximum of 3600 mg, divided into three doses. Fatigue can often be a dose-limiting side effect. Lamotrigine has also been used successfully in the treatment of DLP. This is started at 25 mg daily with a slow titration of 25 mg per

week to decrease the risk of Stevens–Johnson syndrome. Other agents for DLP include carbamazepine, oxcarbazepine, and duloxetine. If the dose of a medication is limited by side effects such as fatigue, one can use combinations of drugs. For example, adding gabapentin, pregabalin, or lamotrigine to amitriptyline can be an effective strategy.

If the pain is localized to a small area, topical agents can be used. This includes lidocaine patches (5%), with up to three patches used at a time. Patients wear the patch for 12 h and then keep them off for 12 h. An alternative is capsaicin cream that can be used three to five times per day. Typically, the patient is started on 0.025% and titrated to 0.075%.

Opiates are not generally useful for treating central neuropathic pain. They also carry a risk for addiction and can adversely affect mental status and coordination, which can worsen existing gait instability.

Cannabis derivatives are among the many other pharmacologic options currently being investigated for treatment of MS-associated pain. Nonpharmacologic approaches can also be used to treat pain in MS patients. Some of these methods include TENS units, acupuncture, and meditation (Table 10.4).

Table 10.4 Dysesthesia Treatments

	Medication	Starting Dose	Typical Dose	Notes
First-line agents	Amitriptyline	25 mg QHS	50–150 mg QHS	Anticholinergic side effects
	Gabapentin	100–300 mg TID	300–1200 mg TID	
Second-line agents	Lamotrigine	25 mg daily	200–400 mg daily	Slow titration due to risk of Stevens–Johnson syndrome
	Duloxetine	30 mg daily	60 mg daily	
	Carbamazepine	100 mg BID	200–400 mg BID	Using extended-release formulation
	Oxcarbazepine	300 mg QHS	300–900 mg BID	Can cause hyponatremia
	Lidocaine patch	On for 12 h, then off for 12 h	Same	
	Capsaicin cream	0.025% 4× per day	0.075% 4× per day	

Impaired gait

Gait difficulties affect 64% of patients at least twice weekly, and of these, 70% reported it to be the most challenging aspect of their MS according to one recent survey. Until recently, there has been no pharmacotherapy, other than that for spasticity, impacting on gait. The potassium channel blocker extended-release dalfampridine (4-aminopyridine) was shown to result in an average 25% increase in walking speed in about 37% of patients overall in phase 3 trials receiving the drug who met prescribed criteria as consistent responders. Among responders, there was significant subjective improvement in gait-related MS symptoms. The most concerning adverse events that have emerged from various dalfampridine trials include seizures, acute encephalopathy, and confusional episodes. In 2010, the USFDA approved the delayed-release formulation of dalfampridine (daily oral dose of 10 mg given about 12 h apart) for use in MS to enhance walking in patients with existing gait impairment. Patients with a history of seizures or impaired renal function should be excluded because of safety concerns. Our approach is to

prescribe a trial period of 2–4 weeks of twice daily dalfampridine, which is usually sufficient to assess individual effectiveness and tolerability in the authors' experience (Figure 10.3).

Spasticity

Spasticity experienced as increased muscle tone, often associated with muscle spasms, is among the commonest and troubling of MS symptoms. Prevalence estimates of spasticity range up to 80% of MS patients. MS lesions interrupt the normal descending inhibitory pathways that synapse on group II spinal interneurons, resulting in overactivity of spinal cord segmental alpha motor neurons. Optimally, a multimodality therapeutic approach should be employed: physical and occupational therapy, stretching, and exercise in addition to pharmacotherapy.

Baclofen is generally the first oral medication recommended in addition to stretching and other physical modalities. It is a GABA$_B$ receptor agonist that inhibits activity of spinal interneurons, resulting in decreased alpha motor neuron activity. It is FDA approved for spasticity with demonstrated efficacy in various clinical trials

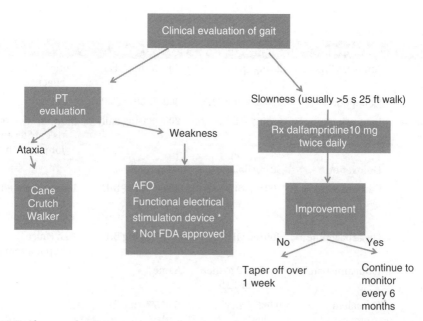

Figure 10.3 Abnormal gait.

in MS. Side effects that limit the effectiveness are daytime sedation and increased muscle weakness that may negatively impact on limb function and especially gait. However, many patients with MS are able to tolerate baclofen doses considerably higher than the 80 mg daily dose recommended by the FDA. The relatively short half-life of baclofen may also limit its effectiveness to 3–4 h. There is a withdrawal syndrome that can occur after chronic use (as little as 1–2 months). The severity depends on the rapidity of drug withdrawal. Symptoms of baclofen withdrawal may include delirium, seizures, and autonomic instability when severe and can be treated more gradual withdrawal of baclofen or benzodiazepines.

The intrathecal (IT) baclofen pump works by directly delivering fractional doses of baclofen to the lower cord through the CSF, thereby avoiding the problem of sedation that occurs with systemic absorption. The IT baclofen pump has been FDA approved for spasticity, and several trials demonstrated efficacy in otherwise intractable cases. Its effectiveness is sustained over time but can be limited by muscle weakness and technical difficulties, such as kinking of the catheter.

Tizanidine is an orally administered centrally active alpha-2-adrenergic agonist that reduces release of excitatory transmitters, effectively reducing muscle tone. It is approved in many countries for reducing spasticity and spasms. Clinical trials in MS patients showed efficacy without the limitation of muscle weakness as may be seen with baclofen. Its effectiveness, however, may be limited by sedation or dizziness that in some cases is associated with orthostatic hypotension. As tizanidine is metabolized by cytochrome oxidase p450 1A2 (CYP 1A2), caution should be used in with concomitant use of CYP 1A2 inhibitors such as fluvoxamine.

Benzodiazepines such as diazepam bind to central benzodiazepine–$GABA_A$ receptors, increasing presynaptic inhibition in the spinal cord. Efficacy in treating spasticity was assessed in several clinical trials and was found to similar to the baclofen effect. In practice, its use is limited both by sedation and its addictive potential in the authors' experience.

The efficacy of gabapentin for spasticity has been suggested in small trials. Although gabapentin has not been specifically FDA approved for this indication, in the authors' experience, it may be most useful in practice as adjunctive therapy for spasms with other spasticity medications such as baclofen. It is not protein bound or metabolized, making it relatively safe to take along with other drugs. Again, its use can be limited by sedation.

BTX blocks presynaptic acetylcholine release at the neuromuscular junction in skeletal muscle. Although not specifically approved for spasticity, efficacy was assessed in several trials. In the authors' experience, its main use in MS is for spasticity in smaller muscles in the hands and feet; however, BTX has demonstrated benefit in the treatment of disabling hip adductor spasticity.

Cannabinoids have also been studied for the treatment of MS in several studies. Nabiximols is a 1:1 mixture of delta-9-tetrahydrocannabinol and cannabidiol administered as an oromucosal spray. It is approved for treatment-resistant MS-related spasticity in the UK, Canada, New Zealand, and several European countries; it is not FDA approved for use in the USA (Table 10.5).

> ★ **TIPS AND TRICKS**
>
> - Patients with MS-associated spasticity frequently tolerate oral baclofen doses above the 80 mg recommended dosage.
> - Botulinum toxin can be useful for focal and disabling hip adductor spasticity.

Tremor

Tremor is a common symptom that can be severely disabling while causing both social embarrassment and profoundly diminished performance of even the simplest activities of daily living. Unfortunately, tremor is often unresponsive to pharmacotherapeutic intervention.

Table 10.5 Pharmacologic Management of Spasticity

Agent	Dosage	Frequency	Side Effects
Baclofen	10–120 mg	TID (may be individualized from single HS dose to q 3 h)	Somnolence; daytime drowsiness; muscle weakness/flaccidity
Tizanidine	6–36 mg	TID	Somnolence; hypotension; dizziness
Clonazepam	0.25–2 mg	HS	Somnolence; daytime drowsiness
Gabapentin	300–3600 mg	TID	Somnolence
Nabiximols* (cannabinoids)	Oromucosal spray	2–12 sprays/day	Dizziness, drowsiness, disorientation

*Approved for treatment of spasticity in the United Kingdom, Canada, New Zealand, and several European countries; not FDA-approved.

Table 10.6 Pharmacologic Management of Tremor

Agent	Dose	Frequency	Side effects
Clonazepam	0.25–2 mg	Start HS and may titrate to TID	Sedation
Propranolol	40–320 mg	Start 40 mg once or twice daily and titrate usually to 120–320 mg in two to three divided doses	Lightheadedness, fatigue, impotence, bradycardia
Primidone	Up to 750 mg starting at 25 mg with slow titration	Start HS and may titrate to 250 mg TID	Sedation
Isoniazid	Up to 1200 mg	QD Can be coadministered with 10–50 mg/day pyridoxine	Hepatic toxicity

Among the drug treatments that are commonly attempted are benzodiazepines such as clonazepam and beta-blockers; the effectiveness of both drug classes may be limited by sedation. Other agents that are sometimes employed are primidone and levetiracetam (may also be limited by sedation or other behavioral effects). Isoniazid was demonstrated in a small trial to be of benefit, but its utility is limited by liver toxicity. Nonpharmacological approaches to treatment include physical means to dampen the tremor such as joint stabilization maneuvers and limb weights. In addition, compensation strategies such as large-handled utensils may be employed (see rehabilitation chapter). Surgical approaches have been employed at selected centers. Stereotactic thalamotomy of ventral intermediate nucleus (VIN) has shown benefit reported in several case series. Some of the concerning adverse effects that have been report are hemiparesis, dysphasia, and dysphagia. Deep brain stimulation has been achieved through stereotactic implantation of microelectrodes in VIN and has shown some efficacy. Potential advantages include reversibility and adjustability. Disadvantages have been adverse effects such as paresthesias reported by many patients and sometimes short-lived effectiveness (Table 10.6).

Further Reading

Awad, R.A. (2011) Neurogenic bowel dysfunction in patients with spinal cord injury, myelomeningocele, multiple sclerosis and Parkinson's disease. *World Journal of Gastroenterology*, **17** (46), 5035–5048.

Boviatsis, E.J., Kouyialis, A.T., Korfias, S. & Sakas, D.E. (2005) Functional outcome of intrathecal baclofen administration for severe spasticity. *Clinical Neurology and Neurosurgery*, **107**, 289–295.

Bywater, A. & While, A. (2006) Management of bowel dysfunction in people with multiple sclerosis. *British Journal of Community Nursing*, **11** (8), 333–334, 336–337, 340–341.

Courtney, A.M., Castro-Borrero, W., Davis, S.L., Frohman, T.C. & Frohman, E.M. (2011) Functional treatments in multiple sclerosis. *Current Opinion in Neurology*, **24** (3), 250–254.

Finnerup, N.B. (2008) A review of central neuropathic pain states. *Current Opinion in Anaesthesiology*, **21**, 586–589.

Fowler, C.J., Miller, J.R., Sharief, M.K., Hussain, I.F., Stecher, V.J. & Sweeney, M. (2005) A double blind, randomised study of sildenafil citrate for erectile dysfunction in men with multiple sclerosis. *Journal of Neurology, Neurosurgery & Psychiatry*, **76** (5), 700–705.

Fowler, C.J., Panicker, J.N., Drake, M. *et al.* (2009) A UK consensus on the management of the bladder in multiple sclerosis. *Journal of Neurology, Neurosurgery & Psychiatry*, **80** (5), 470–477.

Goodman, A.D., Brown, T.R., Krupp, L.B. *et al.* (2009) Sustained-release oral fampridine in

multiple sclerosis: a randomised, double-blind, controlled trial. *Lancet*, **373**, 732–738.

Mills, R.J., Yap, L. & Young, C.A. (2007) Treatment for ataxia in multiple sclerosis. *Cochrane Database of Systematic Reviews*, **1**, CD005029.

O'Connor, A.B., Schwid, S.R., Herrmann, D.N., Markman, J.D. & Dworkin, R.H. (2008) Pain associated with multiple sclerosis: systematic review and proposed classification. *Pain*, **137**, 96–111.

Podda, G. & Constantinescu, C.S. (2012) Nabiximols in the treatment of spasticity, pain and urinary symptoms due to multiple sclerosis. *Expert Opinion on Biological Therapy*, **12** (11), 1517–1531.

Pollmann, W. & Feneberg, W. (2008) Current management of pain associated with multiple sclerosis. *CNS Drugs*, **22**, 291–324.

Samkoff, L.M. & Goodman, A.D. (2011) Symptomatic management in multiple sclerosis. *Neurologic Clinics*, **29**, 449–463.

Smith, C.R., LaRocca, N.G., Giesser, B.S. & Scheinberg, L.C. (1991) High-dose oral baclofen: experience in patients with multiple sclerosis. *Neurology*, **41**, 1829–1831.

United Kingdom Tizanidine Trial Group (1994) A double-blind, placebo-controlled trial of tizanidine in the treatment of spasticity caused by multiple sclerosis. *Neurology*, **44** (11 suppl 9), 70–78.

11

Invisible Symptoms of MS: Fatigue, Depression, and Cognition

Leigh E. Charvet[1], Benzi Kluzer[2], and Lauren B. Krupp[1]

[1]Department of Neurology, Stony Brook Medicine, Stony Brook, NY, USA
[2]Department of Neurology, University of Colorado, Denver, CO, USA

Introduction

Fatigue, cognitive dysfunction, and depression are often referred to as the *invisible* symptoms of multiple sclerosis (MS). These symptoms each have the potential to be the most disabling symptoms of the disease but can be missed on routine physical examination. Further, patients may not mention these symptoms unless specifically questioned. Therefore, it is critical for the clinician to directly address each of these symptoms in the MS patient and manage them appropriately. This chapter will review the prevalence, impact, physiology, recognition, and management of each of these symptoms.

Fatigue

Fatigue is the most common symptom reported by MS patients, affecting approximately three-fourths of all patients, and is a leading contributor to decrements in quality of life. Fatigue is also reported by 40% of patients to be their most disabling symptom, more so than any other symptom including weakness or ataxia, and can contribute to unemployment as well as early retirement. It has been associated with feelings of loss of control over one's environment. Fatigue in MS occurs among all MS subtypes, can persist over years, but can also be seen acutely during relapses. Like other MS symptoms, it can be exacerbated by heat.

Assessment

Fatigue is typically viewed as a subjective feeling of exhaustion that cannot be fully explained by limb weakness or mood. It is associated with the sense that increased effort is required to perform activities. Fatigability, a closely related concept, refers to objective measurable declines in motor or cognitive function during continuous performance of a task. It is important to distinguish fatigue from related symptoms such as depression and sleepiness as the management is different. Studies have shown that MS subjects have both increased subjective fatigue complaints and objective fatigability of motor and cognitive performance. However, subjective fatigue is not adequately explained by reduced motor or cognitive performance. Clinically significant fatigue and fatigability in MS differ from the normal fatigue seen in healthy individuals in that they may have several of the following features: (1) provoked by minimal or no exertion, (2) unpredictably related to activity, (3) poorly responsive to rest or require disproportionate amount of rest, (4) interfere with daily function, and (5) are chronic.

Multiple Sclerosis and CNS Inflammatory Disorders, First Edition. Edited by Lawrence M. Samkoff and Andrew D. Goodman.

While fatigue may be intrinsic to the disease process itself, it is essential to rule out potential secondary causes. When taking a history from MS patients complaining of fatigue, it is important to determine whether fatigue onset correlates with changes in medications, mood, pain, or sleep. Antispasticity medications may occasionally be associated with fatigue. Disease-modifying treatments are less clearly linked to fatigue, and some have been associated with reductions in fatigue. Depressed mood often occurs with fatigue, and fatigue can be a symptom of clinical depression. In these cases, there is severe fatigue upon awakening versus the more common pattern of worsening fatigue as the day progresses. While less studied, anxiety and pain may also be related to fatigue. Sleep disorders commonly seen in MS include insomnia, sleep apnea, nocturia, rapid eye movement sleep behavior disorder, periodic leg movements of sleep, and restless legs syndrome. Sleep studies can help elucidate the cause of daytime fatigue and are probably underutilized in MS. Patients experiencing severe fatigue have twice the frequency of sleep disorders as those without fatigue. Finally, routine laboratory tests should be performed to rule out other common causes of fatigue in the general population including thyroid studies, complete blood count (for anemia), a metabolic panel, and infections.

In clinical practice, fatigue is best detected through a thorough history and a directed interview. Fatigue specific scales, such as the Fatigue Severity Scale or Modified Fatigue Impact Scale, may be used to detect and track fatigue but are typically not needed. Fatigability may also provide an explanation for apparent discrepancies in patients who report difficulties with cognitive or motor function in daily activities but perform well on objective (but brief) bedside testing.

Pathogenesis

The pathogenesis of fatigue in MS is likely multifactorial. Several lines of research have provided insight. Neuropsychological studies have shown some correlations between psychomotor slowing and subjective fatigue complains, suggesting that cognitive effort may partially underlie MS fatigue complaints. Anatomical neuroimaging studies demonstrate that cortical atrophy, rather than total white matter burden, is more likely to be associated with fatigue. White matter lesions involving frontal, parietal, and subcortical connections are also associated with fatigue, supporting a hypothesized role of the basal ganglia and frontal lobes in maintaining effort and parietal lobes in maintaining sustained attention. Functional imaging studies further show that patients with fatigue have increased activity in frontal and motor areas even when starting a task, suggesting that patients with fatigue are utilizing more cerebral resources with all activities and thus more susceptible to decompensation with continued performance.

Management

The first issue in the management of fatigue is to determine the extent to which other potential secondary causes of fatigue are present (Figure 11.1). Pain, depression, anxiety, sleep disorders, anemia, or other metabolic disorders should be treated first if detected before proceeding to other aspects of fatigue management. However, fatigue is frequently a primary symptom of MS and may occur without secondary cause and may persist despite successful treatment of secondary causes.

For the primary treatment of fatigue, there are several pharmacological and nonpharmacological treatments that may be recommended. Despite several positive clinical trials, the effect sizes are generally small, and the benefit to individual patients is variable, with some patients experiencing meaningful benefit but many noting no improvement.

Among nonpharmacological interventions, exercise consisting of either aerobic activity or strength training can reduce fatigue. Patients should be encouraged to start at low levels of intensity and go up slowly to avoid exacerbating

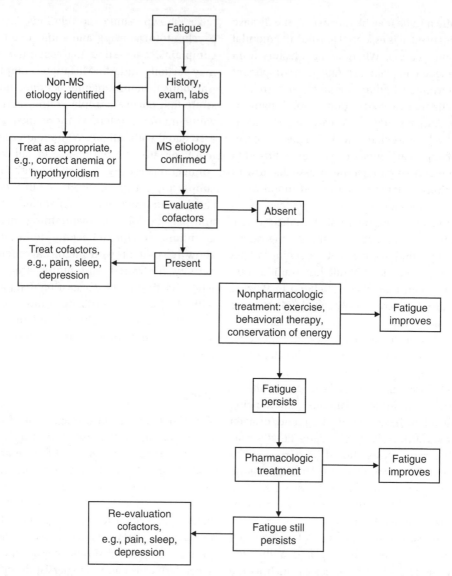

Figure 11.1 Algorithm for the treatment of fatigue.

fatigue. Excessive heat should be avoided, and use of cooling jackets has also been found to decrease fatigue. Psychological and behavioral interventions that have shown efficacy include mindfulness-based meditation, self-efficacy, cognitive behavioral therapy (CBT), and energy conservation strategies.

In patients who fail to benefit or fully respond to nonpharmacological interventions, medications should be considered.

Medications that have been studied for MS fatigue include modafinil, amantadine, and methylphenidate. Although not as commonly used in clinical practice, one study noted benefit with aspirin. With fatigue treatments, significant and sustained benefit is the exception rather than the rule. In patients with prior response, drug holidays should be considered, as benefits over time occasionally can become attenuated.

★ FATIGUE TIPS AND TRICKS

- Fatigue is the most common symptom seen in MS and is the symptom patients most commonly identify as their most disabling symptom.
- While MS is frequently the primary cause of fatigue, patients should be screened and treated for secondary causes if present including sleep disorders, depression, anemia and metabolic disorders.
- Treatment of fatigue may include non-pharmacological interventions and medications.
- For the majority of patients, fatigue treatments result in small to no clinically significant improvements.

Cognition

Problems with cognitive functioning occur in more than half of all patients with MS. Because of the nature of the disorder, areas of impairment can range widely across patients but typically include slowed processing speed, decreased ability to concentrate and reason, and learning and memory problems. Visuomotor integration skills are also often affected.

Cognitive impairment affects all aspects life quality and can be especially debilitating for patients who are trying to maintain employment and household duties. Cognitively impaired patients are less likely to be socially engaged, are at risk for increased mood problems, and have increased problems with activities of daily living. Cognitive impairment has also been shown to increase caregiver burden. For these reasons, it is often listed as the most disabling symptom of the disorder.

Assessment

Cognitive impairment is difficult to detect, in part, because it is not strongly associated with other measurements of neurologic impairment. Studies have demonstrated no significant correlation between EDSS and cognitive impairment when controlling for mood. Cognitive impairment may also take more subtle forms that can be missed in routine examination.

Interview should include questions to both the patient and significant other (if present) about changes in cognitive functioning. Unfortunately, relying exclusively on the patient's complaints can be misleading. For example, summary scores of structured patient-completed questionnaires addressing cognitive functions are much more closely associated with mood than with actual performance on neuropsychological tests. Therefore, objective testing is a much more reliable measure of cognitive performance. The routine mental status examination is too insensitive to identify the deficits routinely experienced by individuals with MS. While we have found that the Montreal Cognitive Assessment to be more sensitive than the MMSE, this assessment tool also fails to detect many impaired individuals. One strategy that has been recommended is to perform a routine screen with cognitive tests that are brief and can be administered by a nurse or physician. The Symbol Digit Modalities Test assesses processing speed and takes only a few minutes to administer. The test contains single digits paired with abstract symbols, and participants must say the number that corresponds to each symbol. If more time is available, then expanding the assessment to include two memory tasks, one assessing visual memory and verbal learning and the other measuring verbal memory, can provide a more comprehensive screen. An expanded screen takes approximately 15–20 min to administer. The normative values that correspond to these tests are available on the Brief International Cognitive Assessment in MS website (bicams.net). When there is any concern that cognitive functioning may be affected, formal neuropsychological evaluation is warranted. This evaluation will provide more in-depth detection of areas of cognitive involvement and also provide a baseline to evaluate for treatment effects or further decline. A neuropsychologist experienced with MS should be helpful in providing recommendations for management.

> ✱ **COGNITIVE ASSESSMENT TIPS AND TRICKS**
>
> - A quick screen for cognitive impairment can be completed during an office visit.
> - The Symbol Digit Modalities Test takes only a few minutes to administer.
> - The Brief International Cognitive Assessment in MS website, bicams.net, provides recommendations and normative values for brief office-based screening
> - Consult with a clinical neuropsychologist experienced with MS when cognitive difficulties are present

Pathogenesis

Cognitive impairment occurs in all MS subtypes. Subtle deficits can even be identified in individuals with the *radiologically isolated syndrome*. Among those with MS, the frequency of impairment ranges is estimated as 20% for clinically isolated syndrome (CIS) and is highest among those with secondary progressive MS, affecting more three-quarters of patients in some studies. Fortunately, the progression of cognitive deficits over time is gradual, and it can take 4–10 years to detect declines. Of note, a 10-year follow-up of participants from a clinical trial by Schwid and colleagues (2007) for relapsing MS in which participants were assessed with a neuropsychological test battery showed little to no worsening in the majority of subjects.

The neuroradiologic markers of MS that have been linked to cerebral dysfunction include lesion burden and global atrophy. Early work demonstrated a strong link between third ventricle width and cognitive deficits. Regional atrophy assessments have demonstrated that atrophy to the thalamus and hippocampus is particularly important. Cortical gray atrophy is also linked to cognitive impairment. Diffusion tensor imaging has linked cognitive impairment to disruption of white matter tracts and in particular thalamocortical pathways. Longitudinal studies of neuroimaging and cognitive functioning have shown that as cerebral atrophy increases, test performance declines.

Treatment

There is some evidence that treatment with disease-modifying therapy is beneficial for cognition. Theoretically, positive clinical trials would demonstrate that the treated group shows less cognitive decline than the placebo group. However, due to the strong practice effect, in which simply by retaking the test patients improve, the clinical trials that demonstrated positive effects on cognition show relative improvement on cognitive outcome. The most comprehensive study of cognition with a disease-modifying therapy involved interferon-beta-1a IM, which showed significant benefit on a composite of cognitive measures related to speeded processing and memory compared with placebo. In a follow-up study of patients with CIS randomized to interferon-beta-1b or placebo, in which the placebo group was crossed over to active treatment after 2 years, at 5 years, there was relative improvement among the early versus delayed treated group on the Paced Auditory Serial Addition Test (PASAT), a measure of working memory. The controlled trial with natalizumab was also associated with relative increases in PASAT performance among the actively treated relative to the placebo-treated group. On the other hand, possibly due to methodological issues including relatively intact cognitive functioning at baseline, the trial with glatiramer acetate was not associated with any differences in outcome with respect to cognition between the placebo-treated and actively treated groups.

With these considerations, cognitive impairment must be managed symptomatically. No medications have been clearly established to improve cognitive impairment. An early study showed some improvement in memory with donepezil treatment, but this was not confirmed with a second larger study. Post hoc analyses suggest that patients with greater memory impairment may gain the most benefit. Others have found that l-amphetamine can improve certain aspects of cognitive functioning, including memory, in patients with relatively greater impairment. However, there are significant concerns with the use of stimulants, and no lasting benefit has yet been demonstrated.

Nonpharmacological options include consultation with an occupational therapist. Patients can be provided with suggestions and assistive devices (e.g., automated reminders) to better navigate their day-to-day activities. Preliminary evidence has suggested that targeted cognitive remediation with a trained provider can also be useful.

Depression

Depression is a frequent and often debilitating MS symptom. Depression can be a presenting symptom of the disorder or occur in the context of any other symptom presentation. Depression in MS can exact a major toll on relationships, work performance, and other measures of quality of life. It can exacerbate fatigue, cognitive impairment, lower pain threshold and lead to increased utilization of healthcare services. It has also been associated with poorer disease management and medication compliance.

Assessment

Lifetime prevalence of depression in MS is estimated to be at about 50%. Population-based studies suggest that up to 42% of MS patients exhibit some depressive symptoms at any one time and 29% experience more severe symptoms. However, studies typically measure the severity of self-reported depressive symptoms rather than the more stringent criteria of whether patients meet full DSM-IV-TR diagnostic criteria for depressive disorder.

All MS patients should be screened for depression, ideally at each visit. Direct questioning concerning mood and outlook is often a sufficient first step. As a general rule, the greatest risk factor for depression is history of a previous episode of depression. A brief self-report questionnaire can supplement the screening procedure, preferably a measure that has been developed with a medical population and validated for use with MS patients. One approach is to have patients complete the questionnaire while in the waiting room, as they take only several minutes to complete. If a patient screens positive for elevated symptoms, a follow-up interview is necessary to establish a diagnosis of major depression. A screen should be selected to minimize the contribution of somatic symptoms, as these may be related to MS rather than depression. Frequently recommended scales include the Beck Fast Screen for depression and the Hospital Anxiety and Depression Scale. Other measures, such as the Center for Epidemiologic Depression Scale (CES-D) and the Hamilton Rating Scales, are more biased toward somatic symptoms.

In cases of depression, the potential for suicide should also be evaluated. It has been estimated that approximately one in four patients with MS may consider suicide at some point, having anywhere between a two and seven times greater risk for completed suicide. Males, those younger in age, and diagnosis within 5 years are all associated with increased risk. Elevated risk has been associated with social isolation and alcohol abuse.

> **⚠ CAUTION: RISK FOR SUICIDE**
> - MS patients are at greater risk for suicide.
> - Males are at greater risk.
> - Risk factors also include those younger in age and recent (within 5 years) MS diagnosis.
> - Also watch for social isolation and alcohol abuse.

While most formal studies have not shown that depression is a major side effect of disease-modifying medications, exceptions do exist. Patients with clear depression, who are resistant to pharmacologic or nonpharmacologic interventions for depressed mood, should be carefully monitored when treated with one of the interferon-beta medications. Symptomatic therapies such as benzodiazepines or antispasticity agents should be reviewed with respect to the risk for increasing symptoms such as mental fogging or apathy that might overlap with depression.

Sleep history is also an important aspect of the assessment of the depressed MS patient. Self-reported poor sleep quality and objective measures of sleep dysfunction are more common in MS relative to the general population and can be result from a variety of factors associated with MS. Impaired sleep may in itself be a cause of depression and exacerbate a patient who is otherwise vulnerable for the development of mood disorder, and disturbed sleep is often a symptom of a major depressive episode.

Current level of social support is also a consideration, as well as discussion of ongoing stressors in the patient's life. Increasing their awareness of the role of stress in their experience depression may be useful.

Pathogenesis

Depression in MS has been associated with a wide range of factors, sometimes in combination. Depression may occur independently from MS, as a reaction to illness and disability, or be directly related to the disease process. Overall, disease severity (as measured by the EDSS) appears to be more strongly related to depression than the pattern of disease progression.

Patients earlier in the course of their disease also appear to be more at risk. Understanding this elevated risk for depression in MS is complicated. Factors related to living with a progressive illness and with disability clearly contribute MS-related depression. However, there also appear to be disease-specific factors that suggest risk from underlying neurological process as well.

Imaging studies have linked structural findings of both lesion location and atrophy and with the presence of depression and severity of depressive symptoms. Studies have shown that lesions in temporal lobe regions and markers of atrophy have been associated with severity of depressive symptoms in MS patients. Hippocampal atrophy has also been linked to elevated depressive symptoms in MS, possibly linked to hyperactivity of the hypothalamic–pituitary–adrenal (HPA) axis system. Measures of with immune dysregulation, such as the numbers of circulating or the production of interferon-gamma, have also been associated with depression and MS.

Psychosocial factors also clearly play a role in depression in MS as well. Studies have demonstrated that reaction to illness and coping styles can be factors in mediating depression risk. Additionally, stressors such as unemployment and poor social support have also been associated with depression in MS patients.

Treatment

While the problem of depression in MS is often observed, there are few studies or recommendations that are specific to the MS patient. Therefore, once the assessment is complete, clinicians follow general guidelines for the management of depression.

Antidepressant medication can be effective, based on its use in otherwise healthy patients with major depressive disorder. In some cases, situational factors change and the antidepressant therapy need not be necessary lifelong. On the other hand, for individuals with recurrent depressive episodes, prophylaxis with pharmacologic or nonpharmacologic interventions may be necessary. Psychiatric referral may be useful. Unfortunately, few controlled trials have evaluated antidepressant use in MS samples, and of those, neither a tricyclic (desipramine) nor an SSRI (paroxetine) led to significantly greater improvement than a placebo and is not superior to nonpharmacological approaches. When considering antidepressant therapy options, side effects should be carefully reviewed to avoid exacerbating problems that are often associated with MS such as fatigue or sexual dysfunction.

CBT, including telephone delivery of the service, has shown promise in trials with MS participants. Similarly, mindfulness-based stress reduction programs represent another intervention which has had growing evidence of success. However, both therapies may only be appropriate for certain patients who are open and motivated to this type of intervention. Similarly, for selected patients, a program of exercise can relieve depressive symptoms.

Summary

In summary, fatigue, cognitive functioning, and depression can each affect the overall symptom presentation and should not be evaluated or managed in isolation. Fatigue is often considered to be the most disabling symptom of MS and is correlated with depression. Fatigue is a symptom of depression. Both fatigue and depression can independently contribute to cognitive impairment. Also, self-reported cognitive impairment is closely linked to depressive symptoms (more strongly than to actual cognitive performance). The stress of living with the burden of fatigue and/or cognitive impairment can contribute to the risk of depression.

Care of an MS patient should include proactively assessing for the presence of these symptoms. Managing the experience of fatigue, depression, and cognitive impairment can greatly enhance the quality of life for a patient with MS.

Reference

Schwid, S.R., Goodman, A.D., Weinstein, A., McDermott, M.P. & Johnson, K.P. (2007) Cognitive function in relapsing multiple sclerosis: minimal changes in a 10-year clinical trial. *Journal of the Neurological Sciences*, **255** (1–2), 57–63.

Further Reading

Amato, M.P. & Portaccio, E. (2012) Management options in multiple sclerosis-associated fatigue. *Expert Opinion on Pharmacotherapy*, **13** (2), 207–216.

Arnett, P.A. & Strober, L.B. (2011) Cognitive and neurobehavioral features in multiple sclerosis. *Expert Review of Neurotherapeutics*, **11** (3), 411–424.

DeLuca, J. & Nocentini, U. (2011) Neuropsychological, medical and rehabilitative management of persons with multiple sclerosis. *NeuroRehabilitation*, **29** (3), 197–219.

Feinstein, A. (2011) Multiple sclerosis and depression. *Multiple Sclerosis*, **17** (11), 1276–1281.

Fredrikson, S., Cheng, Q., Jiang, G.X. & Wasserman, D. (2003) Elevated suicide risk among patients with multiple sclerosis in Sweden. *Neuroepidemiology*, **22** (2), 146–152.

Grossman, P., Kappos, L., Gensicke, H. *et al.* (2010) MS quality of life, depression, and fatigue improve after mindfulness training: a randomized trial. *Neurology*, **75** (13), 1141–1149.

Koch, M.W., Glazenborg, A., Uyttenboogaart, M., Mostert, J. & De Keyser, J. (2011) Pharmacologic treatment of depression in multiple sclerosis. *Cochrane Database of Systematic Reviews*, **2**, CD007295.

Krupp, L.B., Serafin, D.J. & Christodoulou, C. (2010) Multiple sclerosis-associated fatigue. *Expert Review of Neurotherapeutics*, **10** (9), 1437–1447.

Langdon, D.W. (2011) Cognition in multiple sclerosis. *Current Opinion in Neurology*, **24** (3), 244–249.

Mohr, D.C., Hart, S.L., Julian, L. & Tasch, E.S. (2007) Screening for depression among patients with multiple sclerosis: two questions may be enough. *Multiple Sclerosis*, **13** (2), 215–219.

12

Rehabilitation

Nesanet S. Mitiku[1,2], Alexius E. G. Sandoval[3], and George H. Kraft[4]

[1]Departments of Rehabilitation Medicine and Neurology, Icahn School of Medicine at Mount Sinai, New York, NY, USA
[2]Corinne Goldsmith Dickinson Center for Multiple Sclerosis, Icahn School of Medicine at Mount Sinai, New York, NY, USA
[3]Maine Rehabilitation Outpatient Center, Bangor, ME, USA
[4]Department of Rehabilitation Medicine and Neurology, Institute for Stem Cell and Regenerative Medicine, University of Washington, Seattle, WA, USA

Introduction

While immunomodulatory and immunosuppressive treatments for multiple sclerosis (MS) are available, none of these treatments provide a cure. Current disease-modifying treatments (DMTs) primarily reduce the frequency of exacerbations and slow disease progression. As a result, the comprehensive management of MS must not only involve optimal DMT selection but also include maximization of *current function*. Tailoring a program to maximize the current function of an individual is at the heart of MS rehabilitation. Currently, rehabilitation remains the best available way to improve function in MS patients (Kraft 1999).

Given the episodic nature of clinical relapses, the uncertain and incomplete extent of neurologic recovery with each relapse, and the gradual progression of disease in a subset of patients, the immediate targets of rehabilitation will change over time. Therefore, the ideal rehabilitation program for any given patient is dynamic so as to best address the evolving disease process, secondary complications, and changing patient goals. Furthermore, even when DMTs fail to adequately restrain disease activity, rehabilitation strategies can improve patient quality of life (QOL).

EVIDENCE AT A GLANCE

- Exercise programs improve QOL, increase physical capacity, enhance ADL performance, help with depression and reduce perceived fatigue.
- Cognitive rehabilitation can improve cognitive performance; correlated fMRI changes are undergoing investigation.
- Though management strategies exist, bladder and bowel incontinence continue to be a source of disability and interfere with community participation in MS patients.
- Caregiver strain correlates not only with MS severity, but also relates to other features of the person with MS such as depression, anxiety, and perceived QOL.

Physical rehabilitation

The physical manifestations of MS are manifold, and the observed deficits may result from a combination of sensory, motor, coordination,

Multiple Sclerosis and CNS Inflammatory Disorders, First Edition. Edited by Lawrence M. Samkoff and Andrew D. Goodman.

and cognitive dysfunction. Perhaps nowhere is the confluence of deficits in these systems more prominent than in ambulation.

> ⚠ **CAUTION!**
>
> Dalfampridine is contraindicated in individuals with a history of seizure disorder or moderate to severe renal dysfunction (CrCl < 50 ml/min).

Preservation and maximization of ambulation has many benefits, both in the physical (i.e., mobility, maintenance of bone density, and cardiovascular fitness) and psychological realms.

Ambulation: Principles and perturbations

The goal of ambulation is to move from point A to point B in an energetically efficient fashion. Ambulation not only encompasses typical bipedal walking but also includes locomotion via other means such as with a manual or power wheelchair.

At a minimum, successful bipedal ambulation requires sufficient antigravity strength to clear the foot during the swing phase of each step together with stability across the ankle, knee, and hip joints. A review of the most common gait abnormalities in MS is provided in the following text, beginning distally with the ankle and progressing proximally to the hip.

Ankle dorsiflexion

Insufficient ankle dorsiflexion (ADF) is the most common manifestation of lower extremity pathology in the MS patient. The common abnormal gait patterns associated with this deficit are the foot slap (Figure 12.1a) and steppage gait patterns (Figure 12.1d). In both cases, the usual cause is ADF weakness, but excessive plantar flexion tone or contracture can also produce these gait patterns. When ADF weakness is mild, a foot slap pattern is observed. In contrast, severe ADF weakness will often present with a steppage gait pattern (provided hip flexion strength is preserved). In the former, initial contact will usually occur with the heel, and a loud sound will be heard as the rest of the foot comes down. In the latter, the patient will raise the knees as if marching, and initial contact will be quiet and occur with the front of the foot. Such ADF weakness may not fully manifest on manual motor testing. Indeed, some patients with full strength on manual motor testing may exhibit a foot slap only after walking for some distance. Often, a spouse or family member will endorse *loud walking* by the patient. The ADF deficit may be uncovered by having the patient walk multiple laps of an office hallway. Suspicion of this type of weakness should be high in a patient who experiences actual or near falls when walking, especially when faced with tasks requiring divided attention. Detection of such weakness is of paramount importance as insufficient foot clearance puts the patient at risk for further injury. Furthermore, there are interventions to compensate for this weakness.

Knee control

Knee instability secondary to quadriceps weakness (Figure 12.1b) can also prove challenging to the ambulatory MS patient. In order to compensate for this, shortly after the foot makes initial contact with the floor, the patient will snap the knee backward, at times even hyperextending the knee. This maneuver places the ground reaction force closer to the knee axis, increasing stability at that joint. Sometimes, the patient will achieve this rapid extension of the knee by keeping the hand in the ipsilateral pocket and providing a knee extension force by pushing back on the femur with the hand. Chronic forced hyperextension of the knee can lead to permanent ligamentous laxity, increased risk of degenerative changes within the knee joint, and chronic knee pain.

Hip girdle stability

Hip girdle weakness can occur in the MS population. Hip abduction weakness produces an excessive pelvic drop during ambulation (Trendelenburg sign, Figure 12.1c) and, when severe, can complicate maintenance of balance. To compensate, a patient may throw the trunk

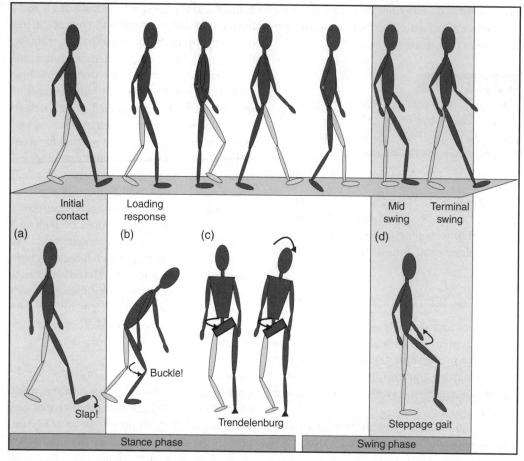

Figure 12.1 Common gait abnormalities in MS patients. (a) Foot slap due to mild ADF weakness, (b) knee instability with buckling leading to a fall, (c) Trendelenburg (compensated on the right) finding secondary to hip abduction weakness, and (d) steppage gait with moderate to severe ADF weakness. Each abnormality is aligned with its corresponding phase of the gait cycle.

toward the side of weakness during stance phase (compensated Trendelenburg, Figure 12.1c); this strategy produces increased strain on the lumbar spine. In the context of normal gait, hip flexor strength is not overly critical; antigravity strength is all that is required. However, in an MS patient who also has ADF weakness, increased hip flexion strength can help with foot clearance (see steppage gait under Ankle Dorsiflexion). In contrast, hip flexor tightness can be problematic during ambulation as it induces excessive lumbar lordosis, translates the center of mass anteriorly, and, as a result, increases the muscular forces required to stabilize both the knee and the ankle.

The influence of spasticity

It is common in individuals with upper motor neuron disease to face barriers to better ambulation as a result of excessive muscular tone. In addition to its biomechanical effects, insufficiently managed spasticity can make walking energetically costly.

Plantar flexion spasticity is common in MS. Excessive plantar flexion spasticity can antagonize ADF during the swing phase of ambulation. Additionally, patients with plantar flexion spasticity may have difficulty transferring weight onto the affected leg during the loading response of the gait cycle.

Spasticity involving musculature crossing the knee can adversely impact limb clearance during swing phase and limb stability during stance phase. Quadriceps spasticity can prevent adequate knee flexion during swing phase and functionally lengthen the swinging leg, making limb clearance more difficult. Hamstring spasticity may prevent adequate knee extension at the terminal portion of swing phase, leading to early weight transfer onto a leg with a bent knee. Landing with an overly bent knee at loading response will not only shorten the step length but also increase the risk of knee buckling and a subsequent fall (Figure 12.1b).

At the hip, patients with excessive adductor tone or spasticity may exhibit a scissoring gait. This gait pattern is characterized by a narrow base of support, placing the patient at increased fall risk.

A thorough assessment of spasticity in the context of ambulation is complementary to a manual assessment of spasticity such as with the Modified Ashworth Scale (Bohannon & Smith 1987). The latter will provide a joint-by-joint numerical measure of velocity-dependent tone and can be useful in quantifying treatment response over time. However, gait assessment highlights those muscles contributing most significantly to gait pathology. These muscles will be prime targets for botulinum toxin or phenol injection when normalization of gait is the desired goal.

Improving ambulation

Rehabilitation interventions for the locomotion deficits described earlier fall into six general categories: bracing, functional electrical stimulation (FES), assistive devices (ADs), reduction of spasticity, exercise-based strategies, and pharmacologic intervention.

Bracing

In addition to providing an external limit to movement across joints exhibiting instability, bracing can slightly enhance movement in selected directions. For ADF weakness, an ankle foot orthosis (AFO) can provide adequate foot clearance either by fixing the ankle at an angle that will ensure foot clearance or by providing an assistive force (such as with a spring or its equivalent, Figure 12.2a) to achieve that same foot clearance. If there is additional mediolateral instability of the ankle, the brace should be designed to capture both malleoli so that stability is restored. If there is fluctuation in limb edema or concern about skin integrity, an AFO can be constructed in the context of an orthopedic shoe (i.e., double metal upright AFO, Figure 12.2b). For individuals with mild quadriceps weakness, the ankle joint of the AFO can be placed in slight plantar flexion, or a ground reaction force model (Figure 12.2c) can be used. Patients are often concerned about the comfort, profile, visibility, and/or weight of the brace.

(a) (b) (c) (d)

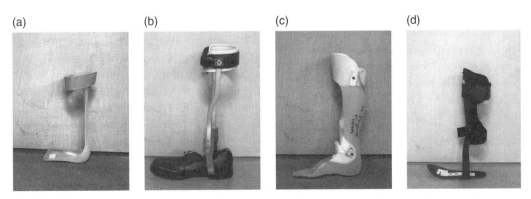

Figure 12.2 AFOs. (a) Posterior leaf spring, (b) double metal upright, (c) ground reaction force, and (d) carbon fiber AFOs.

AFOs are highly customizable with respect to fit and are available in light materials such as carbon fiber (Figure 12.2d). Most AFOs can fit under a straight-legged pant.

For more complex bracing needs (i.e., in the setting of multiple joint instability), the MS patient must be referred to an experienced provider, such as a physiatrist or orthopedist specializing in the management of patients with concomitant joint and upper motor neuron dysfunction.

Functional electrical stimulation

In MS, the lower motor neuron, while intact, is not being driven in a manner to achieve optimal strength. As a result, electrical stimulation of nerves supplying key muscles of ambulation at the appropriate time during the ambulatory cycle can improve ambulatory capacity. Commercially available lower extremity FES devices have been traditionally geared toward assisting ADF through stimulation of the common fibular nerve (Bioness L300 Foot Drop System™, WalkAide®, Odstock Dropped Foot Stimulator®). However, recently, models have become available that have the capacity to address knee instability (Odstock Two Channel Stimulator®, Bioness L300 Plus™) and provide more user customizability as to the target nerve of stimulation (Odstock Two Channel Stimulator®).

> ✋ CAUTION !
>
> FES devices are contraindicated in individuals with pacemakers, uncontrolled epilepsy, cancer (local stimulation may increase blood flow to the tumor), skin breakdown in the area of stimulation, and peripheral nerve injury as the cause of weakness being treated.

FES devices are contraindicated in individuals with pacemakers and in those with lower motor neuron injury as a cause of the weakness being corrected (i.e., fibular nerve dysfunction, L4–L5 nerve root injury, or plexopathy). MS patients can have coincident peripheral nerve injuries, radiculopathies, and plexopathies, and these diagnostic entities should be ruled out on physical examination prior to referral for an FES trial. Should ambiguity as to the cause of lower extremity weakness exist, electrodiagnostic testing should be employed for a definitive diagnosis. Once a referral is made for an FES device, the patient will work with an experienced prosthetist or physical therapist on the fitting and programming of the device. Optimization of stimulation and fit may require multiple visits. There are many considerations in deciding between an FES device and a functional brace; in parallel with our caveat earlier on bracing multiple joints, we advise that a referral to an experienced clinician be made before these are prescribed.

Assistive devices

Handheld ADs increase the patient's base of support and in so doing improve ambulatory stability. The simplest AD is a single-point cane (Figure 12.3a). A cane should be held opposite to the side of greatest weakness. An extended base cane such as a quad cane (Figure 12.3b) or a hemiwalker can provide even greater unilateral support. In the patient with bilateral weakness or in whom gait instability is not adequately corrected with a unilateral device (i.e., cane), bilateral crutches or a walker should be considered. Forearm crutches (Figure 12.3c) are preferred over axillary crutches (Figure 12.3d) in those who require less weight bearing through the hands.

Walkers are highly customizable with variable height, optional wheels, with or without a seat, with different braking systems, and of different materials of construction. A walker with wheels (Figure 12.3f–h) will require less energy during use as the patient avoids picking up the walker in order to advance forward. A built-in seat (Figure 12.3g and h) provides an instant opportunity for rest; this is particularly important for patients in which fatigability is an issue. A passive braking system in which the default brake setting is *on* (i.e., the patient depresses the

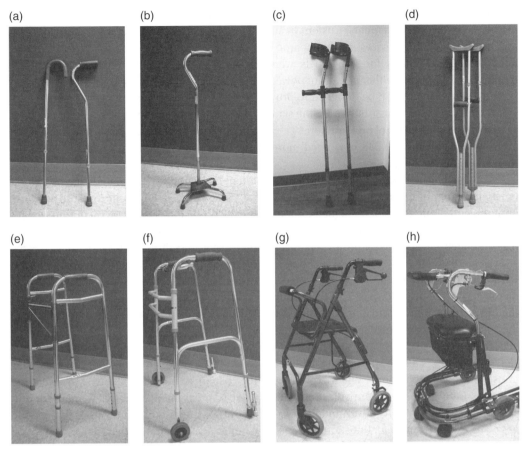

Figure 12.3 ADs for ambulation. (a) Single-point canes, (b) quad cane, (c) forearm crutches, (d) axillary crutches, (e) four-point folding walker, (f) front-wheeled walker, (g) four-wheeled walker with seat and active braking system, and (h) four-wheeled walker with seat and passive braking system (U-Step walker).

brake lever to walk and releases the lever to stop, Figure 12.3h) is also preferred as this provides the greatest amount of support should sudden imbalance arise. With a passive brake system, the walker will not roll away from the individual trying to avert a fall.

Wheelchairs may be prescribed for patients with more severe ambulatory dysfunction. They can be of the manual or power variety. A manual chair is a good option for individuals with moderate trunk control, sufficient upper limb strength and coordination, and adequate cardiovascular fitness. A manual wheelchair can serve as a backup option for MS patients who are only able to ambulate over short distances;

they can use the manual chair for outings where longer distances need to be traversed. An electric scooter is another option for the MS patient with limited ambulatory capacity but with good trunk control. Some manual chairs and scooters can be folded or dismantled and transported in the trunk of a car.

A power chair is more appropriate for individuals who lack the either the upper extremity (UE) function or cardiopulmonary capacity to propel a manual chair, have reduced trunk control, and/or lack the capacity to perform pressure releases for skin protection. Power chair users must have the cognitive ability to drive a chair safely and demonstrate the physical reliability to drive safely. Power chairs can be driven by hand, mouth, chin, or eye movements. Custom head and trunk positioning devices can be incorporated into power chairs for individuals who require extra support. In either manual or power systems, seat cushions can be designed to provide adequate pressure distribution for the skin so as to minimize the risk of pressure sores.

Of note, a patient with MS may need more than one ambulatory aid.

A cane may be adequate for short distances, but a walker may be needed for longer distances or at the end of the day when fatigue is worse. Powered mobility with a scooter or power chair may ultimately be required for protracted travel.

Reduction of spasticity

As previously mentioned, spasticity can add to the energetic cost of ambulation and increase the risk of falls through its biomechanical effects. However, spasticity may also be beneficial; some patients utilize spasticity to facilitate transfers and ambulation. When spasticity serves a useful purpose, overmedication with spasmolytic agents can result in undue weakness. The examiner must identify both the benefits and challenges associated with spasticity in each MS patient.

If, on ambulatory examination, the predominant pattern of spasticity is focal in nature, a targeted spasmolytic approach is desirable. Chemodenervation of the specific muscles impeding ambulatory efficiency avoids the systemic side effects of oral medications. Botulinum toxin injections are most effective in combination with an aggressive stretching program, and the initial injection series should be coupled with a supervised stretching and exercise program involving particular attention to the muscles injected. Should the patient require long-term assisted stretching, a caregiver should be identified prior to completion of the supervised therapy program so that the caregiver can be trained directly by the therapist.

Phenol neurolysis may be appropriate for individuals in whom spasticity has not responded adequately to botulinum toxin or in whom the single-session upper limit cumulative dose of botulinum toxin is being approached. Phenol is particularly useful for adductor spasticity as targeted neurolysis of the anterior branch of the obturator nerve can produce reduced spastic activity of the entire obturator group. An additional advantage of phenol neurolysis is its long duration of 8–9 months. This is in contrast to botulinum toxin that has a duration of action of 2–3 months. Furthermore, the proceduralist can determine the effect of a phenol injection almost immediately as it works by rapid demyelination and/or destruction of the target nerve. However, the promise of a longer duration of action is tempered by an increased procedure duration (with associated increased patient discomfort) and by a 10% risk of persistent dysesthesias. In individuals where spasticity is widespread, oral spasmolytics or a baclofen pump may be better alternatives.

Exercise-based programs

Exercise programs are geared toward improving the patient's intrinsic abilities. A balanced exercise program involves maintenance or pursuit of adequate flexibility, strengthening, and cardiovascular fitness. Joint range of motion deficits identified on examination should be the focus of targeted stretching programs; this will serve to ameliorate the adverse biomechanical effects of inflexibility. Furthermore, prolonged stretching several times daily is the foundation of a good spasticity management program. Strengthening programs should be designed to correct deficits identified on clinical examination while working toward larger functional goals such as improving balance, increasing independence with transfers, achieving normalization of gait, and increasing stair-climbing tolerance. Cardiovascular fitness ought to be incorporated into every exercise program. Early identification of an enjoyable activity that elevates the patient's heart rate and can be performed regularly once the individual has graduated from the supervised therapy environment is critical.

In some individuals, core temperature elevation with exercise may induce Uhthoff's phenomenon, a transient episode of neurologic dysfunction secondary to heat-associated conduction block in previously demyelinated segments. Either internal cooling (ingestion of an iced drink) or external cooling strategies (i.e., formal cooling garments, air conditioning, etc.) may be utilized in order to make exercise feasible. Pools selected for aquatic exercise should not be overly heated.

Lastly, significant levels of disability do not necessarily preclude exercise. With a little bit of creativity, an exercise program can be created for most individuals. Overall, the benefits of exercise extend beyond physical fitness and increased functional capacity; there is evidence to support a positive impact on both mood and fatigue (Dalgas et al. 2010).

A pharmacologic approach

So far, we have discussed strategies that alter the biomechanics of walking through focal interventions or through device substitution. In contrast, 4-aminopyridine (4-AP) works to improve walking by addressing one of the hallmarks of MS: demyelination. It improves conduction through demyelinated pathways by influencing voltage-gated potassium channels. While 4-AP has been available in compounded format for some time, its use was limited by its side effect profile, which included a substantial seizure risk. Dalfampridine, a sustained-release version of 4-AP with an improved side effect profile, was shown to improve walking speed in about one-third of patients with MS (Goodman et al. 2009) and was approved by the FDA for this indication in 2010. Increased walking speed has practical benefits (i.e., safely crossing the street, getting to the bathroom in time).

Upper extremity function

While the lower extremities are often more severely affected, the UEs are also at risk in MS, particularly in those with heavy disease involvement of the cervical spine. Particularly disabling is the combination of upper limb intention tremor and dysmetria. Tremor occurs in 20–60% of individuals with MS (Koch et al. 2007). The amplitude of tremor can be minimized through distal weighting of the affected extremity. Deep brain stimulation (DBS) and/or thalamotomy may improve both postural and intentional tremor associated with MS. However, the results do not appear to be sustained, and there is a risk of additional neurologic disability with surgery (Bittar et al. 2005; Hassan et al. 2012).

Loss of UE function has greater implications for the performance of activities of daily living (ADLs). ADLs include items such as eating, bathing, grooming, dressing, toileting, transferring, shopping, telephone use, computing, writing, bill paying, and driving. As with lower extremity function, interventions for UE function fall into similar categories: bracing, FES, ADs, reduction of spasticity, and exercise-based strategies. However, the nature of bracing, nerves targeted by FES, goals of the ADs, muscles considered for chemodenervation, and prescribed exercises will be specific to the UE. Ongoing collaboration and communication with an occupational therapist experienced in neurologic disorders will expedite successful individualized solutions for MS patients with UE deficits. In individuals with severely limited UE function, the use of voice-activated environmental control systems will greatly enhance independence and reduce the amount of caregiver supervision required.

Home modifications

Alterations to the home according to the needs of the patient can improve QOL greatly. For the wheelchair-enabled individual, the entrance to the home may need to be ramped, doorways widened to accommodate wheelchair width, countertops adjusted to wheelchair height, and bathrooms equipped with a rolling shower chair, no-lip or low-lipped shower, and the appropriate item(s) to ensure safe transfers (grab bars, transfer pole, Hoyer lift).

For the ambulatory individual, double handrails should accompany all stairwells. If foot clearance during ambulation is a problem, home floors should be clear of rugs, exposed wires, and other items that could initiate a fall. Organized areas for cooking and grooming can be created so that these processes are as efficient as possible, thus reducing the energetic cost to the individual. Voice-activated controls within the home can increase independence, particularly for those with limited UE function. Enlisting an occupational therapist in the process of determining the most feasible modifications for a particular individual is highly recommended. The modifications that are possible will be guided by the patient's social, financial, and insurance resources, but additional resources may be obtained through local and national MS support groups.

Organ rehabilitation: Bladder and bowel management

Bladder dysfunction in MS is often characterized by urgency, frequency, and at times incontinences. The most common etiologies are detrusor hyperreflexia and detrusor-sphincter dyssynergia (DSD). In detrusor hyperreflexia, the bladder contracts before it has reached a normal filling volume; the patient is often faced with frequent small-volume voiding. This bladder hyperactivity can be mitigated by the use of antimuscarinic agents such as tolterodine, solifenacin, or oxybutynin; an adequate trial of at least 4 weeks should be given with dose titration during that period. In DSD, coordination between bladder contraction and sphincter opening is compromised; the bladder may at times contract against a closed sphincter producing hesitancy or the urinary sphincter may open in the absence of contraction leading to unanticipated incontinence. Antimuscarinics and catheterization provide the mainstay of DSD treatment; when these strategies are insufficient, referral to a urologist for further workup and treatment options is warranted.

Less frequently, a hyporeflexic bladder will be encountered; this may occur in the setting of reduced bladder sensation where the urge to void is not transmitted. As a result, the bladder becomes markedly distended and over time loses its contractility. In men, particularly in those of advancing age, the overall picture may be complicated by urethral obstruction secondary to enlarged prostatic size. A postvoid residual (PVR) provides a quick in-clinic assessment as to whether urinary retention is a problem. The voided volume should also be measured. If the PVR is low and the voided volume is low and the patient has urgency and/or frequency, detrusor hyperreflexia is most likely. If the PVR is low and the voided volume is high, the patient may have a mildly abnormal voiding reflex but retains good detrusor contractility; this patient should be encouraged to void more often in order to avoid overstretching the bladder. If the PVR is high, regardless of whether the voided volume is low or high, retention is present and problematic. This could be due to DSD, reduced detrusor contractility, or sphincter obstruction. Urodynamic testing could distinguish among these possibilities. In men, a trial of an alpha-2-adrenergic agent may be helpful to ascertain the contribution of urethral constriction. If retention persists, a reliable method of emptying the bladder should be employed to avoid increased urinary tract infections, ureteral reflux, and upper tract damage such as hydronephrosis. Effective bladder emptying methods include clean intermittent catheterization and use of an indwelling catheter.

Like bladder dysfunction, bowel dysfunction is common in MS and most frequently presents as constipation. In addition to disease-related reduction in bowel motility, extrinsic factors such as low fluid intake, low fiber intake, and medication side effects (i.e., anticholinergic medications, opiate medications) contribute to the overall picture. A thorough investigation of the patient's current bowel pattern (frequency, regularity, and consistency), dietary practices, and current medications should be undertaken prior to pharmacologic management of bowel symptoms. Modification of dietary practices or substitution of anticholinergic medications may provide an adequate solution. Increased physical activity can also improve bowel motility. If pharmacologic agents are needed, stool softeners (i.e., docusate), bulking agents (i.e., psyllium, calcium polycarbophil), or motility agents (i.e., polyethylene glycol, magnesium hydroxide, magnesium citrate, bisacodyl) can be selected as appropriate for the patient's bowel history. The ideal bowel program is arrived at methodologically and is regular in practice as well as regular in clinical result.

⚕ CAUTION!

Anti-muscarinic agents are contraindicated in individuals with closed angle glaucoma and gastric distension.

★ TIPS AND TRICKS

MS patients often have a long list of medications to take; streamlining medications can enhance compliance and reduce the risks of polypharmacy. When possible, select medications that address multiple symptoms at once. For instance, in carefully selected patients, a tricyclic antidepressant could be used to treat bladder hyperactivity, neuropathic pain, and sleep disturbance.

⚛ SCIENCE REVISITED

Neurologic control over voiding is distributed over multiple regions: the brain (inhibitory), brainstem (integration of descending brain signals and ascending peripheral signals to allow sphincter coordination), spinal cord, and peripheral nerves (hypogastric, pelvic, and pudendal nerves). The location of CNS micturition loop disruption determines the kind of bladder dysfunction observed. Supraspinal lesions produce bladder hyperreflexia with complete emptying due to preserved sphincter coordination. While spinal cord lesions produce a more variable clinical picture, sphincter dyssynergia is often present.

Cognitive rehabilitation

The prevalence of cognitive impairment among persons with MS is estimated to be between 50 and 75% (Rao *et al.* 1991). Predictors of cognitive dysfunction include an aggressive or progressive disease course, childhood diagnosis of MS, and brain atrophy on MRI (Benedict *et al.* 2004), though cognitive impairment is sometimes detected in the clinically isolated syndrome (CIS). Cognitive impairment adversely influences social functioning, independence, and employability. In some cases, its cumulative impact is more profound than the physical sequelae of MS (Patti *et al.* 2010). Comorbidities such as depression, pain, and fatigue, together with the side effects of medications frequently used in the treatment of MS symptoms, may further impede cognitive performance. The cognitive domains most affected in MS are executive function, attention and concentration, information processing speed, memory, communication, and visuoperceptual processing; IQ is usually preserved (Pepping & Ehde 2005).

Challenges in diagnosis

Diagnosing MS cognitive impairment, particularly in the early stages, can be tricky. Initially, verbal fluency and vocabulary are relatively preserved, particularly in the context of casual conversation. Brief, in-office assessments are often insensitive to cognitive impairment unless it is relatively advanced. When obtaining a clinical history, job performance reviews and reports by family members and friends may be more informative as to the patient's cognitive functioning. Preliminary cognitive testing can be obtained quickly through consultation with a speech language pathologist (SLP) experienced in neurologic disorders. An early SLP consult can also jump-start work toward compensatory strategies for the broad areas of dysfunction identified.

However, if employability or the performance of higher-order cognitive tasks is of primary concern, comprehensive neuropsychological testing (NPT) is recommended. Serial NPT results can also be used to objectively assess for interval cognitive decline. The detailed analyses performed by a neuropsychologist will help the managing physician to determine the rehabilitation strategies that would be most effective for the patient. If improved employment performance is desired, the NPT results may point toward workplace modifications that will allow the individual with MS to improve occupational performance. In other instances, test results will indicate that there is an ability–responsibility mismatch at work; in consultation with a vocational counselor, it may be possible to negotiate a different set of employment responsibilities. When the NPT results indicate that successful employment is unlikely, the test results can be used to support the patient's disability application, improve functioning within the context of ADLs, and, when applicable, help identify safe volunteer possibilities.

The case for nonpharmacological treatment

Prevention through minimization of new lesion acquisition should be the foundation upon which rehabilitation is pursued. Fatigue, depression, pain, sleep disturbance, nutritional deficiencies, and other medical causes of cognitive difficulties should all be sufficiently addressed before the entirety of an MS patient's cognitive dysfunction is attributed to the primary disease. A number of currently available agents have been used and/or studied off-label for the symptomatic treatment of cognitive dysfunction in MS (i.e., donepezil, rivastigmine, amantadine, memantine, 4-AP, ginkgo biloba). However, results have been mixed and interpretation complicated by methodological differences and study design limitations (Patti *et al.* 2010).

While the promises of pharmacologic approaches for cognitive dysfunction have not yet been realized, nonpharmacologic strategies can improve cognitive function now. Simple adjustments such as the use of reminders in the way of calendars, memory notebooks, alarms, voice recorders, personal digital assistants (PDAs), and smartphones can augment memory and organization.

Compensatory strategies are not the only rehabilitation tools available to the MS patient with cognitive dysfunction. Through work with an experienced SLP, a patient can build tailored learning strategies (Basso *et al.* 2006), adapt behaviors that allow for better attention and concentration, and develop a cognitive exercise program that may promote beneficial neuroplasticity (Penner *et al.* 2006; Filippi *et al.* 2012). In addition to work in formal therapy, computer-based programs carried out within the home can also positively influence cognitive function in MS (Stuifbergen *et al.* 2012).

Cognitive impairment in MS has emerged from relative obscurity to be recognized as an undeniably prominent determinant of function and QOL. The treatment repertoire for this entity reflects the relatively short period of time that MS cognitive dysfunction has been in the spotlight. Pharmacologic strategies have yet to clearly demonstrate cognitive improvement. Nonpharmacologic strategies involving either compensatory or restorative approaches improve cognitive function, but the mechanisms through which the restorative approaches operate are uncertain. Thus, the field remains wide open for more rigorous research to elucidate the pathophysiology, develop better diagnostic tools, and ultimately design better therapies for MS cognitive dysfunction.

Summary

MS is a complex disease with an undulating, and in some cases progressive, course that heavily impacts patient function. Maximizing function throughout all phases of the disease is critical to the well-being and QOL of MS patients. Through rehabilitation, function can be improved even when disease-modifying therapies fail to arrest disease. Rehabilitation approaches are available for the physical, cognitive, and secondary organ manifestations of the disease. The exact combination of rehabilitation strategies employed will not only vary from patient to patient but also over time according to a patient's evolving needs.

References

Basso, M.R., Lowery, N., Ghormley, C., Combs, D. & Johnson, J. (2006) Self-generated learning in people with multiple sclerosis. *Journal of the International Neuropsychological Society*, **12** (5), 640–648.

Benedict, R.H., Carone, D.A. & Bakshi, R. (2004) Correlating brain atrophy with cognitive dysfunction, mood disturbances, and personality disorder in multiple sclerosis. *Journal of Neuroimaging*, **14** (3 Suppl), 36S–45S.

Bittar, R.G., Hyam, J., Nandi, D. *et al.* (2005) Thalamotomy versus thalamic stimulation for multiple sclerosis tremor. *Journal of Clinical Neuroscience*, **12** (6), 638–642.

Bohannon, R.W. & Smith, M.B. (1987) Interrater reliability of a modified Ashworth scale of muscle spasticity. *Physical Therapy*, **67** (2), 206–207.

Dalgas, U., Stenager, E., Jakobsen, J. *et al.* (2010) Fatigue, mood and quality of life improve in MS patients after progressive resistance training. *Multiple Sclerosis*, **16** (4), 480–490.

Filippi, M., Riccitelli, G., Mattioli, F. *et al.* (2012) Multiple sclerosis: effects of cognitive rehabilitation on structural and functional MR imaging measures—an explorative study. *Radiology*, **262** (3), 932–940.

Goodman, A.D., Brown, T.R., Krupp, L.B. *et al.* (2009) Sustained-release oral fampridine in multiple sclerosis: a randomised, double-blind, controlled trial. *Lancet*, **373** (9665), 732–738.

Hassan, A., Ahlskog, J.E., Rodriguez, M. & Matsumoto, J.Y. (2012) Surgical therapy for multiple sclerosis tremor: a 12-year follow-up study. *European Journal of Neurology*, **19**, 764–768.

Koch, M., Mostert, J., Heersema, D. & De Keyser, J. (2007) Tremor in multiple sclerosis. *Journal of Neurology*, **254** (2), 133–145.

Kraft, G.H. (1999) Rehabilitation still the only way to improve function in multiple sclerosis. *Lancet*, **354** (9195), 2016–2017.

Patti, F., Leone, C. & D'Amico, E. (2010) Treatment options of cognitive impairment in multiple sclerosis. *Neurological Sciences*, **31** (Suppl 2), S265–S269.

Penner, I.K., Kappos, L., Rausch, M., Opwis, K. & Radu, E.W. (2006) Therapy-induced plasticity of cognitive functions in MS patients: insights from fMRI. *Journal of Physiology-Paris*, **99** (4–6), 455–462.

Pepping, M. & Ehde, D.M. (2005) Neuropsychological evaluation and treatment of multiple sclerosis: the importance of a neuro-rehabilitation focus. *Physical Medicine & Rehabilitation Clinics of North America*, **16** (2), 411–436, viii.

Rao, S.M., Leo, G.J., Bernardin, L. & Unverzagt, F. (1991) Cognitive dysfunction in multiple sclerosis. I. Frequency, patterns, and prediction. *Neurology*, **41** (5), 685–691.

Stuifbergen, A.K., Becker, H., Perez, F., Morison, J., Kullberg, V. & Todd, A. (2012) A randomized controlled trial of a cognitive rehabilitation intervention for persons with multiple sclerosis. *Clinical Rehabilitation*, **26**, 882–893.

13

Psychosocial Adaptation to Multiple Sclerosis

David J. Rintell

Partners Multiple Sclerosis Center, Brigham and Women's Hospital, Boston, MA, USA
Partners Pediatric MS Center, Massachusetts General Hospital, Harvard Medical School,
Boston, MA, USA

Introduction

Although the specific focus of treatment in multiple sclerosis (MS) is the reduction of inflammatory attacks and MRI lesions, the overall treatment goal can be articulated more broadly as the prevention and reduction of disability. If we define disability as impairment in one's ability to engage in activities and relationships, which are meaningful and important to the patient, psychosocial factors need to be taken into account. Neurologists and other clinicians who work with people with MS and their families have long observed that disability is determined not only by inflammatory disease activity but also by psychosocial functioning. One patient may have limited use of limbs or impairment in mobility, but she works full time, engages with family members, and maintains important social connections, while another patient with minimal CNS damage may be confined to home and lives a constrained, limited life. One marker of those patients who remain active and productive is that they have more effectively adapted to life with MS.

Coping and adaptation

Although the terms *coping* and *adaptation* are often used interchangeably, there are important differences in the function of coping and adaptation. Coping is a short-term process by which an individual reacts to a new stressor or crisis with the goal of survival and stabilization. Adaptation is a term utilized in biology and other fields, referring to a continuous process by which an individual makes substantive changes, over time, to accommodate for changing life circumstances and to maintain maximal functioning. Adaptation efforts are usually sustained over time, and old and new resources and strategies are employed to progressively reduce vulnerability to a stressor or threat.

Stages and phases in the adaptation process

Stage theories have been proposed to describe the process of adaptation to chronic illness, based on the stages of grief, as described by Kubler-Ross. There is, however, no evidence for the presence of such stages in adaptation to MS; the repetitive and cyclical nature of loss associated with this type of illness suggests otherwise.

Time phases, descriptive of the challenges to the patient's coping and adaptive processes in chronic illness, have been described by Rolland (1994) (Figure 13.1) and in MS by Antonak and Livneh (1995). As the physical illness changes and evolves, psychosocial demands and challenges evolve as well. The concept of time phases of illness enables neurologists, mental health providers, and patients and their families to appreciate that the illness is a longitudinal process, with changing demands during different time periods (Rolland & Williams 2006).

Multiple Sclerosis and CNS Inflammatory Disorders, First Edition. Edited by Lawrence M. Samkoff
and Andrew D. Goodman.

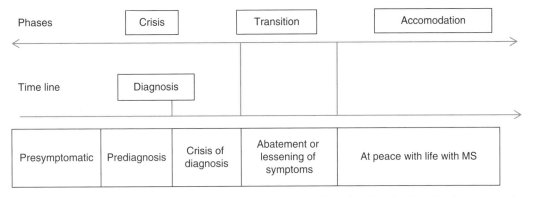

Figure 13.1 Time phases of MS. Source: Adapted from Rolland (1994) and Rolland and Williams (2006).

The phases are not intended to be presented as discrete, ordered steps; as the process of adaptation proceeds, elements of each phase may be experienced at any moment in time. For example, the unpredictable and changing nature of MS can create a crisis during any phase and, with it, a return to some of the challenges of the crisis phase. In addition, some psychosocial concerns occur during all of the phases. It is within this perspective that phases in the process of psychosocial adaptation to MS are here described.

The adaptation process results, in most cases, in successful adjustment, individual and family growth, and accommodation to life with chronic illness. There is a clear role for the neurologist and other healthcare providers to help facilitate this process. Interventions, which further the process of adaptation and address obstacles to successful adaptation, have been highlighted below.

Prediagnosis phases

Presymptomatic

The presymptomatic phase precedes awareness of neurological deficits, although subclinical inflammatory activity may be present in the CNS. Psychosocially, this period serves as a reference point for the events that follow. It retrospectively represents not only what the patient had already accomplished in life but also his or her plans and hopes for the future that were present before even the idea of chronic illness entered the patient's consciousness. When meeting a patient who has lived with MS for any period of time, it is useful to learn about the presymptomatic period to assess his or her premorbid level of functioning, skills, interests, and hopes for the future.

Symptomatic

The symptomatic phase is the period between the onset of symptoms and confirmation of the diagnosis. Prior to the availability of the MRI, this period could last years. In some cases, the medical record would indicate the diagnosis of MS but patient and family were not informed, as there were no treatments approved for use in MS. This phase has a number of common scenarios. First, there are still many patients who live with symptoms for some time, with no definitive medical explanation. Sometimes, these patients are referred to mental health professionals because their symptoms do not appear to be explained through medical tests. These patients may be relieved when they receive the diagnosis, as they learn "it was not all in my head." The next group of patients also responds with relief, because a tumor had been suspected. A third group of patients began experiencing neurological symptoms, received a diagnosis of MS within days, and went from thinking of themselves as completely healthy to learning that they had a serious, potentially disabling chronic illness without much time to process this major life change. One example is the patient with a slight visual disturbance who consults an ophthalmologist, who orders and

MRI and offers the diagnosis of MS on the same day as the consult. These patients are particularly unprepared upon learning of their diagnosis.

The crisis phase

The period following diagnosis is one of vulnerability as the patient and family members struggle to understand the diagnosis and its short- and long-term implications. Patients often report feeling overwhelmed. In the words of one, "I felt my world come crashing down." Even the most thoughtful and sensitive neurologist will provoke uncertainty and anxiety in patient and family because it is not possible to give an individual prognosis (Lansink *et al.* 2004). Not only must the patient confront life-changing news that he or she has a chronic, potentially disabling neurological illness, but must also find a way to gain an understanding of complex and confusing medical information. It is not uncommon, for example, for a newly diagnosed patient to ask for a pill that will *cure* his or her MS or to mistake MS for an immune deficiency. Upon learning that there is no cure for MS, some patients respond with disappointment, anger, hopelessness, and despair.

⭐ **TIPS AND TRICKS**

It is important for neurologists to recognize that some patients may be unable to comprehend and process much information during the diagnostic interview and, should therefore schedule a follow up appointment shortly after the first meeting. At the follow-up, the neurologist can provide a fuller explanation of MS, questions asked and answered, and disease-modifying treatment discussed and, chosen.

The patient's partner experiences the impact of the diagnosis as life changing for him or herself, as well. Support partners in MS tend to be parenting young or school-age children, building their own careers, and younger, as compared to caregivers of later life diseases such as stroke. Partners may experience their own sense of the loss of certain hopes and dreams in the face of MS. Although the life of the support partner is challenging, many report benefits, such as personal growth and closer relationships. Over time, the partner's life will be impacted by a number of factors: the course of the illness, decisions about treatment, adherence to treatment, and participation of the patient in health-promoting programs and behaviors, to mention a few. The partner has an investment in the patient doing as well as possible and can be an important ally and source of information and insight for the neurologist in the treatment of an MS patient. As such, the patient's partner should be included in all treatment decisions.

⭐ **TIPS AND TRICKS**

Include the patient's partner or primary family members in all meetings and exams, particularly when decisions about treatment, rehabilitation, mental health, and other health issues.

During the crisis phase, the patient and support partner are in need of the following interventions from the neurologist:

Education

Educated patients have better overall medical outcomes and improved adherence to medication. The patient's partner and family members should be included in patient education efforts. Family members are likely experiencing similar anxiety and struggle to understand the illness. In particular, it is important to distinguish the objectives and desired outcome of disease-modifying treatment (DMT) from the goals of symptomatic treatment. It is often difficult for the patient and family to grasp that the objective of DMTs is *no change*, that is, no new lesions or clinical attacks, rather than reversal of accrued disability or symptomatic relief.

Instillation of hope

At this moment in time, patients frequently feel that *their life has come to an end*. They fear that their goals and aspirations will no longer be attainable and may feel terror at the image of themselves as a severely disabled person in a wheelchair. They are eager to know how MS will affect their lives in both the short term and also the long term. Given the heterogeneous nature of the illness, however, the neurologist will be unable to make an accurate prediction of the patient's prognosis. Neurologists should ask patients what they fear most and then try to address fears and to correct myths and assumptions about MS head-on with realistic, accurate information and perspective. For example, if the patient's greatest fear is the eventual need to use a wheelchair, the neurologist could cite a recent study that stated that only 20% of patients with a wide age range and duration of illness used a power wheelchair, scooter, or walker (Iezzoni *et al.* 2010). Additionally, it may be of comfort for some newly diagnosed patients to know that patients diagnosed in today's era of DMTs are more likely to have improved outcomes over most existing studies that included patients who had not had the benefit of DMTs early in the disease course. It is advisable to present an optimistic assessment at this point, as the patient has had little time to address her or his anxieties. While there may be a risk in being too optimistic, leading to disappointment down the road, being too pessimistic will potentially increase anxiety and interfere with the patient's successful resumption of premorbid activities and responsibilities (Boeije & Janssens 2004). Furthermore, higher levels of hope have been observed to be protective against patient distress.

It is also important to normalize the reaction of the patient and family. During the crisis of diagnosis, there is often a sense of separation and even alienation from others who are living life without facing such a high level of challenge. Patients and families often feel *abnormal*, which serves to further alienate them from their community. The neurologist can reassure the patient and family that it is normal to have an extreme reaction to the diagnosis and onset of a serious lifelong neurological illness. It is also helpful to assure the family that they will likely find their way through the crisis and that in time they will have greater confidence in their ability to live their lives much as they did before. Lastly, the neurologist should encourage the patient and her/his partner to avoid making major life decisions hastily at this time, such as whether to have children, until they have had more time to process the meaning of the diagnosis in their lives.

The initial shock of the diagnosis often gives way to sadness, anger, depression, and anxiety. Sadness and anger are common reactions to the loss of normal life and previous plans for the future. In addition, uncertainty about future disability can result in a great deal of anxiety. Depression and anxiety can and do occur early in MS. These conditions can be very disabling, and depression can be life threatening. Depression is found early in MS and in CIS. In patients experiencing a first demyelinating event or new diagnosis, 32% of patients experienced depression (Glanz *et al.* 2004). Family members can also experience depression and anxiety soon after diagnosis and may also experience guilt when they experience anger toward the person with MS (Rolland 1994; Holland *et al.* 2007).

The incidence of suicide among people with MS is considerably higher than the general population and in other chronic illnesses (Sadovnick *et al.* 1991). MS patients should be regularly screened for depression, anxiety, and suicidality, and treatment provided through a referral to a mental health professional or by the neurologist if mental health resources are not available.

MS patients have an increased rate of suicide as compared to the general population and matched populations. Sadovnick *et al.* (1991) found that suicide accounted for 15% of all deaths in an MS clinic population. Feinstein (2002) studied 140 serial patients in an MS clinic and found that 28.6% had experienced suicidal intent and that 9 of the 140 had actually attempted suicide. The presence and severity of depression, alcohol abuse, and social isolation had an 85% predictive accuracy for suicidal intent in the MS patients studied.

Neurologists should screen for acute (active in the present) thoughts about suicide and whether the patient has a plan that would result in self-harm. Suicidal ideation accompanied by a method or plan raises concern for the patient's safety. When there is any concern whatsoever about a patient's safety, she or he should be evaluated immediately by a mental health professional, always available at hospital emergency rooms. It is not advisable to release such a patient to family members, who may be unable to keep the patient safe. Regular screening for depression, alcohol abuse, and social isolation can reduce loss to suicide.

It should also be noted that depression, anxiety, and anger at self and others may actually be components of eventual adaptation. This can be reassuring and can be communicated to families concerned about these understandable reactions.

It is during the crisis phase that the experience of grief begins. The losses experienced after the diagnosis of MS are quite different than the loss of a loved one, which occurs within a finite moment in time. The newly diagnosed MS patient experiences the initial loss of a sense of health and then faces additional losses as energy level and abilities become impaired, as compared to premorbid level of functioning, even if slightly or temporarily. One significant loss experienced by MS patients and their families is the loss of their sense of the future. Most individuals and couples nurture long-term plans. The diagnosis of MS initially seems to imply an interruption of future plans. This loss is complicated, as it is sometimes only when hopes for the future are threatened that the individuals and couples become aware of them.

Healthcare professionals can help by telling patients that their experience of loss is natural and expectable and that they need time to grieve these losses. It is also important to inform the patient and family members that as they will work through these losses, they will likely begin to feel better after a time.

The period of crisis following diagnosis also provokes existential questions in the patient and family. Most patients ask, "Why me?," in an effort to put the illness into some context. This, of course, is an inherently unanswerable question, as MS has never been linked to any life choice, lifestyle, diet, or activity. Sometimes, this question is evidence of a patient's sense of being punished and may be linked by the patient to a past choice or action that the patient deems unacceptable. It is a question that is likely beyond the scope of the neurologist to adequately attempt to address. If it can be determined that the patient has a relationship with a member of the clergy, it is advised that the patient be directed to discuss this question with that individual. Patients with a strong sense of faith and spirituality are often among the most successful at coping and adapting to medical illness (Brooks & Matson 1982). Alternatively, individuals may be referred to a mental health professional experienced with MS or other chronic illnesses.

Following the diagnosis, patients and families have the task of regaining control and coping with the initial emotional reaction to the diagnosis. Patients should be encouraged to continue with their usual activities and work, as they will soon learn that their capabilities have not been altered or are altered only slightly or intermittently. They should be informed that virtually all patients make it through this period and go back to living their lives, engaging in usual activities, and achieving their goals—and in doing so, the sense that they can live their lives in spite of the MS is regained. Patients and family members often feel that they need to rethink important future goals immediately, with regard to such issues as family planning, geographic location, and home design.

★ TIPS AND TRICKS

When patients appear to be rapidly rethinking important life decisions with regard to employment, decisions about having children, and changes in location or nature of housing, it is important to advise them to temporarily "table" such decisions until they "get a better handle" on MS.

Disclosure

Soon after diagnosis, patients and partners begin to confront the question of disclosure of their illness to family members, friends, and employers. This is a complex and highly personal decision, with potential errors made by disclosing too prematurely or openly, as well as the mistake of concealing the illness from possible supportive others. There is no single approach or guide regarding disclosure. Some patients conceal their diagnosis and demand that their family members do the same. One patient, 10 years into her MS, had not disclosed outside her nuclear family, because she "didn't want to be that woman with MS." This position makes it impossible for the patient's partner to seek support for their role and forces family members to be untruthful with relatives. On the other hand, disclosure at work should be carefully considered. Although the patient should be protected by the Americans with Disabilities Act, there are many instances of discrimination against patients who disclose without planning. The neurologist and other healthcare providers would be wise to discuss disclosure issues with the patient and partner and refer the patient to a counselor or the MS Society for further discussion.

Defenses

Effective coping during the crisis phase often involves utilization of mechanisms that reduce distress and blunt the full impact and implications of the diagnosis. Patients begin to employ denial, repression, and deferral, which allow room for more positive thinking about the illness.

Hope, expressed as early optimism, could be thought of as a step toward eventually confronting the reality of the situation. Taylor and colleagues studied how an individual develops an optimistic vision of the future. They observed that in cancer, cardiac disease, and HIV, positive illusions, while not related to a patient's actual prognosis, were nevertheless effective in maintaining mental health, mediating the effects of stress, and were associated with successful adjustment to those adverse conditions. Positive illusions contribute to effective coping and positive psychological adjustment to illness. Although there may be some discomfort for the physician, positive illusions voiced by a patient should be accepted rather than challenged, unless, of course, such a perspective threatens treatment compliance.

★ TIPS AND TRICKS

While neurologists can become concerned that the use of denial and other defenses may negatively impact treatment adherence, it is also important to recognize that the use of these defenses and coping mechanisms are a means to reduce the intrusive and frightening thoughts about the possibility of significant disability. It is helpful to remember that the use of these defenses is usually transitional.

Social support

With regard to relationships with others, the crisis phase resembles an acute illness. While the patient may feel a sense of alienation from others who are not facing a potentially disabling illness, a supportive network of family and friends helps to ward off a feeling of isolation and can prevent or reduce depression in early MS. Support groups might be helpful at this time, but many patients in the crisis phase do not elect to participate, feeling unready to meet others with MS who might be visibly disabled. One alternative is to set up one-on-one conversations with other MS patients who are also early in their disease course, but further along in their process of adaptation, through mutual consent.

The interim/transitional phase

For patients with RRMS, there is often a period of stabilization when the symptoms of the initial inflammatory attack abate and the patient is physically much like before. This can be reassuring to the patient and is a marker of the interim/transitional phase. For PPMS patients, this phase occurs during an extended period when symptoms stabilize and no new symptoms emerge. Patients and their families, during this phase, ideally *get back on their feet* and reintegrate into work, activities, and family. It is a period of time when hopefulness emerges. However, because the disease process is more hidden, this period can also be a time when denial and other mechanisms that blunt the impact of the diagnosis can first be observed.

Some patients view the remission or reduction in progression as proof of the belief that the diagnosis was mistaken, that they can *beat MS*, or that DMT is not necessary after all. These ideas and attitudes could put the patient at increased risk of renewal of disease activity.

> ★ TIPS AND TRICKS
>
> Neurologists need to emphasize the need for treatment during remissions and periods of low disease activity, through patient education, reminders, and by predicting the emergence of these ideas before they occur.

Chronic phase

The chronic phase is characterized by a fuller experience of loss and better understanding and acceptance of the unpredictability of MS. During this phase, patients, partners, and family members have begun to experience their own sense of strength and resilience, as they learn to create a meaningful life. The chronic phase is when much of the work of adaptation to MS takes place. Patients, partners, and families are faced with a number of complex, psychosocial issues, and successful adaptation involves effectively addressing these challenges.

Identity

MS is a threat to identity. The challenge to one's personal identity begins soon after diagnosis, but the work of reconsidering identity is largely done during the chronic phase. This work involves resolution of a seeming contradiction: "I am the same person but I am not the same." We tend to think of ourselves in terms of our capabilities, intellect, and relationships. As these factors change, there is a sense that MS has made the patient *not the same person*. Men with MS have a particularly difficult time with the challenge to their former sense of identity. Men tend to define themselves by what they can do, and if there are new limitations on activity, they feel that they are no longer the men they had been. On the other hand, the patient clearly is the same person, although their life has changed significantly. The patient must reconsider her/his goals, self-concept, and core values, in a process that has been called *identity reconstitution*. During this process, the patient regains the sense of the continuity of identity through relationships and meaningful activities. Remarkably, most patients are able to redefine themselves and regain a sense of stable identity, although the process can be challenging and may take some time.

Social isolation and social support

During the crisis phase, relatives, friends, and coworkers tend to provide substantial emotional support to the patient and her/his family. With time and chronicity, however, not only do these support systems fade, but many patients report a reduction of contact with their social network. This may be due to the fact that we have few culturally defined supportive behaviors for chronic illness. Does the neighbor continue to drop off a casserole? Send a get well card? The patient and family often respond to the reduction of social contact and social support with anger, resentment, and bitterness. Pride, and sometimes shame, prevents them from reaching out to social contacts, and the patient and family become socially isolated. Not only is social isolation a well-established health risk, but social support is essential for positive adaptation to MS.

The benefits of social support in MS have been well documented. Social support has been linked to overall adaptation to MS and protection from depression. Social support has been shown to buffer the effects of stress and has been linked to improved medical outcomes in cancer, coronary heart disease, and stroke and better psychological adjustment in MS. Consequently, neurologists should encourage patients to maintain their social support networks, to reconnect with friends with whom they have lost touch, and to participate in support groups sponsored by the MS Society and other groups. This is especially true for men with MS, who are typically less likely to seek social support outside their primary relationship and family. While some patients continue to choose to avoid contact with other people with MS, others become very involved and identified with the illness and choose to participate in many MS-related activities, which are often socially supportive in nature. A social support network, which involves the MS community as well as people untouched by MS, has been described as most effective.

Couples issues

Although many in the MS community believe that the divorce rate is higher among couples living with MS, data reveal that the divorce rate in MS is equivalent to the national average. MS does, however, often put strain on relationships. Couples generally work out a *division of labor* regarding roles and responsibilities, and MS may interrupt established patterns. The well spouse often takes on additional tasks, in addition to his or her own. Changes in employment patterns can put additional financial and interpersonal strains on the couple, as well. These changes are not maladaptive, however, and couples often find their own path to a new equilibrium. A husband with MS who had been the primary wage earner, who might have to reduce or end his employment, might find great satisfaction managing the household and having increased contact with the children.

Changes in intimacy patterns and sexuality are common in couples living with MS. Sexual dysfunction among both men and women is common in MS, with estimates of prevalence of sexual dysfunction ranging from 40% to 90%. Sexual dysfunction in MS has a significant downward impact on quality of life, and sexual problems can contribute to discord and unhappiness in couples living with MS. Patients may experience primary sexual dysfunction, caused by neurological deficits; secondary sexual dysfunction, when other MS symptoms, such as fatigue, dysesthesias, or mobility problems interfere with the sexual relationship; or tertiary sexual difficulties, which are psychological or attitudinal in origin. Patients who take SSRIs for depression may experience decreased sexual desire, difficulty with arousal, and delayed orgasm.

Some neurologists do not screen for sexual dysfunction in their MS patients, because they lack time, resources, and referral sources needed to address sexual issues. Since sexual dysfunction in MS is often treatable and has a significant impact on the couple relationship, neurologists should strive to openly and sensitively address these issues with patients and develop resources and referrals.

Personality issues and personal history

Although the process of adaptation during the chronic phase involves changes in behavior and in relationships, personality variables and life history are also relevant. Patients and families who have confronted adversity in the past tend to be able to more effectively apply previously acquired coping and adaptive strategies to MS. Importantly, these individuals and families have learned that it is possible to overcome obstacles successfully. Those who have a high expectation of success in all their endeavors, or who have never experienced significant failure or insurmountable obstacles in their lives, will more likely be at a disadvantage. Personality characteristics are also relevant. Patients who are flexible and optimistic are comfortable with and well suited for the adaptive process. Conversely, patients who are rigid and inflexible and view the illness as a narcissistic injury tend to be more prone to anger at themselves and others and less capable of mustering their resources for adaptation. A strong sense of self and the ability to use a range of defenses and coping mechanisms, such as humor, can further the adaptive process. Above all, strong social skills and relatedness, which are helpful in maintaining and strengthening social supports, are essential.

Partners and family members will at times report that the patient has experienced a *personality change* as a result of MS. Personality tends to be stable through the lifespan, so the family's report may indicate the presence of a psychiatric problem such as depression. Many MS patients, who had been very attentive and interested in others, become self-focused. Gans (1983) suggests that the patient deinvests in relationships because she needs to invest her attention and energy to managing life. Complaints suggesting a patient's personality change are often an indication that a mental health referral is appropriate.

Risks in the chronic phase

Patients and partners tend to be very invested in reducing exacerbations and forestalling progression. Patients and partners sometimes view progression as a personal failure, evidence of personal weakness, or punishment. It is important to normalize disease progression and encourage the patient to continue efforts to manage the disease medically and psychosocially.

With increasing disability, the patient must learn to accept care and assistance from others. This can be particularly difficult for those patients whose sense of identity is tied to a strong sense of independence. Accepting personal care from one's partner can alter interpersonal boundaries and sometimes reduce the couples' sense of being romantic partners. Receiving personal care from a professional aide presents its own challenges. Accepting help from others can be quite difficult, and this is sometimes evident in a patient's level of anger and frustration.

The accommodation phase

The concept of accommodation comes from the work of Piaget. Accommodation refers to the process of altering one's thinking to conform to external reality. It is in this phase that patients and families have become accustomed to life with MS and, to varying degrees, have made peace with its consequences. In the accommodation phase, patients become comfortable with receiving personal care and accept the loss of privacy and boundary ambiguity.

Considering the extensive literature documenting mental health problems experienced by people with MS, one might assume that few if any MS patients can achieve lives free of psychopathology. However, half of patients never experience a major depressive episode, and many patients are free of mental health problems despite their illness. Many patients report being able to manage the multiple demands of their illness and live happy, productive lives. Successful adaptation to MS does not seem to be dependent on level of physical impairment.

Many patients in the accommodation phase are positive when reflecting on their lives with MS. One gentleman, a power wheelchair user left with only the use of one hand, stated, "I am blessed," referring to the love he receives from family and his important friendships. Patients often report that they have learned valuable life lessons from their experience, to value relationships, to maintain perspective, and to appreciate their own strengths and the kindness of others. Some years ago, this attitude, in which a patient did not appear upset by her disability, was mistakenly characterized as *La Belle indifference*. Currently, this type of positive reflection has been labeled benefit finding, or posttraumatic growth, referring to the ability to identify positive growth in the midst of adversity. One third of the patients in a study by Pakenham reported that they had experienced personal growth as a result of their MS. They also reported benefits accrued in interpersonal relationships, appreciation of life, health gains, and alteration of life priorities and goals. Patients often report that their life *has* changed, but in some ways, for the better. They refer to having a greater sense of themselves as strong and resilient. Priorities have changed and their sense of what is most important in life has become.

Of note, patients in the accommodation phase sometimes opt to discontinue or decrease contact with their neurologist. This may be related to acceptance of the illness, the perception that neurologists do not have much to offer for patients who have lived with MS for many years, or a declining interest in disease-modifying medication.

☆ **TIPS AND TRICKS**

It is important for the neurologist to maintain contact at patients in the accommodation phase. Despite patient perceptions, the neurologist can help to manage troublesome symptoms, thereby improving quality of life, monitor mental health, and provide support to the patient and family.

Acknowledgments

The author wishes to acknowledge the assistance of J. Simpson and P. McCann in the preparation of this chapter.

References

Antonak, R.F. & Livneh, H. (1995) Psychosocial adaptation to disability and its investigation among persons with multiple sclerosis. *Social Science & Medicine*, **40** (8), 1099–1108.

Boeije, H.R. & Janssens, A.C. (2004) 'It might happen or it might not': how patients with multiple sclerosis explain their perception of prognostic risk. *Social Science Medicine*, **59** (4), 861–868.

Brooks, N.A. & Matson, R.R. (1982) Social-psychological adjustment to multiple sclerosis: a longitudinal study. *Social Science & Medicine*, **16** (24), 2129–2135.

Feinstein, A. (2002) An examination of suicidal intent in patients with multiple sclerosis. *Neurology*, **59** (5), 674.

Gans, J.S. (1983) Psychosocial rehabilitation. *Seminars in Neurology*, **3** (2), 201–211.

Glanz, B., Holland, C., Rintell, D. *et al.* (eds) (2004) The impact of social support on depressive symptoms in patients with early MS. Consortium of Multiple Sclerosis Centers, Toronto.

Holland, N.J., Murray, T.J. & Reingold, S.C. (2007) Multiple Sclerosis: A Guide for the Newly Diagnosed. Demos Medical Publishing, New York.

Iezzoni, L.I., Rao, S.R. & Kinkel, R.P. (2010) Experiences acquiring and using mobility aids among working-age persons with multiple sclerosis living in communities in the United States. *American Journal of Physical Medicine & Rehabilitation*, **89** (12), 1010.

Lansink, K.W., Cornejo, C.J., Boeije, T., Kok, M.F., Jurkovich, G.J. & Ponsen, K.J. (2004) Evaluation of the necessity of clinical observation of high-energy trauma patients without significant injury after standardized emergency room stabilization. *Journal of Trauma*, **57** (6), 1256–1259.

Rolland, J.S. (1994) Families, Illness, and Disability: An Integrative Treatment Model. Basic Books, New York.

Rolland, J.S. & Williams, J.K. (2006) Toward a psychosocial model for the new era of genetics. In: S.M. Miller, S.H. McDaniel, J.S. Rolland & S.L. Feetham (eds), Individuals, Families, and the New Era of Genetics, pp. 36–75. WW Norton & Company, New York.

Sadovnick, A.D., Eisen, K., Ebers, G.C. & Paty, D.W. (1991) Cause of death in patients attending multiple-sclerosis clinics. *Neurology*, **41** (8), 1193–1196.

14

Transverse Myelitis and Acute Disseminated Encephalomyelitis

Benjamin M. Greenberg

Department of Neurology and Neurotherapeutics and Department of Pediatrics, University of Texas Southwestern, Dallas, TX, USA

Introduction

Transverse myelitis (TM) and acute disseminated encephalomyelitis (ADEM) are immune-mediated conditions that can affect the central nervous system (CNS). While classically described as demyelinating disorders, some patients may also have damage to the underlying axons leading to long-term symptoms. The semantics and nomenclature related to these conditions have been the source of much confusion, and large-scale controlled trials have been lacking. This chapter will address issues related to nomenclature, biology, clinical presentation, clinical evaluations, and treatment issues related to these rare but important conditions.

First, relative to nomenclature, demyelinating disease terminology has been a source of confusion for patients, families, and practitioners. For example, TM is defined as inflammation of the spinal cord. When it occurs in isolation, it is considered primary or *idiopathic* TM. Yet, in some patients, TM can be part of ADEM (when both the brain and spinal cord are affected), or it can occur as a relapse in multiple sclerosis (MS) or neuromyelitis optica (NMO) patients. In general, primary TM and ADEM are considered monophasic events, while other conditions are frequently recurrent. Thus, one schematic for considering these conditions is outlined in Figure 14.1.

The approach to patients with TM and ADEM is quite similar—recognize the condition, treat the inflammation, determine if there is an underlying cause that puts the patient at risk for recurrent events, and manage long-term symptoms. The remainder of this chapter will deal with each condition separately.

Transverse myelitis

Epidemiology

The term TM was first used in 1948 by an English neurologist, Dr. Suchett-Kaye, to describe a case of rapidly progressive paraparesis with a thoracic sensory level, occurring as a postinfectious complication of pneumonia. While the term myelitis had been used in the 1800s to describe a variety of myelopathic events, *transverse* was added to recognize the commonality of sensory changes in a banding pattern. There are approximately 1500 cases of idiopathic TM per year, but no large-scale epidemiology studies have been completed (Bhat *et al.* 2010). Studies that include TM events that are possible first events of MS suggest an incidence

Multiple Sclerosis and CNS Inflammatory Disorders, First Edition. Edited by Lawrence M. Samkoff and Andrew D. Goodman.

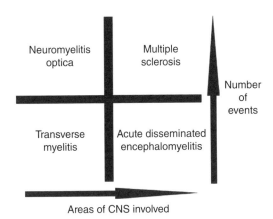

Figure 14.1 Categorization of CNS demyelinating conditions based on temporal course and lesion distribution.

of 24.6 cases per million population or approximately 8100 cases per year in the USA (Young *et al.* 2009). While primary (idiopathic) TM is more common in children than adults, it can occur at any age.

Pathobiology

Pathologically, patients with TM have evidence of inflammation and demyelination within the white matter of the spinal cord. While there are various publications outlining the pathology associated with secondary TM (lupus-associated TM, NMO-associated TM, MS-associated TM, and sarcoid-associated TM), there are few publications of the pathologic findings seen in idiopathic TM from biopsy or autopsy material (Nakano & Ogashiwa 1995; Pittock & Lucchinetti 2006). The majority of evidence suggests a lymphocytic infiltrate enters the spinal cord and coordinates an attack that can lead to abrogation of signal transmission, demyelination, axonal injury, and neuronal cell body injury. While the majority of adult TM cases involve white matter changes in the spinal cord, pediatric patients are increasingly being identified with mixed white matter and anterior horn cell damage (Howell *et al.* 2007).

Clinical presentation

Often, because a condition is rare, its rarity is used to justify delays in diagnosis. Yet, in the case of TM, recognition of the condition starts with recognition of a myelopathy. Evidence of spinal cord dysfunction, regardless of cause, should be recognized as a potential neurologic emergency. The most common presenting symptoms of a myelopathy include weakness, loss of sensation, pain, bowel or bladder dysfunction, and/or ataxia. A careful history and physical assessment are necessary in order to accurately localize a lesion to the spinal cord. Patients who present with a sensory level or acute urinary retention should be considered to have a spinal cord disorder until proven otherwise. Numerous patients have been sent home from offices or emergency rooms in the early stages of myelitis, only to return with severe weakness that could have been treated earlier.

The most common misdiagnoses for myelopathy and, hence, TM include neuropathy (i.e., Guillain–Barré syndrome), *pinched nerves*, urinary tract infections (in the setting of acute urinary retention), and stroke. Careful consideration of possible spinal cord pathology should be given to all patients presenting with acute or subacute neurologic events.

Differential diagnosis and diagnostic criteria

Once a potential myelopathy is clinically recognized, a standard workup should be initiated to determine if the cause is inflammatory (myelitis). In 2002, a working group proposed diagnostic criteria for TM. These recommendations have been incorporated into Figure 14.2, which outlines the initial management of a patient with suspected myelopathy (Transverse Myelitis Consortium Working Group 2002). Of note, there are no published standard of care guidelines for the timing of studies suggested in Figure 14.2, but based on the need for urgent identification of patients, Table 14.1 lists some suggested time considerations. These recommendations are based on the literature supporting emergent surgical intervention for

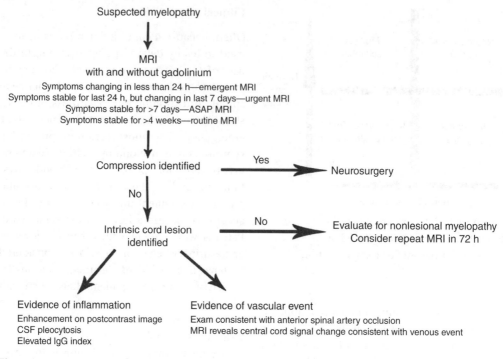

Figure 14.2 Recommended diagnostic pathway for myelopathic patients.

Table 14.1 Timing of MRI Based on the Last Time a Patient's Myelopathic Symptoms Progressed

Timing of Symptom Evolution	Timing of MRI
Less than 24 h	STAT (within hours)
24 h to 7 days	Urgent (same day)
7–30 days	Within 48 h
More than 30 days	Next available

★ **TIPS AND TRICKS**

Patients with a dermatome or myotome level of dysfunction can have abnormalities at *or above* the level of dysfunction. For example, it is important to remember that patients with leg weakness can have cervical spine abnormalities. Thus, imaging of the cervical spine is indicated in patients with isolated leg weakness and normal lumbar and thoracic imaging.

compressive myelopathies and the growing anecdotal evidence supporting early treatment for myelitis (Park *et al.* 2006).

While an MRI is critical for identifying a compressive cause of myelopathy, it is also critical for identifying intrinsic cord pathology categorized as noncompressive. An MRI of the spinal cord (at and above the level of dysfunction) should be obtained with and without gadolinium. The administration of contrast can be useful for determining the etiology of compressive and noncompressive lesions.

If a patient does not have a compressive cause of myelopathy, their workup should then include a lumbar puncture for CSF analysis. TM is suspected in patients with myelopathy and evidence of inflammation, defined as gadolinium enhancement, pleocytosis, or an elevated IgG index (Transverse Myelitis Consortium Working Group 2002, August 27). Of note, these parameters have unknown sensitivity and specificity levels, but are useful tools when evaluating patients. While it is possible for a myelitis patient to have no gadolinium enhancement on MRI and a normal CSF, these features should raise suspicion for alternate explanations. Likewise, patients with vascular events of the cord can have postcontrast enhancement on MRI and abnormal CSF analyses, so the tests are not specific for myelitis (Morimoto *et al.* 1996). Finally, it is worth noting that an isolated elevated CSF protein is the least specific test in myelopathy patients as it can be abnormal in most CNS disorders making its significance difficult to interpret.

Once acute therapy is initiated, practitioners should pursue a workup to try and identify the underlying cause of spinal cord inflammation. The majority of secondary myelitis cases are caused by MS, but NMO, sarcoidosis, systemic lupus erythematosus (SLE), Sjögren syndrome, antiphospholipid syndrome, and copper deficiency should be considered. A typical workup is summarized in Table 14.2.

Acute treatment

Once a patient is suspected of having TM, a healthcare provider is responsible for initiating therapy quickly while continuing to evaluate the patient for underlying causes. The historical standard of care for acute and subacute myelitis is the use of high-dose corticosteroids. There are few, if any, contraindications to high-dose corticosteroids; thus, practitioners should feel comfortable giving doses while evaluations are in progress.

> ### ☝ CAUTION
> Infections of the spinal cord are exceptionally rare. As such, steroids are rarely if ever contraindicated in patients with suspected transverse myelitis. If there are significant concerns for a spinal cord infection it is worth noting that plasma exchange could be pursued without complicating an infection.

There have been no large-scale controlled trials of treatment in acute TM, but small trials and retrospective analyses have supported the use of corticosteroids, plasma exchange, and chemotherapeutic agents (e.g., cyclophosphamide). Intravenous immunoglobulin (IVIG) has been used for myelitis but with little published data. A recent American Academy of Neurology evidence-based guideline for TM found evidence supporting the use of steroids and plasma exchange in myelitis patients but a lack of evidence for IVIG (Scott *et al.* 2011). One retrospective study of a mixed cohort of TM patients identified a benefit to combination steroids and plasma exchange compared to steroids alone in patients without an underlying rheumatologic condition. For patients with SLE or Sjögren syndrome, there was an independent benefit from cyclophosphamide (Greenberg *et al.* 2007). Thus, the current standard of care would call for myelitis patients to

Table 14.2 Standard Evaluation of TM Patients

Test	Reason
Brain MRI	Multifocal brain lesions suggest MS
NMO-IgG	NMO
SSA/SSB	Sjögren-associated TM
ANA	Lupus-associated TM
Anticardiolipin antibody	Antiphospholipid syndrome-associated TM
Copper	Copper deficiency-associated myelopathy
Vitamin B12	Subacute combined degeneration
RPR	Tabes dorsalis
Chest CT scan	Sarcoidosis
CSF oligoclonal bands	Associated with MS

receive early corticosteroid treatment with consideration given for plasma exchange therapy. If research reveals a correlation between response and time to therapy, then early aggressive intervention will become necessary, similar to what is done for acute compressive myelopathy.

Outcomes and long-term management

Many chapters and articles about TM cite a breakdown of outcomes as follows: one third of patients have a good recovery, one third of patients have a fair recovery, and one third of patients have little or no recovery. This pronouncement is based on a 1981 epidemiology study of acute TM patients in Israel that analyzed patients evaluated between 1955 and 1975 (Berman et al. 1981). It does not take into account any patients treated in the modern era of diagnosis and treatment. Yet, these data are repeatedly cited by patients and practitioners as dogma. There is growing evidence to suggest that outcomes are significantly better if patients are diagnoses and treated in a timely and appropriate fashion.

After acute therapy has been concluded, patients should be evaluated for physical and occupational therapy needs. A comprehensive, inpatient, rehabilitation program is preferable for anyone with weakness, ambulation difficulty, or dexterity deficits. Symptomatic improvement occurs via the reduction in inflammation, remyelination, and neurogenic compensation for damage. Proper therapy is essential for retraining patients in appropriate gait and arm use. The nervous system's capability to compensate for damage has historically been significantly underrated, leading to many patients being told that their recoveries would be limited. The improvement from TM can occur over months to years with motor function usually improving more than sensory function (Pidcock et al. 2007). During recovery, patients often have to be managed for spasticity, pain, and urologic dysfunction. A multidisciplinary team is essential for comprehensive care and successful rehabilitation.

Acute disseminated encephalomyelitis (ADEM)

Epidemiology

ADEM is an acute inflammatory event of the CNS that can affect the optic nerve, brain, and/or spinal cord. While the spinal cord can be involved, patients must have brain involvement to be classified as ADEM. There are no large-scale epidemiology studies of ADEM. The estimated prevalence of ADEM in pediatric patients is between 0.2 and 0.8/100,000 per year (Tenembaum et al. 2007; Banwell et al. 2009). There is some evidence to suggest seasonal variation with higher rates in the winter and spring compared to summer and fall (Leake et al. 2004). While most cases are thought to be postinfectious events, there has been some concern for ADEM being triggered by vaccination (Stuve et al. 2005). The data for this is controversial and cases are difficult to prove. The risk benefit data for vaccination strongly favor the use of vaccinations.

Pathobiology

ADEM is notable for a predominantly demyelinating pathology. Brain biopsy specimens often identify demyelination with relative preservation of axons in the presence of a lymphocytic cellular infiltrate. These pathologic features directly influence treatment decisions and expected outcomes. Pathologically, there have been multiple studies that attempt to differentiate the microscopic findings that differentiate demyelination due to ADEM (a monophasic demyelinating disease) and MS (a polyphasic demyelinating disease). In one study, published in 2010, Young et al. (2010) determined that demyelination restricted to the perivenous space was associated with a monophasic course of demyelination as compared to demyelination that was diffuse. The inflammatory cellular infiltrate consists of mostly lymphocytes with occasional granulocytes and plasma cells. Pathologic changes in the brain include astrogliosis, microglial activation, and cortical demyelination (Young et al. 2010).

Clinical presentation

Best described in children, ADEM can present with weakness, sensation changes, vision changes, fever, headache, vomiting, neck stiffness, cognitive changes, changes in mental status, and/or seizures (Table 14.3) (Tenembaum *et al.* 2007). Symptoms can evolve over hours to days and usually reach a nadir within weeks. Given the lack of highly specific clinical signs or symptoms, ADEM should be considered in any patient presenting with acute or subacute neurologic dysfunction. MRI reveals multifocal white matter changes with the predominance of lesions having associated postgadolinium enhancement (Figure 14.3). Spinal cord involvement is seen in 11–28% of patients (Tenembaum *et al.* 2007). CSF analysis usually will identify a lymphocytic pleocytosis and/or an elevated CSF protein.

Patients can sometimes have neurologic damage significant enough to necessitate ICU monitoring or cause respiratory insufficiency

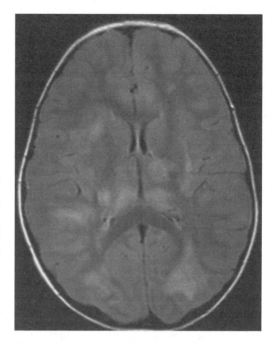

Figure 14.3 FLAIR MRI sequence from a pediatric patient with ADEM.

requiring intubation. Patients need to be monitored carefully for signs of increased intracranial pressure, which should be managed aggressively. Some patients with herniation as a result of ADEM have been successfully managed with hemicraniectomy (Dombrowski *et al.* 2011).

Table 14.3 Clinical Presentations of ADEM Patients

Clinical Sign/Symptom	Prevalence (%)
Fever	52–67
Headache	45–62
Vomiting	35–57
Neck stiffness	15–26
Impaired consciousness	44–77
Seizures	10–34
Ataxia	23–65
Cranial nerve deficit	13–55
Hemiparesis	23–76
Language disturbance	5–26
Paresthesias	2–3

Differential diagnosis and diagnostic criteria

Early evaluations of patients commonly focus on differentiating ADEM from antibody-mediated or infectious encephalitis. Complicating the diagnosis of ADEM, patients can often have fever early in the course of their condition leading to concerns for CNS infections and a delay in diagnosis of an immune-mediated CNS event. A list of conditions commonly considered in the differential diagnosis of ADEM include limbic encephalitis, viral encephalitis, bacterial encephalitis, protozoan encephalitis, toxic exposures, recreational drug exposure, hypoxic–ischemic injury, neoplastic processes, and recurrent demyelinating diseases (i.e., MS).

Patients presenting with encephalopathy and focal neurologic deficits and/or seizures are routinely evaluated for possible CNS infections. This workup should occur simultaneously with an evaluation for ADEM. Typical testing includes an MRI of the brain and spinal cord (as CNS infections rarely cause spinal cord changes). Typical MRI changes in ADEM include T2 hyperintense lesions involving both gray and white matter (Figure 14.3). CSF is usually abnormal with a lymphocytic pleocytosis and elevated protein. CSF should be sent for viral PCRs including HSV, West Nile virus, and Enterovirus testing. Serum and CSF should be tested for antibodies that react against the NMDA receptor.

high-dose corticosteroids (methylprednisolone 30 mg/kg/day up to a maximum of 1 g) as soon as ADEM is suspected. Adjunctive therapy options include plasma exchange (1.1–1.5 volumes per session for 5–7 sessions), cyclophosphamide (500–1000 mg/m^2), and IVIG (2 g/kg divided over 3–5 days) (Nishikawa et al. 1999; Keegan et al. 2002; Marchioni et al. 2002; Khurana et al. 2005). There are no prospective randomized trials validating the superiority of these agents. Patients should be treated with prolonged steroid tapers as multiple cases of transient worsening have been witnessed in the first 30 days of treatment when steroids are tapered quickly.

★ TIPS AND TRICKS

Autoimmune encephalitis has multiple potential underlying pathologic processes. In ADEM multiple lymphocyte subsets infiltrate the brain and cause demyelination. In anti-NMDAR encephalitis there are antibodies produced that bind to CNS antigens and cause neuronal dysfunction. The treatment for this condition often requires more than steroids and/or plasma exchange. Frequently patients require drugs such as cyclophosphamide or rituximab.

✋ CAUTION

After high dose steroids (methylprednisolone 30 mg/kg/day up to a maximum of 1 g) have been completed over 3–5 days, most patients should be treated with an oral prednisone taper. There are no official guidelines, but patients tapered over 2 weeks or less often have transient relapses. Thus, tapers as long as 4–6 weeks are not uncommon and should be considered on a case by case basis.

Differentiating ADEM from a first event of MS is important but complicated. Studies of children after a first episode of demyelination have identified disease onset in adolescence, the presence of intrathecal oligoclonal bands, and optic neuritis as associated with a higher MS risk, whereas early onset and presence of encephalopathy have been associated with a lower risk of subsequent MS (Dale et al. 2009).

Acute treatment

Once diagnosed, the treatment of ADEM requires adequate suppression of CNS inflammation. The standard of care is to initiate therapy with

Outcomes and long-term management

In general, patients with ADEM have profound recoveries with the minority of patients having substantial deficits. Some data suggests that if untreated, 50–70% of patients recover slowly over time (Tenembaum et al. 2007). Children recover more than adults. Less than 25% of patients have long-term cognitive changes on testing, but the sample sizes for these studies are small (Kuni et al. 2012). Patients with brainstem involvement tend to have worse outcomes. A variant of ADEM, acute hemorrhagic leukoencephalitis, has a dramatically worse prognosis than ADEM.

References

Bhat, A., Naguwa, S., Cheema, G. & Gershwin, M.E. (2010) The epidemiology of transverse myelitis. *Autoimmunity Reviews*, **9** (5), A395–A399.

Young, J., Quinn, S., Hurrell, M. & Taylor, B. (2009) Clinically isolated acute transverse myelitis: prognostic features and incidence. *Multiple Sclerosis*, **15** (11), 1295–1302.

Nakano, H. & Ogashiwa, M. (1995) Complete remission of narcolepsy after surgical treatment of an arachnoid cyst in the cerebellopontine angle. *Journal of Neurology, Neurosurgery & Psychiatry*, **58** (2), 264.

Pittock, S.J. & Lucchinetti, C.F. (2006) Inflammatory transverse myelitis: evolving concepts. *Current Opinion in Neurology*, **19** (4), 362–368.

Howell, K.B., Wanigasinghe, J., Leventer, R.J. & Ryan, M.M. (2007) Concomitant transverse myelitis and acute motor axonal neuropathy in an adolescent. *Pediatric Neurology*, **37** (5), 378–381.

Transverse Myelitis Consortium Working Group (2002) Proposed diagnostic criteria and nosology of acute transverse myelitis. *Neurology*, **59** (4), 499–505.

Park, Y.S., Nakase, H., Kawaguchi, S., Sakaki, T., Nikaido, Y. & Morimoto, T. (2006) Predictors of outcome of surgery for cervical compressive myelopathy: retrospective analysis and prospective study. *Neurologia Medico-Chirurgica (Tokyo)*, **46** (5), 231–238.

Morimoto, T., Yamada, T., Nagata, K., Matsuyama, T. & Sakaki, T. (1996) Intramedullary gadolinium-DTPA enhancement in a patient with cervical spondylotic myelopathy and an associated vascular lesion. Case report. *Neurosurgical Focus*, **1** (6), e3.

Scott, T.F., Frohman, E.M., De Seze, J., Gronseth, G.S. & Weinshenker, B.G. (2011) Evidence-based guideline: clinical evaluation and treatment of transverse myelitis: report of the Therapeutics and Technology Assessment Subcommittee of the American Academy of Neurology. *Neurology*, **77** (24), 2128–2134.

Greenberg, B.M., Thomas, K.P., Krishnan, C., Kaplin, A.I., Calabresi, P.A. & Kerr, D.A. (2007) Idiopathic transverse myelitis: corticosteroids, plasma exchange, or cyclophosphamide. *Neurology*, **68** (19), 1614–1617.

Berman, M., Feldman, S., Alter, M., Zilber, N. & Kahana, E. (1981) Acute transverse myelitis: incidence and etiologic considerations. *Neurology*, **31** (8), 966–971.

Pidcock, F.S., Krishnan, C., Crawford, T.O., Salorio, C.F., Trovato, M. & Kerr, D.A. (2007) Acute transverse myelitis in childhood: center-based analysis of 47 cases. *Neurology*, **68** (18), 1474–1480.

Tenembaum, S., Chitnis, T., Ness, J. & Hahn, J.S. (2007) Acute disseminated encephalomyelitis. *Neurology*, **68** (16 Suppl 2), S23–S36.

Banwell, B., Kennedy, J., Sadovnick, D. *et al.* (2009) Incidence of acquired demyelination of the CNS in Canadian children. *Neurology*, **72** (3), 232–239.

Leake, J.A., Albani, S., Kao, A.S. *et al.* (2004) Acute disseminated encephalomyelitis in childhood: epidemiologic, clinical and laboratory features. *The Pediatric Infectious Disease Journal*, **23** (8), 756–764.

Stuve, O., Nessler, S., Hartung, H.P., Hemmer, B., Wiendl, H. & Kieseier, B.C. (2005) Acute disseminated encephalomyelitis. Pathogenesis, diagnosis, treatment, and prognosis. *Der Nervenarzt*, **76** (6), 701–707.

Young, N.P., Weinshenker, B.G., Parisi, J.E. *et al.* (2010) Perivenous demyelination: association with clinically defined acute disseminated encephalomyelitis and comparison with pathologically confirmed multiple sclerosis. *Brain*, **133** (Pt 2), 333–348.

Dombrowski, K.E., Mehta, A.I., Turner, D.A. & McDonagh, D.L. (2011) Life-saving hemicraniectomy for fulminant acute disseminated encephalomyelitis. *British Journal of Neurosurgery*, **25** (2), 249–252.

Dale, R.C., Brilot, F. & Banwell, B. (2009) Pediatric central nervous system inflammatory demyelination: acute disseminated encephalomyelitis, clinically isolated syndromes, neuromyelitis optica, and multiple sclerosis. *Current Opinion in Neurology*, **22** (3), 233–240.

Keegan, M., Pineda, A.A., McClelland, R.L., Darby, C.H., Rodriguez, M. & Weinshenker, B.G. (2002) Plasma exchange for severe attacks of CNS demyelination: predictors of response. *Neurology*, **58** (1), 143–146.

Nishikawa, M., Ichiyama, T., Hayashi, T., Ouchi, K. & Furukawa, S. (1999) Intravenous immunoglobulin therapy in acute disseminated encephalomyelitis. *Pediatric Neurology*, **21** (2), 583–586.

Marchioni, E., Marinou-Aktipi, K., Uggetti, C. *et al.* (2002) Effectiveness of intravenous immunoglobulin treatment in adult patients with steroid-resistant monophasic or recurrent acute disseminated encephalomyelitis. *Journal of Neurology*, **249** (1), 100–104.

Khurana, D.S., Melvin, J.J., Kothare, S.V. *et al.* (2005) Acute disseminated encephalomyelitis in children: discordant neurologic and neuroimaging abnormalities and response to plasmapheresis. *Pediatrics*, **116** (2), 431–436.

Kuni, B.J., Banwell, B.L. & Till, C. (2012) Cognitive and behavioral outcomes in individuals with a history of acute disseminated encephalomyelitis (ADEM). *Developmental Neuropsychology*, **37** (8), 682–696.

15

Neuromyelitis Optica

Marcelo Matiello[1] and Brian G. Weinshenker[2]

[1]Department of Neurology, Massachusetts General Hospital and Brigham and Women's Hospital, Harvard Medical School, Boston, MA, USA
[2]Department of Neurology, Mayo Clinic, Rochester, MN, USA

Introduction

Neuromyelitis optica (NMO) is a severe idiopathic autoimmune disease of the central nervous system (CNS). For reasons not completely understood, NMO preferentially affects the optic nerves and spinal cord causing relapses of optic neuritis (ON) and of transverse myelitis associated with a long lesion in the spinal cord, typically extending three or more spinal segments (longitudinally extensive transverse myelitis, LETM).

For a century since its original recognition as a clinical entity by Devic (1894) and Gault (1894), NMO was regarded as a monophasic disease characterized by near-simultaneous bilateral ON and myelitis in quick succession without recurrence, but with increasing understanding of its pathogenesis and improved ability to differentiate it from prototypic multiple sclerosis (MS), it is now believed to be a relapsing disease in the majority of affected individuals. Whether these two forms are the same disease or pathophysiologically different is a matter of debate. The boundaries between the monophasic form and the relapsing form are unclear, which complicates an analysis of this issue.

Most NMO patients are seropositive for the highly specific autoantibody NMO-IgG. NMO-IgG targets aquaporin-4 (AQP4), leading to complement-dependent cytotoxicity, extensive demyelination, and necrosis, although inflammatory cells, including neutrophils and eosinophils, seem to play an important role. In vitro and animal studies have now shown that NMO-IgG is not just a diagnostic biomarker for NMO; it is an essential component of NMO pathophysiology.

In this chapter, we discuss the current status of the diagnosis and treatment of NMO. It is likely that the rapidly increase in understanding of NMO-IgG-driven pathophysiological mechanisms may lead to specific therapies in the near future.

Diagnosis

Demographic features

Although considered a rare disorder, NMO is vastly underrecognized. Many cases now regarded to be NMO spectrum disorders are diagnosed as MS, isolated or recurrent transverse myelitis, idiopathic or recurrent ON, ADEM, or connective tissue disease-associated myelitis (e.g., lupus or Sjögren myelitis). Population-based studies have recently estimated the incidence and prevalence. In the French Indies, NMO has an incidence of 0.20/100,000 (95% CI, 0.05–0.35) and prevalence of 4.2/100,000 (95% CI, 3.7–5.7). In

Multiple Sclerosis and CNS Inflammatory Disorders, First Edition. Edited by Lawrence M. Samkoff and Andrew D. Goodman.

Southern Denmark, the yearly incidence rate of NMO was estimated to be 0.4 per 100,000 person-years (95% CI, 0.30–0.54) and the prevalence was 4.4 per 100,000 (95% CI, 3.1–5.7) in a largely white population. While MS prevalence differs markedly from country to country, likely due to a combination of genetic and environmental factors, NMO prevalence seems to be similar throughout the world.

NMO typically begins in late middle age, but it may also occur in children. The relapsing form of NMO is eight times more frequent in women than in men, while the monophasic form affects women and men equally.

NMO patients infrequently have relatives with this condition, but familial occurrence is more common than expected from its frequency in the general population. Based on clinical symptoms and frequency of NMO-IgG, the familial form of the disease is indistinguishable from sporadic NMO detection. In a series of 14 families with NMO, no more than 2 generations were affected in any family, and all but 1 family with multiple cases of NMO had only 2 affected members.

Clinical characteristics

Acute attacks

The core clinical features of NMO are acute attacks of ON and myelitis, which are usually more disabling than when they occur as manifestations of prototypic MS.

The occurrence of bilateral simultaneous ON or sequential ON in rapid succession is more suggestive of NMO than MS. Also, the persisting visual deficits are more severe in NMO. Other clinical characteristics of the NMO ON attacks, that is, pain, pattern of visual loss, occurrence of positive visual phenomena, and funduscopic findings, do not distinguish MS- and NMO-related ON.

Myelitis attacks are frequently accompanied by longitudinally extensive (longer than three vertebral segments) lesions on MRI scan and more frequently cause *complete* (symmetrical and with motor, sensory, and sphincter involvement) than *partial* myelitis-related deficits.

Lhermitte's symptom (paresthesias in the spine or limbs elicited by neck flexion), paroxysmal tonic spasms, and radicular pain often accompany the myelitis. Paroxysmal dystonic spasms that respond to carbamazepine occur much more frequently and severely in patients with NMO than in those with MS. Pain is also much more frequent in NMO than in MS.

Brainstem syndromes are also common, as are hypothalamic lesions, and this likely reflects areas of high expression of AQP4 in the CNS. Attacks of severe and intractable hiccough and of nausea and vomiting lasting weeks to months are particularly characteristic of NMO. These may be the presenting symptoms, and result from inflammation of the area postrema. Respiratory failure due to acute cervical myelitis or brainstem demyelination is the most common cause of NMO-related death. Death in this context has become less frequent due to improved prophylaxis of attacks with long-term immunosuppression and improved management of acute relapses (see section Treatment).

Hypothalamic manifestations of NMO include narcolepsy, associated with hypocretin deficiency, and syndrome of inappropriate antidiuretic hormone (SIADH). SIADH accompanied 16% of NMO attacks in a series of 43 NMO cases; SIADH occurred in 12% of initial NMO attacks.

Symptomatic brain lesions are compatible with a diagnosis of NMO, but are unusual at disease onset. Occasionally, NMO patients may develop encephalopathy due to transient vasogenic brain edema and may be diagnosed as having posterior reversible encephalopathy syndrome.

Long-term course/disability

The clinical course of NMO is characterized by the stepwise deterioration in the visual, motor, sensory, and bowel/bladder functions as the result of collective attack-related neurological disability. Unlike MS, a progressive course of gradually worsening disability rarely supervenes in the later phases of NMO. Therefore, if attacks can be prevented, the prognosis may be good.

Benign cases of NMO do exist but are much less common after lengthy follow-up than in patients with MS. Eleven of 175 (12%) of NMO patients had a score of 3 or lower on the Expanded Disability Status Scale after a 10-year follow-up. Nonetheless, 3 of these 11 patients experienced a disabling attack of NMO after 15 years of follow-up.

Chronic pain is also more common in NMO than MS. In a comparative study of 37 patients with NMO and 51 with MS, the percentage of patients who reported pain was higher in NMO (83.8%) than in MS (47.1%) ($p=0.0004$). The Pain Severity Index score was greater in NMO than in MS (NMO 3.8 ± 2.8, MS 1.6 ± 2.1, $p<0.0001$) when the analysis was confined to patients with a history of myelitis.

Association with autoimmunity

Patients with NMO have other autoimmune diseases more frequently than do patients with MS. The most common is autoimmune thyroiditis. However, NMO has been associated convincingly with myasthenia gravis and quite convincingly with celiac disease, lupus, and Sjögren syndrome. The clinical features of the neurological syndromes in connective tissue-associated NMO are similar to those seen in uncomplicated NMO. NMO patients with concomitant autoimmune diseases had similar frequency of NMO-IgG seropositivity as did those without such diseases. In contrast, patients with other autoimmune diseases without clinical features of NMO were consistently seronegative for such autoantibodies. The immunological basis of the association of NMO and other diseases is unknown but is likely due to common genetic and/or environmental susceptibility factors.

Diagnostic criteria

NMO

The diagnosis of NMO has been facilitated since diagnostic criteria were defined. The most recent set of criteria incorporates NMO-IgG testing, which has become available worldwide. The diagnostic criteria no longer specify an arbitrary interval between episodes of ON and transverse myelitis. However, because occurrence of ON and myelitis do not differentiate between NMO and *opticospinal MS*, the criteria included

specificity criteria that usually distinguish between NMO and prototypic MS. The most important clinical criterion for such differentiation is the presence of a longitudinally extensive spinal cord lesion (MRI T2 signal lesion extending over three or more vertebral segments, in the context of an acute myelitis attack). The most important nonclinical criterion is the presence of autoantibodies directed to AQP4. Symptomatic brain lesions are compatible with a diagnosis of NMO but are unusual at disease onset.

NMO DIAGNOSTIC CRITERIA

Optic neuritis
Acute myelitis

At least two of three supportive criteria:
1. Contiguous spinal cord MRI lesions extending over ≥3 segments in the context of an acute myelitis attack
2. Brain MRI at initial presentation not meeting diagnostic criteria for MS
3. NMO-IgG seropositive status

Source: Wingerchuk *et al.* (2006)

NMO spectrum disorder

NMO-IgG serology allows the identification of conditions named NMO spectrum disorders. Patients that are NMO-IgG positive and have one of the conditions listed below likely have similar clinical course and response (or lack of response) to therapy as do patients meeting criteria for NMO.

1. Limited (or inaugural) forms of NMO:
   a. Idiopathic single or recurrent events of LETM
   b. Isolated, recurrent or simultaneous bilateral ON
2. ON or LETM associated with systemic autoimmune disease
3. ON or myelitis associated with brain lesions typical of NMO (hypothalamic, corpus callosum, brainstem)

Opticospinal MS

Uncertainty persists, at least in some circles, as to whether Asian opticospinal MS is distinct from NMO, even after NMO diagnostic criteria and discovery of NMO-IgG have been reported. Some reports suggest that as currently defined (ON, myelitis, no brain lesions, or perhaps only minor brainstem lesions), opticospinal MS is heterogeneous and probably an admixture between NMO and MS. Multiple studies have shown that regardless of whether patients are labeled as having NMO or OSMS, those who have LETM (isolated or recurrent), intractable vomiting, and hiccough and are seropositive for NMO-IgG have a worse prognosis, higher frequency of severe visual loss, and poor response to interferon-beta. Patients with this clinical and serological profile should be treated with immunosuppressive drugs rather than immunomodulatory MS therapies. Interferon-beta has been convincingly shown to be ineffective for attack prevention in NMO. Recent studies suggest that natalizumab is ineffective, and possibly harmful, possibly because it does not prevent the influx of neutrophils that seem to play an important role in the pathogenesis of NMO.

Differences in relapsing versus monophasic NMO

Contemporary studies classify NMO as either monophasic (no further attacks after ON and TM index events) or relapsing. Predicting monophasic versus relapsing disease course is important, since monophasic NMO patients do not require long-term immunosuppression. Prototypic monophasic disease patients develop uni- or bilateral ON and myelitis within a very short interval, typically within a month or two, but the limits of monophasic disease and its distinction from relapsing disease are not entirely resolved. In a large series of NMO patients, demographic factors (female sex, older age of disease onset), less severe motor impairment with the first myelitis attack, and a longer interval between the first and second attacks were associated with relapsing rather than monophasic disease. In prospective studies, the presence of NMO-IgG also predicted recurrences after a single episode of LETM and of recurrent ON.

☆ TIPS AND TRICKS

NMO-IgG seropositive predicts recurrence

In a patients with a single episode of transverse myelitis, or of ON, a positive result for NMO-IgG predicts recurrence of attacks. Patients seropositive for NMO-IgG after a first demyelinating event should be treated with long term immunosuppression.

Association of NMO with other autoantibodies and autoimmune conditions

NMO patients may have other autoimmune diseases (e.g., myasthenia gravis, SLE, Sjögren syndrome). NMO patients frequently have other non-specific autoantibodies (e.g., ANA, SSA and SSB) and they frequently are not accompanied by clinical evidence of their clinical counterparts (e.g., SLE and Sjogren's syndrome).

Spinal cord LETM

While detecting a longitudinally extensive spinal cord lesion is strongly suggestive of NMO diagnosis, if the spinal cord MRI is not performed during the acute event or a patient is taking immunosuppressants, the lesion may not meet the three spinal cord length criterion. In contrast, MS patients who have multiple clinical or subclinical episodes of transverse myelitis may have aggregated lesions that may be confused as a longitudinally extensive transverse myelitis lesion; typically these lesions do not enhance with gadolinium and are an aggregate of peripheral and central lesions in the cord. Other considerations aid in the differential diagnosis between NMO and MS (e.g., NMO-IgG serology; brain MRI).

Monitoring immunosuppressant treatment

There is insufficient evidence that NMO-IgG antibody titers correlate with disease activity, and therefore monitoring titer is not currently advisable in reaching treatment decisions, such as intensifying or terminating immunosuppressive treatment. If a patient develops a severe relapse while on full dose of the medication, a second line drug should be started.

Investigations

Serology

NMO-IgG was the original name given to the disease antibody biomarker found in serum of NMO patients. In 2004, Mayo Clinic investigators identified a specific immunofluorescence pattern when testing sera from NMO patients using a protocol to detect paraneoplastic disorders. Subsequently, a larger prospective study was performed with sera of NMO and opticospinal MS patients, of individuals with high-risk syndromes (recurrent LETM and recurrent ON), and of MS patients and individuals with other neurological or autoimmune disease. The sensitivity of the autoantibody was 73% (95% CI, 60–86) and specificity was 91% (79–100) for NMO. Several independent investigators have confirmed the presence of NMO-IgG using a variety of different assays for anti-AQP4 antibodies detection, such as immunoprecipitation assay, ELISA, and cell-based assays.

CSF

Spinal fluid examination may provide important supportive information for NMO diagnosis. While MS is usually associated with a normal cell count or slight pleocytosis, acute attacks of NMO, particularly myelitis, will be accompanied by a marked elevated cell count, ranging from 50 to 1000×10^6 WBC/l in roughly a quarter of individuals and occasionally with predominance of neutrophils. Another useful although incompletely sensitive or specific finding is the presence of oligoclonal bands (OCB): 80% of MS patients have OCB compared to only 20% of NMO patients. Albumin CSF/serum ratios, total protein, and CSF L-lactate levels correlate with disease activity and with the length of the acute myelitis lesion.

MRI

In the context of an acute attack of NMO, the spinal cord MRI usually demonstrates a lesion extending over three or more continuous vertebral segments, usually centrally located and associated with patchy gadolinium enhancement. Acute lesions are hypointense on T1- and hyperintense on T2-weighted images (Figure 15.1). In subsequent evolution stages of

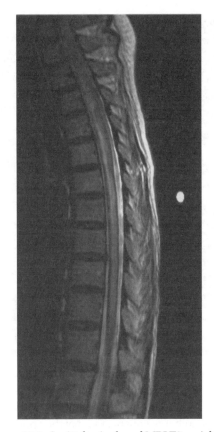

Figure 15.1 Sagittal spinal cord MRI T2-weighted sequence of an NMO patient with acute myelitis. A longitudinally extensive thoracic lesion is present.

the lesion, central cavities or extensive cord atrophy may develop, although occasionally lesions may regress completely, and this is more commonly seen in those with *benign* course.

In the context of an ON, gadolinium enhancement of the optic nerve(s) or of the optic chiasm may be detected (Figure 15.2).

Brain MRI lesions are detected in approximately 60% of NMO patients throughout the disease course. Most brain lesions observed in NMO are nonspecific and asymptomatic; however, lesions in the brainstem and hypothalamus appear to be characteristic. As mentioned previously, some NMO patients may develop posterior reversible encephalopathy-like lesions with characteristics suggestive of vasogenic edema, perhaps due to impairment of AQP4 function.

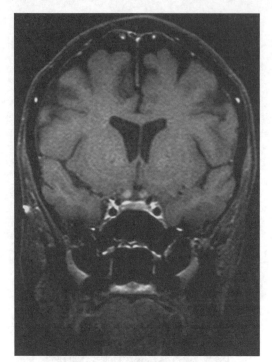

Figure 15.2 Coronal brain MRI T1-weighted sequence after gadolinium administration of an NMO patient with acute bilateral ON. Swelling and gadolinium enhancement of the optic nerves and optic chiasm is visible.

OCT and VEP

Recently, optical coherence tomography (OCT) has been suggested to be a useful tool for differential diagnosis between NMO and MS. In a large study, 26 NMO spectrum patients with a history of ON, 17 patients with isolated LETM without ON, 378 patients with RRMS, and 77 healthy controls were studied. Greater retinal fiber layer thinning was detected in NMO ON eyes (mean retinal nerve fiber layer thickness 63.6 micron) relative to both RRMS ON eyes (88.3 μm, $p < 0.0001$) and control eyes (102.4 μm, $p < 0.0001$). A first episode of NMO ON was estimated to cause 24 μm more loss of RNFL thickness than MS ON. Eyes in the LETM group and unaffected NMO eyes were not significantly different from controls. Whether OCT reveals anything more than the well-known fact that NMO-associated ON is more severe is unclear. Overlap between OCT findings in NMO and MS probably does not offer the necessary specificity to add greatly to the differential diagnosis between NMO and MS.

Visual evoked potentials (VEP) findings tend to show more prominent abnormalities in NMO than in MS. In a comparative study, patients with NMO more frequently had lack of response or lower amplitude of the P100 component than those with MS.

Differential diagnosis

Patients with NMO typically present with either transverse myelitis or ON; each syndrome has a very extensive differential diagnosis. Early and accurate NMO diagnosis is critical to allow optimal attack-prevention treatment especially considering the propensity to severe attack-related disability. The details of the differential diagnosis of isolated ON or myelitis are beyond the scope of this chapter, and readers are referred to the following reviews: ON (Burton *et al.* 2011) and myelitis (Jacob & Weinshenker 2008).

The most common differential diagnosis to consider for combined ON and TM is MS, and the neurologist should pay special attention to the NMO-distinguishing clinical, neuroimaging, and laboratorial characteristics. As previously mentioned, compared to MS, NMO-related ON is more severe and more often bilateral and will more often lead to permanent visual impairment. The presence of MS-typical brain MRI lesions at the time of the first or recurrent ON makes a diagnosis of MS more likely than if MRI scan of the brain is negative for parenchymal lesions; however, brain lesions may occur in NMO, and some brain lesions that are nonspecific for demyelinating disease occur in healthy individuals. Transverse myelitis in MS typically results in asymmetrical clinical findings that are not as disabling as occurs in NMO. MRI lesions in MS typically extend over one or two vertebrae segments and are localized to the lateral or dorsal parts of the cord; in contrast, lesions in NMO typically are centrally located in the cord and extend over three or more spinal segments, although the long length of lesions may be mitigated by immunosuppressive treatment.

Other conditions that mimic NMO are less common. Sarcoidosis can cause optic neuropathy and myelopathy accompanied by inflammatory lesions, although the evolution of the myelopathy is typically not as acute as that in transverse myelitis where the nadir of neurological deficit occurs within 3 weeks, as required by the current diagnostic criteria for transverse myelitis. Factors that raise significant index of suspicion for sarcoidosis rather than NMO include the following: insidiously progressive course, persistent nodular enhancement, and pial enhancement in the spinal cord; persistent pleocytosis; elevated angiotensin-converting enzyme level in serum and CSF; and history of cranial nerve palsy, especially seventh cranial neuropathy. If the suspicion for sarcoidosis is high, biopsy of an accessible lesion should be considered. Up to half of patients with Behçet disease have neurological symptoms, most commonly affecting the basal ganglia and brainstem; optic neuropathy and inflammatory myelopathy can also occur. Oral aphthous ulcers, genital ulcers, uveitis, and pathergy reaction are other clinical features that permit a diagnosis of Behçet disease. Paraneoplastic myelopathy, particularly when associated with autoantibodies directed to collapsin response mediator protein 5 (CRMP5), may cause an NMO-like illness with both longitudinally extensive myelopathy and optic neuropathy.

Treatment

EVIDENCE AT A GLANCE

No randomized placebo-controlled clinical trial has been conducted specifically to evaluate NMO treatment. Both the recommendations for treating acute exacerbations and for relapse prevention are based on clinical trials that included patients with a variety of demyelinating diseases or on small open-label NMO series studies.

Acute treatment

Following an attack of NMO, high-dose IV methylprednisolone (1 g IV for 5 days) is considered standard treatment and should be initiated as soon as it is clear that a patient is having an attack. Based on a randomized, controlled trial that included patients with NMO and acute TM

and other nonrandomized experience, plasma exchange (PLEX) is recommended to treat attacks that do not respond to IV steroids. The usual treatment consists of seven exchanges in alternate days (1–1.5 plasma volumes exchange per treatment).

Paroxysmal tonic spasms may follow an attack after days to weeks and, when they occur as the sole manifestation of disease (i.e., unaccompanied by any lasting new weakness or sensory loss), can be managed by low doses of carbamazepine (200 mg twice daily is usually sufficient) without need for additional corticosteroids.

Long-term treatment

For long-term relapse prevention, immunosuppressive drugs are recommended rather than the immunomodulatory agents used for MS patients (e.g., interferon-beta, glatiramer acetate, natalizumab).

Azathioprine (2.5 mg/kg/day) with oral corticosteroids (prednisone beginning at 60 mg daily or every other day for 6–9 months, subsequently decreasing to lowest possible maintenance dose or discontinuation) is a typical, effective, and relatively inexpensive treatment. Early azathioprine initiation and adequate dosage (aiming for 2–2.5 mg/kg/day, accompanied by an anticipated increase in mean corpuscular volume) are necessary to insure adequate efficacy.

Mycophenolate mofetil (2 g/day) with oral corticosteroids is another effective option that may be used as initial or alternative treatment rather than azathioprine.

For refractory cases, the CD20+ B-cell depleting monoclonal antibody, rituximab (1000 mg intravenously twice separated by 2 weeks, repeated every 6–9 months) is the most extensively studied alternative treatment. It acts rapidly and perhaps requires shorter intervals of maintenance treatment with corticosteroids. It has been reported to increase the risk of relapse in the first month, although the frequency of early relapse is unclear. When B cells repopulate, the risk of relapses returns, and awaiting repopulation before retreatment is hazardous; accordingly, many would advise routine retreatment every 6 months even before repopulation occurs, although there are some individuals who are early *repopulators* where even this approach may be inadequate to prevent return of attacks.

A drug that has been reported to be effective in treatment-refractory cases, based on a very small number of cases, is mitoxantrone ($12\,mg/m^2$ every 3 months, with maximum cumulative dose limited to $140\,mg/m^2$, primarily due to cardiotoxicity) and there are some evidence of efficacy in nonrandomized small series of NMO patients.

Future treatment perspectives

Perhaps the most exciting perspective is the potential for disease-specific therapy targeting the major players in the pathogenesis of NMO: AQP4, NMO-IgG, and complement. The initiators of the autoimmune response are almost certainly proximal to NMO-IgG in the pathogenesis of NMO and likely include autoreactive T cells, but after the patient presents with disease, NMO-IgG, AQP4, and complement seem to be the most critical elements and the most obvious targets for intervention. Some new treatments mentioned in the succeeding text illustrate how selective targeting of these disease essential elements has begun.

Four ongoing therapeutic studies for NMO are listed on the ClinicalTrials.gov registry. Two evaluate stem cell transplantation either using autologous hematopoietic or umbilical cord mesenchymal stem cells. One case of NMO has been reported in which autologous stem cell transplant for lymphoma was followed shortly by a severe attack of NMO just months after the treatment, despite previous clinical stability on azathioprine treatment. The results of an open-label study of the effects of eculizumab, a monoclonal antibody directed against the complement protein C5, have been recently reported, and the reports in this open-label study of patients many of whom failed other treatments are very promising; there were 2 minor neurological episodes over one year of treatment in 14 individuals, many of whom had failed other treatments before enrollment in this study (Pittock *et al.* 2013).

Finally, a study on maintenance PLEX will record the feasibility, tolerability, safety, and preliminary efficacy data regarding whether maintenance PLEX can be used to prevent attacks of NMO.

A novel nonpathogenic recombinant human monoclonal anti-AQP4 antibody (aquaporumab) was created to selectively protect AQP4 from binding NMO-IgG. Aquaporumab lacks functionality for complement- and cell-mediated cytotoxicity due to an engineered mutation in the Fc portion of the immunoglobulin. In vitro and in vivo studies showed a reduced complement-mediated cytotoxicity by 90% and prevention of NMO-like lesions.

⚙ SCIENCE REVISITED

Aquaporin-4 (AQP4) is transmembrane protein that functions as a water-selective channel. AQP4 is expressed in several tissues but primarily in the CNS, where it is the predominant aquaporin. It is concentrated in the astrocyte foot processes by the dystrophin cytoskeleton to which it is anchored. AQP4 water channels exist as heterotetramers of M1 and M23 protein isoforms. These tetramers are organized in orthogonal arrays that may be visualized by freeze-fracture electron microscopy. AQP4 is the first molecule to be defined as a specific target for the autoimmune response in any form of CNS demyelinating disease.

Prognosis and follow-up

Measuring disability

Similarly to MS, the Kurtzke Expanded Disability Status Scale (EDSS) has been used to quantify disability in NMO, but it includes a variety of functional systems rarely affected in NMO, which do not contribute greatly to the composite score. A more specific NMO scale (Wingerchuk *et al.* 1999) may be more informative in quantifying optic nerve and spinal cord impairment. Both scales can be used to determine the attack severity and to quantify long-term disability. Disease activity is typically evaluated by the annualized relapse rate (ARR). Because randomized parallel design clinical trials are rarely considered ethical in NMO, typically, before and after treatment, ARR is used to measure treatment success in retrospective and prospective studies, but this is a potentially flawed measure due to regression to the mean and differences in ascertainment of retrospective pretreatment relapse frequency.

Antibody serology and titers

Serum levels of NMO-IgG may correlate with disease course and treatment response. In a study of 96 serum samples from eight NMO-IgG-positive patients, increasing NMO-IgG serum levels appeared to be associated with relapse (vs. remission status) and with the CD19 cell counts in patients being treated with rituximab. In another study, antibody titers were higher in patients with complete blindness in comparison with those with ON who experienced some degree of recovery and in patients with longer compared to shorter spinal cord lesions.

Severity of NMO attacks may be correlated to the degree of complement activation by NMO-IgG. Complement-mediated cell death of AQP4-expressing cells was compared in vitro in serum of NMO patients with mild attacks compared to those with severe attacks. The median percentage of AQP4-transfected cells lesioned was 14% for patients with mild attacks and 54% for patients with severe attacks. This potentially promising test requires more study before it can be applied in clinical situations.

✋ CAUTION!

MS treatments
   Patients with NMO should not be treated with interferon beta, natalizumab, fingolimod nor glatiramer acetate. Patients may worsen if treated with interferon beta, fingolimod or natalizumab.

References

Burton, E.V., Greenberg, B.M. & Frohman, E.M. (2011) Optic neuritis: a mechanistic view. *Pathophysiology*, **18** (1), 81–92.

Devic, E. (1894) Myélite subaiguë compliquée de névrite optique. *Le Bulletin Médicale*, **8**, 1033–1034.

Jacob, A. & Weinshenker, B.G. (2008) An approach to the diagnosis of acute transverse myelitis. *Seminars in Neurology*, **28** (1), 105–120.

Watanabe, S., Nakashima, I., Misu, T. *et al.* (2007) Therapeutic efficacy of plasma exchange in NMO-IgG-positive patients with neuromyelitis optica. *Multiple Sclerosis (Houndmills, Basingstoke, England)*, **13** (1), 128–132.

Wingerchuk, D.M., Hogancamp, W.F., O'Brien, P.C. & Weinshenker, B.G. (1999) The clinical course of neuromyelitis optica (Devic's syndrome). *Neurology*, **53** (5), 1107–1114.

Further Reading

Apiwattanakul, M., Popescu, B.F., Matiello, M. *et al.* (2011) Intractable vomiting as the initial presentation of neuromyelitis optica. *Annals of Neurology*, **68** (5), 757–761.

Gault, F. (1894) De la neuromyélite aiguë. Lyon University, Lyon.

Lennon, V.A., Kryzer, T.J., Pittock, S.J., Verkman, A.S. & Hinson, S.R. (2005) IgG marker of optic-spinal multiple sclerosis binds to the aquaporin-4 water channel. *Journal of Experimental Medicine*, **202** (4), 473–477.

Magaña, S.M., Matiello, M., Pittock, S.J. *et al.* (2009) Posterior reversible encephalopathy syndrome in neuromyelitis optica spectrum disorders. *Neurology*, **72**, 712–717.

Matiello, M., Lennon, V.A., Jacob, A. *et al.* (2008) NMO-IgG predicts the outcome of recurrent optic neuritis. *Neurology*, **70** (23), 2197–2200.

Matiello, M., Kim, H.J., Kim, W. *et al.* (2010) Familial neuromyelitis optica. *Neurology*, **75** (4), 310–315.

Matiello, M., Pittock, S.J., Porrata, L. & Weinshenker, B.G. (2011) Failure of autologous hematopoietic stem cell transplantation to prevent relapse of neuromyelitis optica. *Archives of Neurology*, **68** (7), 953–955.

Papeix, C., Vidal, J.S., de Seze, J. *et al.* (2007) Immunosuppressive therapy is more effective than interferon in neuromyelitis optica. *Multiple Sclerosis*, **13** (2), 256–259.

Pittock, S.J., Lennon, V.A., McKeon, A., *et al.* (2013) Eculizumab in AQP4-IgG-positive relapsing neuromyelitis optica spectrum disorders: An open-label pilot study. *Lancet Neurology*. [Epub ahead of print]

Tradtrantip, L., Zhang, H., Saadoun, S. *et al.* (2012) Anti-aquaporin-4 monoclonal antibody blocker therapy for neuromyelitis optica. *Annals of Neurology*, **71**, 314–322.

Weinshenker, B.G., O'Brien, P.C., Petterson, T.M. *et al.* (1999) A randomized trial of plasma exchange in acute central nervous system inflammatory demyelinating disease. *Annals of Neurology*, **46** (6), 878–886.

Weinshenker, B.G., Wingerchuk, D.M., Vukusic, S. *et al.* (2006) Neuromyelitis optica IgG predicts relapse after longitudinally extensive transverse myelitis. *Annals of Neurology*, **59** (3), 566–569.

Wingerchuk, D.M., Lennon, V.A., Pittock, S.J., Lucchinetti, C.F. & Weinshenker, B.G. (2006) Revised diagnostic criteria for neuromyelitis optica. *Neurology*, **66** (10), 1485–1489.

16

Neurosarcoidosis

Thomas F. Scott

Department of Neurology, Drexel University College of Medicine, Pittsburgh, PA, USA
Allegheny MS Treatment Center, Pittsburgh, PA, USA

Introduction

Neurosarcoidosis (NS) is a rare and enigmatic disorder, essentially idiopathic. The primary substrate or mechanism of multiple organ tissue destruction appears to be a granulomatous inflammatory process. Although new knowledge of the immunopathology is slowly emerging as in other idiopathic inflammatory disorders, NS and even the more common pulmonary or systemic sarcoidosis remain largely mysterious. At present, a genetic predisposition is suggested by familial studies, and environmental triggers are postulated, but we are left with little in the realm of solid scientific evidence to explain the etiology of sarcoidosis.

This summary of the clinical aspects of NS is divided into general principles of diagnosis, treatment, and prognosis, followed by discussions of clinical challenges in treating NS as it typically presents in various anatomical regions in the central and peripheral nervous system.

General principles of diagnosis

NS is sometimes used as the prototypic example of a *zebra*; clinicians should avoid thinking about until all the *horses have been rounded up* for elimination. The consideration of NS usually is appropriately placed near the end of the list of possibilities when encountering a patient with one of the typical presentations (e.g., subacute myelopathy, CPA tumor, peripheral neuropathy (PN), isolated cranial neuropathy). Roughly half of NS is diagnosed prior to any knowledge of systemic sarcoidosis. A large proportion of patients presenting initially with neurological symptoms due to NS will have systemic sarcoidosis diagnosed as part of the workup for their neurological complaints. A consideration of NS should alert physicians to review a patient's medical history for systemic evidence of diagnosis (dry cough, skin lesions, other organ involvement). Biopsy of non-CNS tissues is often possible and generally preferred to biopsy of nervous tissue. Applying the widely used Zajicek criteria, or similar criteria, the term *definite NS* is reserved for patients who have undergone biopsy of nervous tissue found to have granulomatous inflammatory pathology. Many or most patients are ultimately classed as only *probable NS*, after obtaining evidence of granulomatous inflammatory in non-nervous system tissue, and empirical treatment is undertaken rather than risking biopsy of CNS tissue. A minority of cases in large series met criteria for *definite NS*.

The physician's tools for arriving at a diagnosis of NS include a standard array of history taking and physical examination skills combined with targeted laboratory testing, essentially unchanged over the last two decades. Concerning all the various presentations of NS, the diagnosis is obviously much easier when a diagnosis of systemic sarcoidosis has already been established by tissue biopsy.

Multiple Sclerosis and CNS Inflammatory Disorders, First Edition. Edited by Lawrence M. Samkoff and Andrew D. Goodman.

If radiographic and other paraclinical evidence for NS is accompanied by typical clinical manifestations, a biopsy of the nervous tissue can generally be avoided in patients with well-established systemic disease. Given a lack of any such history, a search for evidence of systemic disease is undertaken as soon as NS is suspected. History taking and review of systems should include particular attention to stigmata of systemic sarcoidosis, and physical examination should include a skin examination. Initial laboratory studies, including imaging, are directed according to clinical localization of lesions (e.g., electromyography and nerve conduction studies for peripheral NS, cerebral or spinal MRI for central nervous system sarcoidosis; see Table 16.1). Initial studies also include a search for asymptomatic disease (e.g., CT of the chest, abdomen, and pelvis) (Figure 16.1).

Table 16.1 Selected Differential Diagnosis for NS According to Localization

1. Nonbacterial meningitis/meningeal: infection (in particular fungal), neoplasm (carcinomatous meningitis), and Vogt–Koyanagi–Harada disease, vasculitis
2. Cerebral intra-axial lesions: neoplasm (in particular lymphoma or glioma), demyelinating disease, vasculitis and other vascular disorders, histiocytosis. Extra-axial intracranial: meningloma, idiopathic hypertrophic pachymeningitis
3. Pituitary area: pituitary hypophysitis, histiocytosis, lymphoma, infectious disease, germ cell tumor
4. Myelopathy: demyelinating disease, neuromyelitis optica, and vasculitis
5. PN (particularly mononeuritis multiplex and polyradiculopathy): vasculitis, diabetes, toxic/metabolic disorders, Lyme disease

★ **TIPS AND TRICKS**

A tool box for diagnosis and staging of NS
1) Physical examination.
2) History including family history and review of systems.
3) Imaging: CT chest, abdomen, and pelvis, gallium scan, spinal and cerebral MRI.
4) Blood work: complete metabolic profile including calcium and electrolytes, serum oligoclonal bands and IgG, angiotensin converting enzyme, erythrocyte sedimentation rate.
5) Electrophysiology: electromyography, nerve conductions, evoked potentials.
6) Tissue biopsy.
7) Minimum cerebrospinal fluid examination: differential, cell count and oligoclonal bands, total protein, IgG concentration, and glucose (note: consider cerebrospinal fluid angiotensin converting enzyme, although no laboratory can claim to have rigorously determined cutoffs for normal values, consider cultures and stains for infectious illness and cytology).

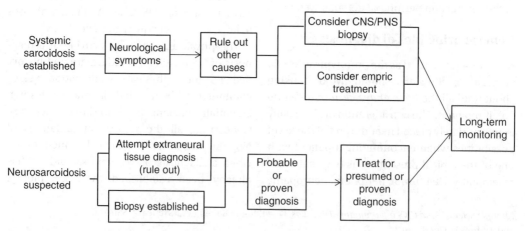

Figure 16.1 Algorithm for diagnosis of neurosarcoidosis.

The tendency for an initial misdiagnosis of NS as multiple sclerosis (MS) has been discussed in many reports, involving 8 out of 50 patients in one large series of NS (see Figure 16.2 for a representative case). Many of these patients present with acute or subacute complaints related to optic neuropathy or myelopathy, clinically indistinguishable from a clinically isolated syndrome due to MS, and with evidence of systemic sarcoidosis emerging only years later. Combining the clinical picture with the typical laboratory findings of NS, namely, rounded deep white matter lesions often seen on MRI, and cerebrospinal fluid (CSF) with immune activation, we see that NS can be the ultimate mimic for MS (for detailed description of CSF abnormalities, see succeeding text). Thus far, there has not been a detailed biopsy or autopsy description of a patient with both diseases simultaneously, although there have been descriptions of tissue studies of deep white matter lesions in NS being pathologically distinct from MS.

General principles of treatment

Corticosteroids and alternative immunosuppressant agents constitute the mainstay of treatment for most cases. Treatments are aimed at either quickly reducing inflammation-mediated injury to the nervous system or relieving mass effect caused by granulomatous tissue surgically. Initial stabilization is followed usually by an empiric attempt to prevent relapse by slowly withdrawing immunologically active agents over months or years. One exceptional situation in which urgent evaluation for possible lifesaving surgery is required can be seen in patients who develop hydrocephalus (either communicating or noncommunicating).

Due to the rarity of NS, there have been no randomized controlled comparative studies of any treatments (no class I or class II evidence is available). The readily apparent response to steroids in most cases combined with the seriousness of potential neurological deficits occurring in NS makes standard placebo trials

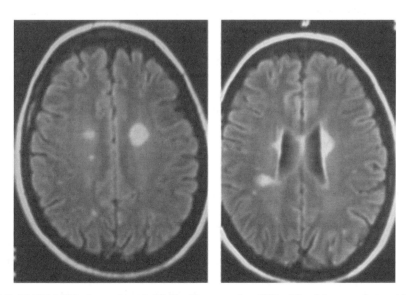

Figure 16.2 FLAIR MRI of a patient initially diagnosed as MS with a history of steroid-responsive optic neuritis in 1989 followed 2 years later by a right internuclear ophthalmoplegia. The patient developed biopsy-proven pulmonary sarcoidosis 6 years after her optic neuritis and stopped beta-interferons at that time due to a strong suspicion of NS. The patient was then followed long term for a total of 19 years from onset without further relapse or change in MRI.

Table 16.2 Reported Treatments

Various corticosteroid regimens, often prolonged
Azathioprine
Methotrexate
Cyclophosphamide
Mycophenolate
Chlorambucil
Low-dose radiation therapy
Cyclosporin
Infliximab
Combinations of the above

impractical in the acute setting. It is foreseeable that a multicenter trial might be able to compare different treatment regimens involving steroids plus other agents in NS during long-term care (perhaps following patients for many months or years).

Two basic treatment strategies have emerged from small and large case series of treated patients: (1) initial treatment with corticosteroids (moderate- or high-dose regimens), weaning over weeks or months and reserving alternative therapies for relapsing or refractory cases. (2) Initial treatment may be tailored to the severity of the initial presentation (e.g., using alternative immunosuppressive agents *up front* in conjunction with corticosteroids in patients with symptomatic intracranial or spinal NS and using corticosteroid steroids alone in patients with mild isolated cranial nerve disorders or PN). Small case series expound the virtues of stepwise treatments moving toward more novel treatments in refractory cases, with some patients requiring three or more attempts to arrive at a regimen resulting in disease control. There are rare reports of low-dose radiation therapy allowing preservation of optic nerve function in refractory disease. If relapse occurs, which is often years after initial control, it is reasonable to return to previously used medications to induce another remission (Table 16.2).

Dosages

Optimal dosages are not determined (refer to specific recommendations of the limited studies available for each medication, but typical dosages for Cytoxan might involve monthly pulses at 700 mg/m^2 for 6 months, methotrexate 10–20 mg once weekly for several months, mycophenolate 1000 mg bid for several months, and azathioprine 2–2.5 mg/kg for several months. Note that since these immunosuppressants all have serious toxicity profiles, they should only be prescribed by experienced physicians who have special expertise in neuroimmune disorders.

Specific presentations

Aseptic meningitis

CSF analysis is often part of the workup for suspected NS, for example, as part of the workup for cranial neuropathy, yielding the designation of *aseptic meningitis*, as the investigative process evolves. In fact, most neurologic presentations for sarcoidosis might be expected to justify consideration of CSF analysis. The aseptic meningitis picture of NS is typically seen with a CSF formula of mild to moderately elevated white blood cells, usually lymphocyte predominant. Other typical CSF findings may sometimes help differentiate NS from MS, although considerable overlap exists (see Table 16.3). When NS meningitis is seen in association with headaches or other symptoms of increased intracranial pressure, physicians should consider the possibility of evolving hydrocephalus, a rare but life-threatening complication. Frequent imaging and CSF analysis in these patients are suggested. Unfortunately, we have had experience with a few cases of extreme increased intracranial pressure leading to death in the setting of only minimal or no signs of hydrocephalus radiographically, making management in these cases difficult. Extremely high CSF protein levels may be a clue in identifying life-threatening aseptic meningitis. On the other hand, many cases of aseptic meningitis due to NS seem to be easily managed with only moderate doses of corticosteroids. Therefore, in a relatively uncomplicated setting, we generally treat aseptic meningitis with corticosteroids alone.

Myelopathy

Myelopathy due to NS usually presents as a subacute process with subtle symptoms and examination findings evolving over months

Table 16.3 CSF in NS versus MS

Test	NS	MS
Oligoclonal bands, high IgG concentration	Often	Often
Polymorphonuclear cells, eosinophils	Often	None
Lymphocytosis	May be mild or moderate	Mild
Glucose	Sometimes low	Normal
Total protein	Occasionally very high	Normal or mild increase

(spastic weakness, sensory complaints). The diagnosis is often made in the setting of known systemic disease, typically with nonspecific intramedullary abnormalities seen on MRI, which may or may not enhance. MRI lesions may be small or span multiple segments. In the absence of systemic disease, biopsy is often undertaken to make a diagnosis, especially if the lesion radiologically mimics a neoplasm with enhancement and expansion of the spinal cord. MS is not suspected when prominent nerve root enhancement and meningeal enhancement are seen. Myelopathy can occasionally be related to compression from extra-axial lesions of sarcoidosis involving paraspinal tissues or bone.

More subtle presentations can easily be mistaken for a form of MS (often primary progressive) or a *clinically isolated syndrome*, especially in the setting of nonspecific MRI findings and spinal fluid abnormalities (e.g., oligoclonal bands, increased IgG concentration). A moderately elevated CSF leukocyte count, low CSF glucose, and very high CSF may all point away from a diagnosis of MS (see Table 16.3). Alternatively, spinal fluid may be normal.

Cerebral neurosarcoidosis

Intra-axial lesions of NS mimic a wide variety of disorders. Multifocal intracranial lesions might present with headache, seizures, encephalopathy, ataxia, or focal signs and symptoms. Lesions may be seen on MRI as subtle and nonspecific abnormalities of cerebral white matter or very rounded and ovoid *Dawson's fingers*, mimicking MS. Rarely, deep white matter lesions are seen in the setting of vasculitis related to sarcoidosis. Deep enhancing or nonenhancing lesions of the brainstem and diencephalon may mimic lymphoma, MS, histiocytosis, or glioma. Occasionally,

large parenchymal lesions can mimic glioblastoma. A search for systemic disease is often negative, leading to diagnostic biopsy. In some cases of NS presenting with clinical, MRI, and CSF findings all consistent with NS, a diagnosis of MS is given but changed years later after systemic disease becomes apparent. Very high CSF leukocyte counts and protein levels are among the red flags that should point clinicians away from MS.

Several reports of parenchymal cerebral hemorrhages, including severe brainstem hemorrhages, have called attention to the tendency of the granulomatous inflammation of NS to invade and disrupt small blood vessels. Ischemic strokes are also rarely seen, sometimes in the setting of widespread intracranial leptomeningeal inflammation. Reports of both intracerebral hemorrhage and ischemic stroke are among the rarest available, making up only 0–2% of patients in large series.

> ⭐ **TIPS AND TRICKS**
>
> Consider sarcoidosis when a patient presents with disease clinically and radiographically similar to multiple sclerosis or lymphoma.

Cranial neuropathy

All cranial nerves can be affected by NS. Cranial nerve VII palsy is perhaps the most frequently seen and often is the sole manifestation of essentially a benign form of the disorder. Bilateral eighth nerve disease can cause devastating hearing loss and deserves aggressive treatment. Optic nerve disease is also fairly common and can be very disabling. The optic nerve can be compressed by granulomatous lesions, and biopsy reports have also verified granulomatous inflammation within the optic nerve in a few patients. Other cases involve loss of vision due to granulomas of other ocular structures such as the retina and uvea. Although prospective studies are lacking, it has been noted that low-dose corticosteroid regimens are often sufficient to handle cranial nerve lesions. Notably exceptional cases have been reported to involve refractory optic neuropathy failing steroids and seeming to require immune suppression and even low-dose radiation therapy to halt or reverse loss of visual function.

Peripheral neuropathy and myopathy

PN due to NS can appear in many different forms, including mononeuropathies, mononeuritis multiplex, polyradiculopathy, and acute and chronic symmetrical polyneuropathy. Most cases present with subacute complaints and respond well to corticosteroids alone. Histologically, the PN of NS is primarily an axonopathy, presumably due to granulomatous infiltration in and around nerve tissues. Sarcoid myopathy usually has a slow onset with proximal predominant weakness and may vary from mild to severe. Diagnosis requires EMG and may be assisted by finding elevated serum CK level, ACE level, or ESR. Biopsies have revealed granulomatous inflammation invading muscle tissues. Remission is usually obtained through immunosuppression. Myopathy was found in a small proportion of patients in most large series but is likely present in a mild asymptomatic or minimally symptomatic form in many patients.

Prognosis and long-term monitoring

After initial remission, it is expected that more than half of NS patients will remain disease-free during long follow-up periods (5–15 years) and perhaps lifelong (data limited). It is generally recommended that at least a few years of MRI follow-up be performed on patients with intracranial disease, as asymptomatic progression may be easily detected in rare patients. Other forms of NS will usually be immediately apparent to patients, though perhaps subtle. Physicians should caution patients to report all new or recurrent symptoms, including headaches (which may herald severe relapse relating to meningeal NS, mass lesions, and increased intracranial pressure with or without hydrocephalus). Relapses tend to respond similarly to initial attacks, with only rare cases requiring stepwise escalation of therapy.

Further Reading

Gelwan, M.J., Kellen, R.I., Burde, R.M. & Kupersmith, M.J. (1988) Sarcoidosis of the anterior visual pathway: successes and failures. *Journal of Neurology, Neurosurgery & Psychiatry*, **51**, 1473–1480.

Moravan, M. & Segal, B.M. (2009) Treatment of CNS sarcoidosis with infliximab and mycophenolate mofetil. *Neurology*, **72**, 337–340.

Oh, S.J. (1980) Sarcoid polyneuropathy: a histologically proven case. *Annals of Neurology*, **7**, 178–181.

Scott, T.F. (1993) Neurosarcoidosis: progress and clinical aspects. *Neurology*, **43**, 8–12.

Scott, T.F. (2000) Cerebral herniation after lumbar puncture in sarcoid meningitis. *Clinical Neurology and Neurosurgery*, **102**, 26–28.

Scott, T.F., Seay, A.R. & Goust, J.M. (1989) Pattern and concentration of IgG in cerebrospinal fluid in neurosarcoidosis. *Neurology*, **39**, 1637–1639.

Scott, T.F., Yandora, K., Valeri, A., Chieffe, C. & Schramke, C. (2007) Aggressive therapy for neurosarcoidosis long-term follow-up of 48 treated patients. *Archives of Neurology*, **64**, 691–696.

Scott, T.F., Yandora, K., Kunschner, L.J. & Schramke, C. (2010) Neurosarcoidosis mimicry of multiple sclerosis: clinical, laboratory, and imaging characteristics. *Neurologist*, **16**, 386–389.

Stern, B.J., Aksamit, A., Clifford, D., Scott, T.F. & Neurosarcoidosis Study Group (2010) Neurologic presentations of sarcoidosis. *Neurologic Clinics*, **28**, 185–198.

Zajicek, J.P., Scolding, N.J., Foster, O. *et al.* (1999) Central nervous system sarcoidosis – diagnosis and management. *Quarterly Journal of Medicine*, **92**, 103–117.

17

Lyme Neuroborreliosis

Erica Patrick and Eric Logigian

Department of Neurology, University of Rochester Medical Center, Rochester, NY, USA

Introduction

Lyme disease, a tick-borne infection caused by the spirochete *Borrelia burgdorferi*, may cause peripheral or central nervous system (CNS) involvement within days to weeks of onset in 10–15% of patients or months to years of onset in a much smaller percentage. CNS Lyme disease can occasionally mimic multiple sclerosis (MS), and it is important to distinguish the two diseases. This chapter will review nervous system Lyme disease with an emphasis on its diagnosis and treatment.

Borrelia burgdorferi infection

B. burgdorferi sensu stricto is the causative spirochete in North America, while most European cases are caused by *Borrelia garinii or afzelii (B. burgdorferi sensu lato)*.

The spirochetal infection is transmitted by the *Ixodes* tick: *Ixodes scapularis* in the northeastern and central USA, *Ixodes pacificus* in the northwestern USA, *Ixodes ricinus* in Europe, and *Ixodes persulcatus* in Asia. The basic principles of infection are the same for the different tick species. In order for transmission to occur, the tick must feed on an infected reservoir. For example, in northeastern North America, the white-footed field mouse serves as the reservoir host for the larval and nymphal forms, whereas the definitive host for the adult tick is the white-tailed deer.

The spirochetes, which remain in the tick's gut, will then replicate with continued feeding and ultimately migrate to the tick's salivary glands for injection into the new host. Transmission of the spirochete occurs slowly. For example, the process requires approximately 48 h of persistent attachment in the case of the *I. scapularis* tick. Given their smaller size, nymphal ticks are more likely than their adult counterparts to attach for this time period without detection and removal by a human host.

Areas endemic for Lyme disease are those in which both the infected reservoir and the *Ixodes* tick are common and where humans come into contact with the tick. Within the USA, this occurs in rural and suburban areas in the Northeast from Maine to Maryland (particularly coastal regions and the Hudson River valley), in the Midwest in Wisconsin and Minnesota, and in the West in Northern California, and Oregon Lyme disease may also be acquired in central European countries, Scandinavia, Russia, China, or Japan.

Nonneurologic manifestations

Spirochetes injected into the skin of a human host migrate centrifugally, resulting in a slowly expanding erythematous lesion known as erythema migrans. This lesion is typically painless and nonpruritic and may expand to a large size. Untreated, erythema migrans lasts on average about 3–4 weeks before subsiding.

Multiple Sclerosis and CNS Inflammatory Disorders, First Edition. Edited by Lawrence M. Samkoff and Andrew D. Goodman.

Flu-like symptoms may accompany or follow erythema migrans due to the early hematogenous dissemination of the spirochete. Patients in this phase may experience fevers, muscle aches, headache, malaise, or fatigue.

Once introduced into the human host, the *Borrelia* spirochete preferentially migrates to certain organs. In addition to the nervous system, the spirochete tends to infect cardiac and rheumatologic tissues. For example, some patients may develop cardiac complications such as atrioventricular block or a subtle myocarditis during the early phase of infection. Rarely, patients with cardiac involvement may develop a dilated cardiomyopathy. In addition to the heart, *Borrelia* may invade synovial tissue, causing joint inflammation and oligoarticular arthritis, most commonly affecting large joints such as the knee. Occasionally, this results in chronic arthritis.

As a general rule, untreated Lyme disease tends to unfold in stages beginning with early localized disease (erythema migrans) followed by early disseminated disease (early neurologic disease, meningitis, cranial neuritis, and radiculoneuritis, and cardiac manifestations, atrioventricular block and myocarditis) and late disease (oligoarticular arthritis and late neurologic manifestations). However, it is important to note that overlap of these stages is not uncommon and that one or more of them may not occur or may not be noticed.

Early neurologic manifestations

Within days to weeks following early dissemination of the *Borrelia* spirochete, approximately 10–15% of patients develop nervous system involvement. This typically occurs from early spring to late fall with a peak incidence in summer. Early nervous system Lyme disease most commonly presents as lymphocytic meningitis, cranial neuritis, or radiculoneuritis, either alone or in combination (see Figure 17.1).

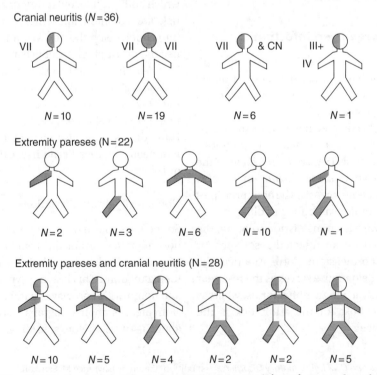

Figure 17.1 The distribution of pareses. Source: Ackerman *et al.* (1984). Reproduced with permission of Yale Journal of Biology and Medicine.

Lymphocytic meningitis often occurs in association with cranial neuritis or radiculoneuritis but can also occur in isolation in approximately 5% of patients, typically 2–10 weeks after onset of infection. As with other forms of meningitis, these individuals may present with a headache, photophobia, or stiff neck. However, meningeal symptoms and signs may be minimal or absent in some patients with Lyme meningitis, and a high index of suspicion is required to perform a lumbar puncture in a patient with other symptoms to suggest the disease. Cerebrospinal fluid (CSF) analysis typically reveals a lymphocytic pleocytosis, an elevated protein, and a normal glucose.

Cranial neuropathies are also relatively common during the early phase of Lyme infection. Cranial nerve VII, the facial nerve, is the most frequently affected cranial nerve (seen in about 50–75% of patients with early neurologic involvement) and may be bilateral in about one-third of patients with facial palsy. Other, less commonly involved cranial nerves are the fifth (trigeminal nerve) and sixth (abducens nerve), with rare involvement of the others.

The optic nerve, cranial nerve II, is not commonly affected by Lyme disease. However, there are published case reports in Europe and North America describing patients with a painful optic neuropathy that develops along with, or shortly following, symptoms typical of early disseminated Lyme disease. These case reports also suggest that optic neuritis observed in this setting may improve with standard treatment for Lyme disease. Optic neuritis may therefore be a rare complication of early neuroborreliosis, and Lyme disease may be considered in the differential diagnosis in the appropriate clinical setting (e.g., after exposure in an endemic area with other neurologic or nonneurologic symptoms of the disease).

An underdiagnosed early manifestation of Lyme disease is radiculoneuritis, which presents as severe radicular pain affecting one or more cervical, thoracic, or lumbosacral dermatomes, often with accompanying motor and reflex changes. This may be confused for a radiculopathy due to structural causes, from diabetes or herpes zoster, or for a primary cardiac or gastrointestinal process. Radiculoneuritis usually presents within 1 month of erythema migrans, if the skin rash is observed, and, like facial palsy, typically resolves spontaneously within several months of onset.

Other peripheral nerve manifestations include a confluent or nonconfluent mononeuritis multiplex, brachial neuritis, or, rarely, a progressive demyelinating polyneuropathy typical of Guillain–Barré syndrome (GBS) but with a CSF lymphocytic pleocytosis rather than the typical GBS findings of elevated CSF protein with normal cellularity.

Later-onset neurologic manifestations

Months to years after disease onset, untreated Lyme disease can result in late neurologic manifestations, such as Lyme encephalitis or encephalopathy, encephalomyelitis, or axonal polyradiculoneuropathy.

A subacute encephalopathy or encephalitis may develop in patients with a preceding symptomatic Lyme infection. This has been a topic of some controversy, but it seems clear that months to years after onset of infection, a small percentage of untreated patients may develop subacute memory loss, sleep disturbance, irritability, headache, or word-finding difficulty. This syndrome complex is nonspecific, as it may be seen in numerous other systemic diseases or in other diseases of the CNS, such as MS. Patients with Lyme encephalopathy, however, invariably have past or present evidence of *Borrelia* infection (e.g., erythema migrans, cranial neuropathy or radiculoneuropathy, oligoarticular arthritis), in addition to objective evidence of memory impairment and elevated serum or CSF Lyme titers. It is unclear if Lyme encephalopathy is due to direct *Borrelia* infection of the brain parenchyma or if the spirochete exerts an extrathecal indirect effect via the diffusion of neuroimmunomodulators into the CSF. Whatever the pathogenesis, these patients respond subjectively and objectively to a 2–4-week course of intravenous (IV) ceftriaxone.

In Europe, and less commonly North America, a syndrome of progressive Borrelial encephalomyelitis has been described. This is characterized by direct involvement of the spinal cord or brain parenchyma. This may occur in patients with Lyme radiculitis with spinal cord involvement at the corresponding spinal level, causing symptoms of a myelopathy at and below those levels (i.e., spasticity, a sensory level, or bladder dysfunction). Rarely, Lyme disease may directly affect the brain parenchyma. This typically occurs in focal areas of white matter and may raise the possibility of MS or brain tumor. CSF findings may be similar to those found in MS, except that these patients should have evidence of intrathecal production of anti-*Borrelia* antibodies. Also, these patients may have had prior symptoms of localized or disseminated Lyme disease.

Transverse myelitis is a rare complication of Lyme disease which typically occurs during the later stages, although it has also been reported during the early stage. Affected patients may experience sensory changes, such as band-like tightness, weakness at or below the affected spinal levels, and possibly urinary tract dysfunction. MRI of the spinal cord typically reveals cord edema with or without contrast enhancement of the involved levels. Several case reports note that the MRI scan appears more severe than the clinical presentation. Transverse myelitis from Lyme disease generally responds well to a course of antibiotics.

Late peripheral nervous system involvement may also occur. In contrast to the early syndrome of cranial neuritis or radiculoneuritis, later-onset neuropathy is milder and less distinctive with features of a subtle radiculoneuropathy or mononeuropathy multiplex that may become confluent over time. It typically presents with symmetric or asymmetric positive and negative sensory symptoms and signs of distal paresthesias, radicular pain, or both. Weakness, if present, is typically slight. Electrodiagnostic testing typically reveals this to be an axonal polyradiculoneuropathy. This is *not* considered to be residual disease from an early-onset Lyme radiculoneuritis.

There are patients with adequately treated Lyme disease who develop various postinfectious sequelae of *Borrelia* infection including generalized fatigue, fibromyalgia, headache, cognitive symptoms, or sensorineural hearing loss. This symptom complex is sometimes termed *post-Lyme syndrome*. Some patients develop diffuse pain and paresthesias with trigger points characteristic of fibromyalgia. In contrast to patients with Lyme encephalopathy, encephalitis, or encephalomyelitis, these patients typically lack objective evidence of nervous system involvement on testing and do not experience sustained improvement after further courses of antibiotic therapy.

Diagnosis

The diagnosis of neurologic Lyme disease is based on clinical criteria, with confirmatory lab testing. Although there are a multitude of tests that can be used to aide in the diagnosis of Lyme disease, most lack the high sensitivity and specificity expected for an accurate laboratory tool. In the appropriate clinical setting (e.g., a high pretest probability of disease), a positive test is confirmatory. By contrast, if the clinical data yield a low pretest probability, then a positive test result is more likely to be a false positive.

★ TIPS AND TRICKS

Currently available laboratory testing for Lyme disease can yield false negative and false positive results and the clinician must interpret the results based on the clinical picture and pre-test probability of disease. In addition, it should be remembered that a positive antibody test for Lyme disease documents exposure to the organism, but not necessarily active infection.

Direct culture of *Borrelia* is difficult. A special medium is required (BSK-II), and the organism's slow reproduction time necessitates several weeks of growth. In addition, the spirochete tends to be tissue bound and is therefore far easier to detect histologically from an erythema migrans lesion than from serum or CSF culture. In one study, CSF cultures were positive in only 10% of cases with clear Lyme meningitis. For unclear reasons, the spirochete has never been convincingly cultured from nervous system tissue itself.

Laboratory support for the diagnosis of *Borrelia* infection most often involves detecting an antibody response in the patient's serum, typically utilizing an enzyme-linked immuno-sorbent assay (ELISA). This antibody response appears within weeks of infection and has almost always occurred by the time of nervous system involvement (see Figure 17.2). Conversely, patients with erythema migrans are often seronegative. As with other infections, the IgM response is the first to appear, which then declines after a few months. After 1 month or so, an IgG response is detectable. To minimize false-positive results, all positive or equivocal IgG or IgM antibody titers from an ELISA should be confirmed with a Western blot. A positive IgM response in the absence of a positive IgG after more than a few months of infection indicates that the IgM result was likely a false positive.

In CNS neuroborreliosis, *Borrelia* antibody titers may be assessed in both serum and CSF to confirm the intrathecal presence of the spiro-chete. If the specific concentration of antibody produced in the CSF surpasses that in the serum (e.g., CSF index > 1), the CNS presence of the organism is confirmed. Importantly, an elevated index does not connote active infection, as the index may remain elevated after antibiotic treatment and resolution of symptoms (the same is true for the serum IgG response). Also, intrathecal production of the antibody may be delayed compared to extrathecal production in the serum, causing false-negative results early in the disease course. Of note, CSF analysis in CNS Lyme disease may reveal an elevated IgG, IgA, or IgM index or elevated oligoclonal bands, laboratory findings typical of other immune-mediated diseases such as MS.

CSF analysis in a patient with suspected neu-roborreliosis may also include PCR analysis. Probes have been developed against the plasmid DNA that encodes the outer surface protein A of the spirochete. Reports show there may be a place for its use in the evaluation of meningitis, but results are variable in both the CSF and serum. PCR is unfortunately not a very useful test, as one study showed less than 50% sensitivity even in Lyme meningitis and other studies report similar findings. False positives also occur, and true positives do not distinguish DNA from viable organisms versus residual nonviable DNA after spirochetocidal antibiotic therapy.

Many attempts have been made to develop better diagnostic tests for the detection of Lyme disease. A Lyme urine antigen test was developed, which was subsequently found to be unreliable. Other unreliable or unvalidated tests include an assay of specific T-cell immunoreactivity against *B. Borrelia*, a measurement of CD57 count, flow cytometry, isolated Western blots, urine reverse Western blots, urine dot blots, and immunoflu-orescence for L-forms of *Borrelia*. Ordering of these tests should be avoided in the absence of further validation, and the results of such tests should be interpreted with caution.

Conversely, some recently developed tests show great promise for increasing diagnostic accuracy. The first is an ELISA of the C6 peptide of the *Borrelia* major-variable protein-like sequence locus. Analysis of serum or CSF C6 peptide ELISA appears to provide a higher sensitivity for early disease than the standard two-step ELISA and Western blot testing. High levels of the chemokine CXCL 13 in the CSF may be useful in the diagnosis of Lyme neurobor-reliosis during the early stages. However, this marker may also be elevated in other immune-mediated diseases such as MS, so results should be interpreted with caution.

Several ancillary tests may be useful in documenting deficits in patients with neurobor-reliosis; however, the findings are typically nonspecific. For example, a brain or spinal cord MRI in individuals with symptoms of encephalomyelitis may show large white matter lesions, while those with encephalopathy may demonstrate numerous small, rounded areas of increased T2 signal intensity. Neuropsychologic testing in patients with Lyme encephalopathy

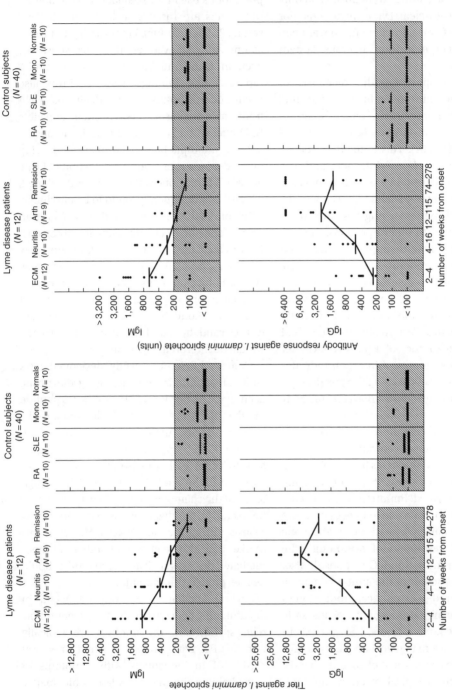

Figure 17.2 Antibody responses to the *I. dammini* spirochete in 41 serial serum samples from 12 patients with different clinical manifestations of Lyme disease, as compared with the responses found in 40 control subjects, determined by ELISA. Antibody titers were determined by serial dilutions of each serum (*left*), and antibody responses, shown in units, were calculated from a single dilution compared with a standard curve (*right*). The horizontal bar indicates the geometric mean response for each group, and the shaded areas indicate the range of responses generally observed in controls. Arth = arthritis, mono = infectious mononucleosis. Source: Craft *et al.* (1984). Reproduced with permission of Oxford University Press.

may reveal memory impairment in patients in whom memory appears intact on the routine neurological exam. Memory is typically affected to a greater extent than problems with attention, psychomotor skills, or visuospatial organization. Minor impairments of language have also been seen. Patients with Lyme encephalopathy have been shown to have temporal lobe hypometabolism on positron emission tomography (PET) studies and multifocal perfusion defects, which were most pronounced in the fronto-temporal regions on single-photon emission computed tomography (SPECT) imaging. Along with neuropsychiatric testing, PET or SPECT may be used as adjunctive diagnostic tools in patients with the nonspecific symptoms of Lyme encephalopathy to help differentiate their etiology from a primary psychiatric condition, but the abnormalities observed are not specific for Lyme neuroborreliosis. Finally, nerve conduction studies and needle electromyography may be helpful in documenting peripheral nerve manifestations of Lyme neuroborreliosis.

Differential diagnosis

Lyme radiculoneuropathy can present similarly to diabetic or herpetic radiculoneuropathy. Neurosarcoidosis may also cause a similar radiculoneuropathy and is one of the diseases associated with bifacial palsy—the others being GBS, HIV, various chronic meningitides, and Tangier's disease. Lymphocytic meningitis can be seen in numerous disorders, including neurosarcoid and zoster radiculitis. Lyme disease can typically be distinguished from these other conditions by the presence of typical extraneurologic manifestations of the disease such as erythema migrans, oligoarticular arthritis, and elevated serum or CSF *Borrelia* antibody titers.

The symptoms, signs, and brain MRI abnormalities of Lyme encephalomyelitis are reminiscent of MS, acute demyelinating encephalomyelitis (ADEM), and other MS mimics such as CNS lupus or Sjögren syndrome. The CSF parameters in Lyme encephalomyelitis may also be indistinguishable from these conditions with positive oligoclonal bands and an elevated IgG index. CNS

Lyme disease is distinguished from these other conditions by a history of exposure in an endemic area, characteristic extraneurologic symptoms, and positive antibody titers.

Lyme encephalopathy should be differentiated from sleep disturbances such as sleep apnea, depression, other systemic diseases such as rheumatologic disorders or other infections, and post-Lyme syndrome. Lyme encephalopathy improves after a course of IV antibiotics, while only transient or no improvement occurs in the other conditions listed.

There is no compelling evidence that Lyme disease causes progressive dementia, Parkinson's disease, or amyotrophic lateral sclerosis. A hypothetical link to MS has been proposed in which *Borrelia* exposure is the trigger that activates the immune system, leading to immunologic *flares*. The regional distribution of MS somewhat mirrors that observed in Lyme encephalomyelitis, but there is currently no definitive data to support this link.

Treatment

Lyme disease responds well to appropriate antibiotic therapy. Practice guidelines for Lyme neuroborreliosis have been established by the Quality Standards Subcommittee of the American Academy of Neurology and by the Infectious Diseases Society of America. Treatment trials in nervous system Lyme disease have shown efficacy of IV penicillin as well as third-generation cephalosporins with good CNS penetration. Ceftriaxone is the most frequently used agent, given the convenience of once daily dosing (as opposed to penicillin administered six times daily). Several European studies have shown that oral doxycycline is equivalent to treat meningitis, facial palsy, or radiculitis caused by the European strains of *Borrelia*. No studies have specifically compared IV antibiotics to oral doxycycline in the USA, but the European data suggests that oral doxycycline would be effective in the USA for these conditions as well. Occasionally patients with a facial palsy from Lyme disease may receive steroids for idiopathic facial palsy prior to diagnosis; the available data shows no clear harmful or beneficial role for corticosteroids in neuroborreliosis.

Acute neuroborreliosis, manifesting as cranial neuropathies, radiculoneuritis, or meningitis, has been shown to respond to a 2–4-week course of IV ceftriaxone 2 g daily, IV cefotaxime 2 g every 8 h, or IV penicillin 20–24 million total units daily in divided doses. The European trials suggest that oral doxycycline 100 mg two or three times daily may be as effective as IV antibiotics. In the USA, oral antibiotics such as doxycycline are used for isolated facial palsy, but in the presence of a severe headache, stiff neck, or CSF pleocytosis, a 2–4-week course of IV antibiotics is often recommended. It is interesting to note that many of the acute neurologic manifestations of Lyme disease, such as facial palsy or radiculoneuritis, are largely self-limited with no significant neurologic sequelae even in the absence of treatment. The benefit of antibiotic therapy in these cases is to shorten the duration of symptoms or prevent the late manifestations of the disease.

Patients with late-onset nervous system Lyme disease also respond to a 2–4-week course of antibiotics, although in general improvement in symptoms is slower and more incomplete than in acute neuroborreliosis. Parenchymal brain or spinal cord involvement, such as that seen in encephalomyelitis or transverse myelitis, warrants IV antibiotic treatment as described for acute disease for a total of 2–4 weeks. Lyme encephalopathy and radiculoneuropathy can also be successfully treated with a 2–4-week course of IV ceftriaxone. No studies have been performed to assess the efficacy of oral agents in late-onset disease; oral antibiotics may successfully treat peripheral nervous system manifestations, but this has not been studied.

As previously noted, nonspecific postinfectious sequelae of *B. burgdorferi* infection do not respond to prolonged antibiotic administration. In numerous studies, prolonged courses of antibiotics beyond 4 weeks have not been shown to improve outcomes and are associated with more treatment-related morbidity and increased cost. For example, ceftriaxone, especially with prolonged administration, has been associated with line infections and biliary sludging.

> **✋ CAUTION!**
>
> Antibiotic treatment courses beyond 4 weeks do not improve outcomes, and expose the patient to potential harmful side effects of treatment. Further, the major reason for lack of improvement after appropriate antibiotic therapy is incorrect diagnosis (e.g., the patient's symptoms are not due to active Lyme disease).

Practitioners in areas endemic for Lyme disease should be aware of methods available for the prevention of Lyme disease. If possible, tick-prone areas such as tall grasses should be avoided to prevent the initial tick bite. In rural areas where entrance into the tick's habitat is unavoidable, long clothes should be worn while outdoors then removed and washed immediately after exposure. At the time of this publication, a vaccine is not commercially available to prevent Lyme disease.

Conclusion

Lyme disease may affect the peripheral nervous system or CNS and may do so during early or late stages of the disease. Care must be taken to appropriately differentiate neuroborreliosis from other central or peripheral nervous system disorders with similar presentations, such as MS or ADEM. A careful history with inquiry about endemic exposure and nonneurologic manifestations (skin rash, myocarditis, or oligoarticular arthritis) in conjunction with knowledge of the clinical spectrum of Lyme neuroborreliosis and judicious laboratory testing will almost always suffice in making the diagnosis of Lyme neuroborreliosis. Initiation of appropriate antibiotic therapy typically results in resolution or improvement of neurologic symptoms.

Acknowledgments

We would like to thank Ahmad Manasra for his assistance during the editing process.

References

Ackerman, R., Horstrup, P. & Schmidt, R. (1984) Tick-borne meningopolyneuritis (Garin-Bujadoux, Bannwarth). *The Yale Journal of Biology and Medicine*, **57**, 485–490.

Craft, J.E., Grodzicki, R.L. & Steere, A.C. (1984) The antibody response in Lyme disease: evaluation of diagnostic tests. *The Journal of Infectious Diseases*, **149** (5), 789–795.

Further Reading

Fung, B.P., McHugh, G.L., Leong, J.M. & Steere, A.C. (1994) Humoral immune response to outer surface protein C of *Borrelia burgdorferi* in Lyme disease: role of the immunoglobulin M response in the serodiagnosis of early infection. *Infection and Immunity*, **62** (8), 3213–3221.

Halperin, J.J. (2005) Central nervous system Lyme disease. *Current Neurology and Neuroscience Reports*, **5**, 446–452.

Halperin, J.J. (2011) Neurologic manifestations of Lyme disease. *Current Infectious Disease Reports*, **13**, 360–366.

Halperin, J.J., Shapiro, E.D., Logigian, E. *et al.* (2007) Practice parameter: treatment of nervous system Lyme disease (an evidence-based review): report of the quality standards subcommittee of the American Academy of Neurology. *Neurology*, **69**, 91–102.

Kaplan, R.F., Meadows, M.E., Vincent, L.C., Logigian, E.L. & Steere, A.C. (1992) Memory impairment and depression in patients with Lyme encephalopathy: comparison with fibromyalgia and nonpsychotically depressed patients. *Neurology*, **42**, 1263–1267.

Logigian, E.L., Kaplan, R.F. & Steere, A.C. (1990) Chronic neurologic manifestations of Lyme disease. *The New England Journal of Medicine*, **323**, 1438–1444.

Logigian, E.L., Kaplan, R.F. & Steere, A.C. (1999) Successful treatment of Lyme encephalopathy with intravenous ceftriaxone. *Journal of Infectious Diseases*, **180**, 377–383.

Steere, A.C. (2001) Lyme disease. *New England Journal of Medicine*, **345**, 115–125.

Wormser, G.P., Dattwyler, R.J., Shapiro, E.D. *et al.* (2006) The clinical assessment, treatment, and prevention of Lyme disease, human granulocytic anaplasmosis and babesiosis: clinical practice guidelines by the Infectious Diseases Society of America. *Clinical Infectious Diseases*, **43**, 1089–1134.

18

Neuro-Behçet Syndrome

Aksel Siva and Sabahattin Saip

Department of Neurology, Cerrahpaşa School of Medicine, Istanbul University, Cerrahpaşa, Turkey

Introduction

Behçet disease (BD), originally described in 1937 by Hulusi Behçet as a distinct disease with orogenital ulceration and uveitis known as the *triple-symptom complex*, is an idiopathic chronic relapsing multisystem vascular inflammatory disease of unknown origin. The disease affects many organs and systems, causing mucocutaneous lesions, uveitis sometimes resulting in blindness, nervous system involvement and major vessel disease that may be fatal, musculoskeletal problems, gastrointestinal involvement, and others.

Epidemiology

The epidemiology of the disease shows a geographical variation, seen more commonly along the Silk Route, extending from the Mediterranean region to Japan. This is coupled by a similar variation in HLA-B51 association, which is strongly associated with the disease in high prevalence areas such as Middle and Far East.

Its prevalence has been reported to be less than $0.5/10^5$ in the USA and between 0.5 and $1/10^5$ in Northern and Central Europe and goes up to $2.5/10^5$ in northwestern Mediterranean region and increases further in the eastern Mediterranean region. Prevalence rates up to $400/10^5$ have been found in population-based studies in Turkey, and rates between 10 and $20/10^5$ have been reported in Japan, China, and Korea, countries at the other end of the ancient trade routes of Silk Road.

The usual onset of the BD is in the third or fourth decade. Although rare, onset in children has also been reported. The gender distribution is almost equal. However, the reported increased tendency to affect men more than women may be explained by the higher incidence of systemic complications and more severe disease in men, possibly bringing them to earlier medical attention.

Diagnosis and systemic manifestations of Behçet disease

Currently the diagnosis of BD is clinical. The most widely used diagnostic criteria are the International Study Group's classification criteria, according to which a definitive diagnosis requires recurrent oral ulcerations plus two of the following: recurrent genital ulcerations, skin lesions, eye lesions, or a positive pathergy test (Table 18.1).

Oral aphthae

The presence of recurrent oral ulcers is required for the diagnosis of BD, and it is quite unlikely to see cases without oral ulcers. However, 1–3% of patients can have several of the other features of the syndrome without ever having aphthae. Aphthae are frequently the first manifestation of

Multiple Sclerosis and CNS Inflammatory Disorders, First Edition. Edited by Lawrence M. Samkoff and Andrew D. Goodman.

Table 18.1 Criteria for Diagnosis of Behçet Disease*

Finding	Definition
Recurrent oral ulceration	Minor aphthous, major aphthous, or herpetiform ulcers observed by the physician or reliably described by the patient, which recurred at least three times over a 12-month period
Recurrent genital ulceration	Aphthous ulceration or scarring observed by the physician or reliably described by the patient
Eye lesions	Anterior or posterior uveitis or cells in the vitreous body on slit-lamp examination or retinal vasculitis detected by an ophthalmologist
Skin lesions	Erythema nodosum, pseudofolliculitis, papulopustular lesions, or acneiform nodules not related to glucocorticoid treatment or adolescence
Positive pathergy test[†]	Test interpreted as positive by the physician at 24–48 h

Source: International Study Group for Behçet's Disease (1990). Criteria for diagnosis of Behçet's disease. *Lancet*, **335**:1078–1080. Reproduced with permission of Elsevier.
*For a definite clinical diagnosis of BD, the patient must have recurrent oral ulceration plus at least two of the other findings, in the absence of any other clinical explanations.
[†]The pathergy phenomenon is a nonspecific skin hypersensitivity that is almost specific for BD. It is performed by inserting an 18 g needle into the dermis of the forearm. The reaction is considered positive if a papule or a pustule forms at the puncture site within 48 h. Presence of erythema only is considered negative.

the syndrome, and it is not uncommon for some patients to have only oral ulcers for many years before other signs appear.

Genital ulceration

External genital ulcers, which have the next highest sensitivity for the diagnosis of BS, usually occur on the scrotum in men and on the labia in women.

Skin lesions

Skin lesions of different kinds are seen in up to 80% of patients with BS. These are folliculitis, papulopustular lesions, and acneiform lesions, which occur more commonly in men, and erythema nodosum, which are more common in women.

Eye involvement

This is one of the most serious manifestations and a leading cause of morbidity in BD. The overall prevalence is about 50%, being more common and more severe in men and young patients. It's bilateral in 90% and consists of a chronic relapsing posterior and anterior uveitis and acute panuveitis, with blurred vision, decreased visual acuity, photophobia, pain in the eye, and conjunctival hyperemia being the common ocular symptoms. Optic nerve involvement can occur but is rare.

The pathergy phenomenon

The pathergy phenomenon, a nonspecific hypersensitivity reaction of the skin, is one of the diagnostic tests that are almost specific to BD, but its sensitivity varies largely between different ethnic and geographical groups (range, 20–80%). It is produced by inserting a 20 gauge needle into the dermis of the forearm of the patients. The reaction is considered positive if a papule or pustule is formed at the site of the puncture within 24–48 h. Erythema alone is considered negative.

Musculoskeletal involvement

A nonerosive, nonmigrating monoarthritis or oligoarthritis, involving the large joints, either in the form of arthritis or arthralgia is reported in about 50% of patients. Another musculoskeletal manifestation associated with BD is aseptic necrosis of the bone. This is possibly related to vasculitis and not necessarily to steroid use.

Gastrointestinal involvement

Although most common in the ileocecal region, ulcers can be seen all along the digestive tract with various clinical symptoms. Gastrointestinal involvement is relatively frequent in Japan, but not in other geographic areas.

Cardiovascular involvement

Major vessel involvement is another serious cause of morbidity and mortality in BD. BD is one of the few vasculitides that can involve both the venous and arterial sides of the circulatory system. Arterial disease is less common (occurring in <5% of cases), but it is of high most importance, as it may manifest itself in the form of arterial aneurysms or occlusions or as pulmonary artery aneurysms with the risk of fatal hemoptysis and death. Deep vein thrombosis and thrombophlebitis are among other large-vessel complications, and all are expected to be seen in 25–30% of the cases, while a possibly higher proportion do have small-vessel involvement, mostly affecting postcapillary venules. In BD, there is also a tendency to develop venous thrombosis after venipunctures. Although rare, myocardial ischemia associated with coronary vasculitis or with inflammation such as endocarditis, myocarditis, and pericarditis may all occur.

Other systems

Other systems reported to be involved through the course of the disease are pulmonary, urinary, and the central nervous system (CNS). Unlike many other systemic vasculitides, glomerulonephritis is uncommon. Amyloidosis of the AA type is seen sporadically.

Laboratory investigations

There are no laboratory findings specific for BS. The moderate anemia of chronic disease and leukocytosis can be seen in some patients. The erythrocyte sedimentation rate is only mildly elevated, as is the C-reactive protein. None of these correlates with disease activity. Autoantibodies are absent, whereas complement levels may be high. However, HLA testing can support the diagnosis in populations where the disease is associated with HLA-B51 phenotype and may help in the differential diagnosis.

Pathology and etiopathogenesis of Behçet syndrome

The core histopathologic phenomenon seems to be a vasculitic involvement in some cases and a low-grade, chronic, nonspecific inflammation in others. Histopathologic changes consistent with vasculitis involving both arterial and venous systems have been shown. However, vascular involvement in BD is predominantly venous in contrast to what is seen in most other systemic vasculitides. Other than vasculitis, involved tissues may show various types of histopathological lesions varying with the age of the lesion according to the time of examination, a nonspecific inflammatory reaction with neutrophilic predominance in early lesions is expected, whereas as lesions age lymphocytes become more predominant. Interestingly, usually a clear-cut vasculitic process cannot be demonstrated in the CNS, and studies on pathology of the CNS involvement indicate that neuro-Behçet syndrome (NBS) may not a cerebral vasculitis, but rather be a perivasculitis.

The etiology of BD is unknown, but clinical and laboratory data suggest that there is dysfunction of both innate and adaptive immune systems, resulting in an exaggerated response to viral or bacterial insults. Debate is ongoing about whether the hyperreactivity reaction seen in BD is an autoimmune phenomenon or as suggested by more recent data an autoinflammatory phenomenon. Autoinflammatory diseases indicate a relatively rare group of heritable disorders that are characterized by seemingly unprovoked episodes of inflammation and relative lack of an obvious autoimmune pathology (i.e., pathogenic high-titer autoantibodies or antigen-specific T cells). These disorders arise from various genetic disorders, which result in a chronic low-grade inflammatory activity with overlapping recurrent inflammatory attacks. However, along with immunological and genetic

Table 18.2 Suggested Diagnostic Criteria for NBS[*]

Fulfilling the International Diagnostic Criteria for BD
Onset of neurological symptoms not otherwise explained by any other known systemic or neurological disease or treatment
Presence of at least two of the following:
1. Objective abnormalities on neurological examination (clinical evidence)
2. Abnormal neuroimaging findings suggestive of NBS (imaging evidence)
3. Abnormal CSF findings suggestive of NBS (laboratory evidence)

Source: Siva, A. and Saip, S. (2009) *Journal of Neurology*, **256**, 513–529. Adapted with permission from Dr. Dietrich Steinkopff Verlag.
[*]Diagnosis of NBS is confirmed when all above criteria are fulfilled.

factors, fibrinolytic defects have been implicated as well (Table 18.1 and Table 18.2).

Nervous system involvement in Behçet disease: *Neuro-Behçet syndrome*

NBS is defined as the occurrence of neurological symptoms in a patient with BD that is not better explained by any other well-known systemic or neurological disease. The prevalence of NBS in BD is between 3% and 9% in large series. However, when BD patients are followed for up to two decades, the frequency of neurological involvement increases to 13.0% in males and 5.6% in females. In a Japanese autopsy series of patients with BD, it was reported that 20% had pathological evidence for neurological involvement.

The mean onset age of BD is about mid-third decade, and neurological involvement occurs after a mean of 5 years. Despite the gender difference being insignificant in BD, neurological involvement occurs more commonly in men, with a male to female ratio of up to 4:1. Such a significant male predominance has also been noted for other severe vascular complications of BS. However, once NBS develops, the severity doesn't show a gender difference.

BD is rare in the pediatric population. About 3% of BD patients present at or before 16 years of age; however, neurological involvement may be seen in up to 10% of them.

Although neurologic involvement is relatively uncommon in BD, when it occurs, it presents with numerous and different neurological problems that are related either directly or indirectly to the disease (Table 18.3). Cerebral venous sinus thrombosis (CVST), parenchymal–CNS

involvement secondary to vascular inflammation, and the neuro-psycho-Behçet variant, in which an organic psychotic syndrome is prominent, are considered direct effects. As all demonstrate neurological manifestations, they will be reviewed here as NBS.

Peripheral nervous system (PNS) involvement is extremely rare, despite that neurophysiological and histopathological studies may demonstrate nonspecific findings in some patients without related symptoms.

Neurologic complications of various BD treatments and neurologic complications secondary to systemic involvement of the disease are among indirect neuropsychiatric consequences of the disease.

The suggested diagnostic criteria for NBS in a patient that fulfills the International Diagnostic Criteria for BD is the occurrence of neurological symptoms not otherwise explained by any other known systemic or neurological disease or treatment, and in whom objective abnormalities are detected either on neurological examination, and/or on neuroimaging studies (magnetic resonance imaging (MRI) disclosing findings suggestive of NBS) and/or abnormal cerebrospinal fluid (CSF) findings consistent with NBS (Table 18.2).

The two major forms of neurological involvement in BD are parenchymal–CNS involvement and CVST. Neurological manifestations clinically are related commonly to brainstem or corticospinal tract syndromes in the former one and to increased intracranial pressure in the second form.

Clinical and neuroimaging evidence also confirms this subclassification of NBS. CNS NBS or *intra-axial NBS* is due to small-vessel disease and

Table 18.3 The Neurological Spectrum of Behçet Disease

Primary Neurological Involvement (Neurological Involvement Directly Related to BD)
CVST (extra-axial NBS)
CNS involvement (intra-axial NBS)
Neuro-psycho-Behçet syndrome
Isolated headache syndrome (migraine-like, nonstructural)
PNS involvement
Subclinical NBS

Secondary Neurological Involvement (Neurological Involvement Indirectly Related to BD)
Neurologic complications secondary to systemic involvement of BD (i.e., cerebral emboli from cardiac complications of BD, increased intracranial pressure secondary to superior vena cava syndrome)
Neurologic complications related to BD treatments (i.e., CNS neurotoxicity with cyclosporine, peripheral neuropathy secondary to thalidomide or colchicine)
Somatoform neurologic symptoms related to psychogenic factors of having a chronic disease

Coincidental: Unrelated (Non-BD) Neurological Involvement
Primary headaches and any other coincidental neurological problem

Source: Siva, A. and Saip, S. (2009) *Journal of Neurology*, **256**, 513–529. Adapted with permission from Dr. Dietrich Steinkopff Verlag.
BD, Behçet disease; CNS, central nervous system; CVST; Cerebral venous sinus thrombosis; NBS, neuro-Behçet syndrome.

causes the focal or multifocal CNS involvement manifested in the majority of patients. The second form, CVST or *extra-axial NBS*, which is due to large-vessel disease presenting with thrombosis of the major cerebral venous sinuses, has limited symptoms, a better neurological prognosis, and generally an uncomplicated outcome. These two types of involvement occur in the same individual very rarely and presumably have a different pathogenesis. Many of the CNS NBS patients with small-vessel inflammation have a relapsing–remitting course initially, with some ultimately developing a secondary progressive course later, and a few will have a progressive CNS dysfunction from the onset.

Extra-axial NBS

CVST is seen in 10–20% of BD patients in whom neurologic involvement occurs. Thrombosis of the venous sinuses may cause increased intracranial pressure with severe headache, mental changes, and oculomotor cranial nerve palsies. In some patients, the only manifestation may be a moderate headache. It is well known that the clinical presentation resulting from thrombosis of the intracranial venous system varies according to the site and rate of venous occlusion and its extent.

Experience suggests that the CVST in BD evolves gradually and a fulminating syndrome with violent headache, convulsions, paralysis, and coma is unlikely. Papilledema and sixth nerve paresis are the most common signs reported, and hemiparesis may develop in some.

There is a tendency for CVST to occur earlier in disease course compared to the parenchymal type of CNS disease, and this difference is significant in male patients. In the pediatric age group affected with BD, the neurologic involvement is mostly in the form of CVST. Any of the sinuses may be affected, but the superior sagittal sinus is the most commonly thrombosed, with a substantial number of these patients also disclosing lateral sinus thrombosis. Intracranial hypertension without any obvious neuroimaging abnormality initially has been reported, with some of these patients developing neuroimaging findings consistent with CVST in further attacks later.

Parenchymal–CNS involvement in BS patients with CVST is unlikely. The extension of the clot into the cerebral veins causing focal venous hemorrhagic infarction is uncommon, and also the occurrence of CVST with primary CNS involvement (coexistence of intra- and extra-axial NBS) is extremely rare. Extra-axial NBS occurs earlier in the disease course compared with the parenchymal–CNS type of neurological involvement. A close association between CVST and systemic major vessel disease in BD has been reported. It is also well established that neurological disease in the form of CVST has a better neurological prognosis. However, since patients with major vessel disease have a higher rate of morbidity and mortality, CVST in a patient with BD may not be associated always with a favorable outcome.

It's likely that the two major forms of neurological disease (intra- and extra-axial involvement) in BD might have different pathogenic mechanisms.

★ TIPS AND TRICKS

Neurological involvement is unlikely prior to the onset of systemic signs and Sx of Behcet's Disease (oral ulcers are most likely to precede) and neuroimaging (Cranial MRI) is highly suggestive for intra-axial NBS.

Intra-axial NBS

Parenchymal–CNS involvement is seen in 75–80% of BD patients in whom neurologic involvement occurs. The most common form of presentation of intra-axial NBS is the onset of a subacute brainstem syndrome that includes ophthalmoparesis and other cranial nerve findings, dysarthria, and uni- or bilateral corticospinal tract signs with or without weakness and ataxia (Table 18.4). The presentation may include all or some of these symptoms and signs, and during the acute stage, a mild confusion may also be seen. The patient most commonly is a young man, and if he is also of Mediterranean (or Middle East, or Oriental) origin, the probability of NBS then should be included in the differential diagnosis. Such a patient (if a reliable history can't be obtained from the patient, than his/her family member/s) needs to be interviewed for the presence of systemic findings of BD. In the case of BD, it will be very likely to obtain a past or present history of oral aphthous ulcers and some other systemic manifestations of the disease. Many patients may be found to have never consulted a physician because of the mild nature of their

systemic symptoms or may be missed because of not reporting a full-blown picture of the disease. It will be quite unlikely to see NBS cases without oral ulcers. The MRI findings of the disease are almost pathognomonic, and this will further support the diagnosis. However, it should be kept in mind that parenchymal NBS (intra-axial NBS) does not always present with brainstem signs and symptoms. Cognitive behavioral changes, emotional lability, a self-limited or progressive myelopathy, urinary sphincter dysfunction, and to a lesser extent other CNS manifestations such as extrapyramidal signs and seizures have been reported. There are also a few cases reported with isolated progressive ataxia (with cerebellar atrophy on MRI), isolated optic neuritis (OP), and recurrent peripheral facial paresis. OP is extremely rare in BD, and most visual symptoms in BD are due to ocular involvement.

Arterial NBS

Arterial disease, both systemically and in the CNS, is rare in BD. Case reports with bilateral internal carotid artery occlusion, vertebral artery thrombosis, vertebral artery dissection, intracranial aneurysms, and intracranial arteritis with their corresponding neurological consequences suggest that arterial involvement may be a subgroup of NBS.

Intracranial hemorrhages may occur but are extremely rare, with most occurring within ischemic lesions.

Neuro-psycho-Behçet syndrome

Some patients with BS develop a neurobehavioral syndrome, which consists of euphoria, loss of insight, disinhibition, apathy, psychomotor agitation, or retardation, with paranoid and obsessive behavior unrelated to glucocorticosteroid or any other therapy. These psychiatric manifestations may be observed either at the onset of other neurological symptoms of NBS or independently.

Cognitive changes in BD

Cognitive changes, including memory and attention impairment, language or visuospatial disturbances, and executive dysfunction, have all been observed in BD. Neuropsychological

Table 18.4 Classical Presentation and Features of a Patient with Intra-axial (Parenchymal) NBS

Demographics:
• Commonly, the patient is a young male of Mediterranean (or Middle East, or Far East) origin!

Clinical presentation of intra-axial NBS

(any of the following is possible!)
• *A brainstem syndrome of subacute onset (most common)*
   o ophthalmoparesis & other cranial nerve findings, dysarthria, ataxia uni or bi-lateral corticospinal tract signs with/without weakness
• *An encephalopathy*
   o with mild confusion and cognitive-behavioral changes, emotional lability
• *A myelopathy*
   o may be severe/paraparesis and urinary sphincter dysfunction likely
• *Rarely*
   o Extrapyramidal signs; optic neuritis; seizures;
• Unlikely to be NBS without past history of oral ulcers

Neuroimaging – MRI

(MRI findings almost pathognomonic)
Distribution and lesion burden:
Brainstem & deep hemispheric structures
• Mesodiensephalic junction upward extension (+)
• ponto-bulbar involvement ± up/downward extension
• Diencephalic region, basal ganglia
Uncommon;
• cerebral hemispheres, cerebellum
• spinal cord – but when seen likely to be LEM; AQP4-antibodies are likely to be negative
Acute phase
• DW-MRI & Proton MRS - consistent with "vasogenic edema"
• Gd - enhancement: (±) & Hemorrhage within the lesions (±)
• Temporal course
   o change in lesion-size/dissapearance of lesions
   o new and asymptomatic lesions
   o atrophy/enlargement of the third ventricule

Abbreviations:

NBS: Neuro-Behçet Syndrome; LEM; longitudinally extensive myelitis; AQP4: Aquaporine-4; MRI: magnetic resonance imaging; MRS: magnetic resonance spectroscopy, DW-MRI: Diffusion weighted MRI; Gd: Gadolinium

status deteriorated insidiously, regardless of the neurological attacks during the follow-up period in most of the patients, and the presence of cognitive decline was not directly related to detectable lesions on neuroimaging at early stages of the disease.

Headache in BS

Headache is the most common neurological symptom seen in patients with BS and may be due to different causes. It can occur as the presenting symptom of NBS either due to CNS involvement or CVST. It can also be seen in association with ocular inflammation. In several studies on headache in BD, the most common type of headache was reported to be migraine (the original sentence may be kept or modified— as some of these patients do have migraine but not all! Others have this migraine-like headaches described in the following text as characterized by bilateral, frontal, moderate paroxysmal throbbing pain). This is not true migraine, since it generally starts after the onset of BS and commonly accompanies the exacerbations of systemic findings of the disease. It may be explained by a vascular headache triggered by immunomediated disease activity in susceptible individuals and may be seen in up to 18% of BD patients. This type of *isolated headache syndrome* isn't specific for migraine, and similar headaches have been described in some other systemic inflammatory disorders such as systemic lupus erythematosus. Such headaches may not have any significant impact in most patients. However, a substantial number of patients with BS may report a severe headache of recent onset without any neurological deficit and not consistent with any coexisting primary headache or ocular inflammatory pain. These patients require further evaluation and follow-up even if they do not have neurological signs, as such a symptom may indicate the early onset of NBS. Finally, coexisting primary headaches such as migraine and tension-type headache in patients with BS also are seen.

PNS involvement

PNS involvement is rare in BD. There are case reports describing BD patients with clinical and electrophysiological findings consistent with mononeuritis multiplex, polyradiculoneuritis, distal sensorimotor axonal neuropathy, and axonal sensory neuropathy with recurrent episodes of myositis. However, some PNS disorders in BD may be related to agents such as thalidomide or colchicines, used to treat the primary disease itself.

Subclinical NBS

The incidental finding of neurological signs in patients with BS without neurological symptoms was reported in some series, with a minority of these patients developing mild neurological attacks later. It was suggested that this group of patients represent a milder form of the disease, since the mortality and disability rate was found to be significantly low when they were followed prospectively. Subclinical CNS involvement was also detected by MRI and in SPECT studies, as well as with brainstem auditory and somatosensory evoked potentials and transcranial magnetic stimulation, but their significance remains unclear.

Diagnostic studies in NBS

Neuroimaging

Cranial MRI is quite specific and sensitive in showing the reversible inflammatory parenchymal lesions of intra-axial NBS. Lesions are generally located within the upper brainstem, occasionally extending to the diencephalic and basal ganglia regions or the pontomedullary structures (Figure 18.1). Hemispheric white matter lesions are not common, and when they are present, they are almost always associated with diencephalic and brainstem lesions. A frequent finding is the resolution or the decrease in the size of the lesions when follow-up imaging studies are available. Such studies may also disclose the appearance of new *silent* lesions without corresponding clinical symptoms and signs. Tumefactive lesions may also be seen. Recent work using susceptibility weighted imaging had revealed that the proportion of lesion detection is significantly larger than that with conventional MRI and most lesions in intra-axial NBS are hemorrhagic supporting the proposed venous theory in pathology.

Spinal cord involvement in NBS is uncommon but usually affects the cervical spinal cord. Longitudinally extensive myelitis-like intramedullary lesions, sometimes extending to the brainstem, reminiscent of neuromyelitis optica, have been described in NBS. However, antiaquaporin antibodies have not been found in NBS.

MR venography is the preferred study to diagnose or confirm CVST in BD, although T1- and T2-weighted MR images often demonstrate venous clot. The yield of conventional cerebral angiography in NBS is low, as vascular pathology is most prominent in postcapillary venules. Besides, it should be kept in mind that not only a neutrophilic infiltration with arterial injury may occur at the site of arteriographic puncture in patients with BS but that there may be more unfortunate consequences related to this procedure (Figure 18.2).

CSF

If performed during the acute stage, CSF studies usually show inflammatory changes in most cases of NBS with parenchymal involvement, with

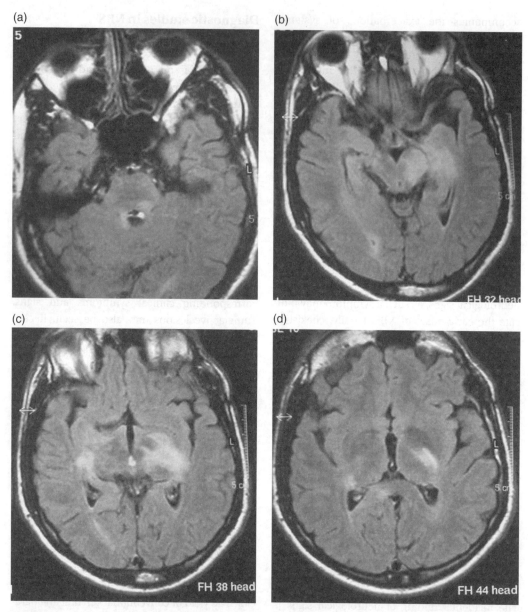

Figure 18.1 (a–d) Flair MR images of a patient with intra-axial NBS showing a brainstem lesion involving the dorsal pons and midbrain and extending to the diencephalic–basal ganglia region on the left.

elevated white cell count and protein (the quantitative information may be kept—as it has a differential value). Although neutrophilic predominance is common during the acute phase of disease, lymphocytosis is characteristic of later stages and chronic NBS. Oligoclonal bands can be detected but are seen in less than 20% of NBS cases. Elevated concentrations of IL-6 in the CSF of patients have also been reported. CSF in patients with CSVT will be under increased pressure, but the cellular and chemical composition is usually normal.

Differential diagnosis

Differential diagnosis of intra-axial NBS

Patients with NBS are young and frequently present with an acute or subacute brainstem syndrome or hemiparesis. Hence, the possibility of BS is often included in the differential diagnosis of multiple sclerosis (MS) and in the stroke of

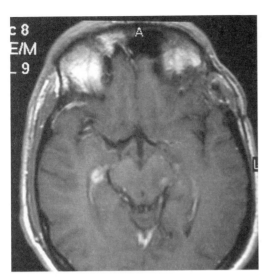

Figure 18.2 T1W images with gadolinium of the same patient showing sparse enhancement in the lesion.

the young adult, especially in the absence of its known systemic symptoms and signs.

MS is more common in women, whereas NBS is seen frequently in men. Onset age is about the same, but OP, sensory symptoms, and spinal cord involvement, which are common in MS, are rarely seen in NBS (Table 18.5). However, sometimes the clinical presentation of NBS may be confused with MS, but the neuroimaging–MRI findings are clearly different. The pattern of brainstem involvement in NBS, which commonly extends to involve basal ganglia and diencephalic structures, is atypical of MS. Furthermore, periventricular, corpus callosum, and ovoid lesions suggestive of MS are uncommon in NBS. Disproportionate brainstem and cerebellar atrophy that is seen in the chronic phase of NBS is unusual in MS. Spinal cord lesions extend no more than a few vertebral segments in MS, contrary to the more extensive lesions that have been observed in the few cases of NBS. The CSF also reveals different patterns, with a more prominent pleocytosis and low rate of positivity for oligoclonal bands in NBS.

An acute stroke-like onset is not common in NBS, and MRI lesions compatible with classical arterial territories are also not expected. The absence of systemic symptoms and signs will serve to differentiate the primary CNS vasculitic

disorders from NBS and the difference in the systemic symptoms and signs from the secondary CNS vasculitides, as well as the MRI findings.

Neuro-Sweet disease, sarcoidosis, and tuberculosis may resemble BD and NBS, but a detailed clinical evaluation and MRI and other diagnostic studies are likely to reveal the true nature of the disease. Due to their ophthalmologic and some other systemic manifestations, rare diseases such as Vogt–Koyanagi–Harada syndrome, Reiter syndrome, Eales disease, Cogan syndrome, and Susac syndrome are other considerations in the differential diagnosis of BD. All may present with nervous system manifestations and therefore are included in the differential diagnosis of NBS. However, a complete ophthalmologic examination will reveal the true nature of eye involvement in each of these syndromes, which have differences from the eye involvement seen in BD. Gastrointestinal symptoms in BD may mimic Crohn disease or chronic ulcerative colitis. Eye disease is rare, and genital ulcers are absent in inflammatory bowel diseases. The diagnosis can be confirmed by intestinal biopsy. Whipple disease may be briefly mentioned here as a disease with gastrointestinal and various nervous system symptoms that may resemble BD too.

Differential diagnosis of extra-axial NBS (CVST)

In patients who present with symptoms of intracranial hypertension and in whom neuroimaging reveals thrombosis in one or more of the cerebral venous sinuses, BD needs to be included in the differential diagnosis. The presence of its systemic findings is the only clue to the association of CVST with BD, and their absence will exclude this possibility. As already mentioned, hemorrhagic venous infarcts or other parenchymal lesions on MRI isn't expected in patients with extra-axial NBS.

Prognosis

Neurological involvement in BD is a remarkable cause of morbidity, and approximately 50% of the NBS patients are moderate to severely

Table 18.5 The Differential Diagnosis of MS and Intra-axial (CNS) NBS

	MS	CNS NBS
Gender	Female > male	Male > female
Symptoms at onset		
Common	ON, sensory, spinal cord, BS/INO, motor, cerebellar	Headache, motor, BS cranial neuropathies
		Dysarthria, cerebellar
Uncommon	Headache, BS cranial neuropathies	ON, sensory, spinal cord, BS/INO
MRI		
PV and SC lesions	(+++)	(±)
Brainstem lesions	Small, discrete, extension (–)	Large, diffuse, extension (+)
Spinal cord lesions	(+++)/less than 3 segments	(±)/more than 3 segments
CSF		
Inflammatory changes	(±)	(+++)
OCB (+)	>90%	<20%

Source: Modified from Siva and Saip (2009) *Journal of Neurology.*
BS, brainstem; CNS, central nervous system; CSF, cerebrospinal fluid; INO, internuclear ophthalmoplegia; MRI, magnetic resonance imaging; OCB, oligoclonal bands; ON, optic neuritis; PV, periventricular; SC, subcortical.

disabled after 10 years of disease. The mortality rate due to all causes is about 10% when patients are followed for up to two decades, with a mortality rate due to neurological involvement remaining around 12%.

Onset with cerebellar symptoms and a progressive course were unfavorable factors, while onset with headache, a diagnosis of CVST, and disease course limited to a single episode were favorable. An elevated protein level and pleocytosis in the CSF were also reported to be associated with a poorer prognosis.

Treatment

Neurological involvement in BD is heterogeneous, and it is difficult to predict its course and prognosis and response to treatment. Currently, there is no evidence for the efficacy of any treatment for any form of NBS, and empirical impressions and expert opinion are the guidelines for management. As in many chronic relapsing inflammatory disorders, the treatment options in NBS consist of relapse treatment, long-term attack-preventing treatment, and symptomatic treatment. Moreover, management of the two major clinical forms of neurological involvement of BD (CNS disease and CVST) slightly differs, as well.

Intra-axial NBS

Acute episodes
Glucocorticoids are used to treat acute CNS involvement, but their effects are short-lived and they do not prevent further attacks or progression. Acute attacks of intra-axial NBS are treated with high-dose intravenous methylprednisolone (IVMP 1 g/day) for up to 10 days or by oral prednisolone (1 mg/kg for up to 4 weeks or until improvement is observed). Both forms of treatment should be followed with an oral tapering dose of glucocorticoids over 2–3 months in order to prevent early relapses (Figure 18.3).

Long-term treatments
After the attack treatment, long-term maintenance treatment with immunosuppressive agents should be considered, since this form may follow a relapsing or secondary progressive

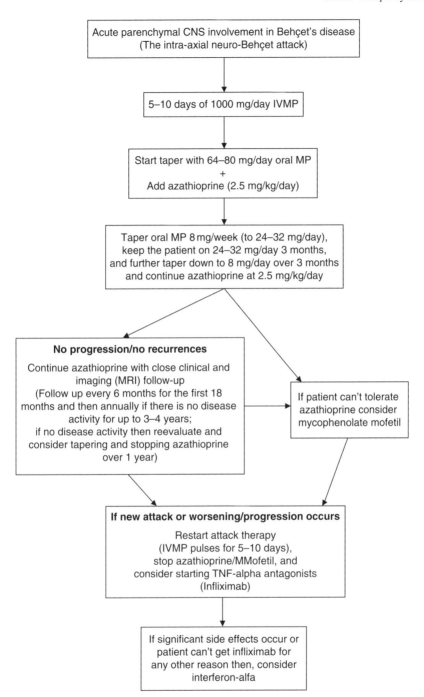

Figure 18.3 (Experience-based) Treatment algorithm for intra-axial neuro-Behçet disease.
MP: methylprednisolone; IVMP, intravenous methylprednisolone.
Source: Modified from Akman-Demir *et al.* (2011). *Current Treatment Options in Neurology*, **13**,
290–310. Reproduced with permission of Current Science.

course and may result in significant physical and cognitive deficits leading to neurological disability. Immunosuppressants, such as azathioprine, mycophenolate mofetil, and cyclophosphamide, and therapies with interferon-alpha or anti-TNF agents have been shown to reduce some of the systemic manifestations of BD and are likely to have some effect despite not having evidence-based efficacy in NBS. Cyclosporine is known to cause nephrotoxicity or to accelerate the development of CNS symptoms, and therefore, its use in NBS is not recommended.

Extra-axial NBS

Cerebral Venous Sinus thrombosis

CVST in BD is also treated with steroids, since clot formation is caused by low-grade endothelial inflammation rather than hypercoagulability.

The addition of anticoagulation, including short-term fractionated heparin, to glucocorticoids is controversial, as these patients have a higher probability of harboring pulmonary or other aneurysms, which may be associated with an increased risk of bleeding.

References

Akman-Demir, G., Saip, S., Siva, A. et al. (2011) Behçet's disease. *Current Treatment Options in Neurology*, 13, 290–310.

International Study Group for Behçet's Disease (1990) Criteria for diagnosis of Behçet's disease. *Lancet*, 335, 1078–1080.

Siva, A. & Saip, S. (2009) The spectrum of nervous system involvement in Behcet's syndrome and its differential diagnosis. *Journal of Neurology*, 256, 513–529.

Index

Note: Page numbers in *italics* refer to figures; those in **bold** to tables.

Multiple Sclerosis and CNS Inflammatory Disorders, First Edition. Edited by Lawrence M. Samkoff
and Andrew D. Goodman.
© 2014 John Wiley & Sons, Ltd. Published 2014 by John Wiley & Sons, Ltd.